General
Orthopaedics

NOTICE

General Orthopaedics

Frank C. Wilson, M.D.

Kenan Professor of Orthopaedics
School of Medicine
University of North Carolina at Chapel Hill
Chapel Hill, North Carolina

Patrick P. Lin, M.D.

Fellow in Orthopaedics
Memorial-Sloan-Kettering Cancer Center
New York, New York

McGraw-Hill
HEALTH PROFESSIONS DIVISION

New York St. Louis San Francisco Auckland Bogotá Caracas Lisbon London
Madrid Mexico City Milan Montreal New Delhi San Juan Singapore
Sydney Tokyo Toronto

McGraw-Hill

A Division of The **McGraw·Hill** *Companies*

GENERAL ORTHOPAEDICS

Copyright © 1997 by The McGraw-Hill Companies, Inc. All rights reserved.
Printed in the United States of America. Except as permitted under the United
States Copyright Act of 1976, no part of this publication may be reproduced or
distributed in any form or by any means, or stored in a data base or retrieval system, without the prior written permission of the publisher.

1234567890   DOC DOC   9876

ISBN 0-07-070757-X

This book was set in Times Roman by Progressive Information Technologies, Inc.
The editors were Martin J. Wonsiewicz and Peter McCurdy.
The production supervisor was Richard Ruzycka.
The cover designer was Bob Freese.
The indexer was K. Unger.
R. R. Donnelley & Sons, Inc. was printer and binder.

This book is printed on acid-free paper.

Library of Congress Cataloging-in-Publication Data

General orthopaedics / [edited by] Frank C. Wilson, Patrick P. Lin.
        p.   cm.
    Includes index.
    ISBN 0-07-070757-X
    1. Orthopedics. 2. Musculoskeletal system—Diseases. I. Wilson,
Frank C.,   II. Lin, Patrick P.
    [DNLM: 1. Musculoskeletal Diseases. 2. Orthopedics—methods.   WE
140 G326 1997]
RD731.G42   1997
617,3—dc20
DNLM/DLC
for Library of Congress   96-35345
                                                                          CIP

This book is dedicated to those present and future physicians
who have been, and are, a continuing stimulus to a better understanding
of the structure and function of the locomotor system.

Contents

Contributors

Louis C. Almekinders, M.D.
Associate Professor of Orthopaedics
School of Medicine
University of North Carolina at Chapel Hill
Chapel Hill, North Carolina

Gary D. Bos, M.D.
Associate Professor of Orthopaedics
School of Medicine
University of North Carolina at Chapel Hill
Chapel Hill, North Carolina

H. Robert Brashear, M.D.
Professor of Orthopaedics
School of Medicine
University of North Carolina at Chapel Hill
Chapel Hill, North Carolina

Thomas G. Braun, M.D.
Clinical Associate Professor of Neurology
School of Medicine
University of North Carolina at Chapel Hill
Chapel Hill, North Carolina

Edmund R. Campion, M.D.
Assistant Professor of Orthopaedics
School of Medicine
University of North Carolina at Chapel Hill
Chapel Hill, North Carolina

Laurence E. Dahners, M.D.
Professor of Orthopaedics
School of Medicine
University of North Carolina at Chapel Hill
Chapel Hill, North Carolina

Douglas R. Dirschl, M.D.
Assistant Professor of Orthopaedics
School of Medicine
University of North Carolina at Chapel Hill
Chapel Hill, North Carolina

Mary Anne Dooley, M.D.
Research Assistant Professor of Medicine
  (Rheumatology)
School of Medicine
University of North Carolina at Chapel Hill
Chapel Hill, North Carolina

Walter B. Greene, M.D.
Professor and Chair, Department of Orthopaedic
  Surgery
University of Missouri Health Sciences Center
Columbia, Missouri

Richard C. Henderson, M.D., Ph.D.
Associate Professor of Orthopaedics
School of Medicine
University of North Carolina at Chapel Hill
Chapel Hill, North Carolina

Patrick P. Lin, M.D.
Fellow in Orthopaedics
Memorial-Sloan-Kettering Cancer Center
New York, New York

Jordan B. Renner, M.D.
Associate Professor of Radiology
School of Medicine
University of North Carolina at Chapel Hill
Chapel Hill, North Carolina

Frank C. Wilson, M.D.
Kenan Professor of Orthopaedics
School of Medicine
University of North Carolina at Chapel Hill
Chapel Hill, North Carolina

Foreword

As the twenty-first century approaches, it is quite apparent that the delivery of health care in the United States has undergone, and is undergoing, major change—perhaps the most profound in the history of medicine. Some have characterized it as the industrialization of medicine, pointing out that there is now a strong mandate for measuring best practices and determining outcomes. Further, an analysis of the work force reveals strong movement towards "primary care"—a term that easily accommodates broad definition. The demands of the work-force under managed care dictate a central role for the "generalist," no matter which specialty. Obviously, this mandate applies directly to orthopaedics, which is a broad interdisciplinary specialty encompassing the recognition, investigation, and management of the diseases and disorders of the musculoskeletal system.

Given such an environment, there exists a vacuum of information for practitioners concerned with disorders and diseases of the musculoskeletal system—those "primary care orthopaedists" who limit their practice to the outpatient arena.

This text has been carefully structured to present a comprehensive coverage of musculoskeletal diseases and disorders from historical landmarks through formation and growth, physiology and biochemistry, biomechanics, physical diagnosis, diagnostic modalities, rehabilitation, genetic and congenital disorders, vascular and epiphyseal disorders, neuromuscular diseases, infections, tumors, traumatic disorders, degenerative and rheumatic diseases, metabolic and endocrinologic disorders, developmental disorders, and finally, a glossary of orthopaedic terms.

Who better to assemble such a timely text than Frank C. Wilson, M.D., Kenan Professor of Orthopaedics at the University of North Carolina, who has devoted a professional lifetime to advancement of the understanding and teaching of the disorders of the musculoskeletal system. He recognized the need for this book and, with Patrick P. Lin, M.D., and a cadre of expert authors, provided the understanding, dedication, and perseverance necessary to bring *General Orthopaedics* to publication. The result of this collective effort is a comprehensive, lucidly illustrated work that is highly relevant to our times and the times that lie ahead. It will serve as a rich source of information for the practitioner of primary care orthopaedics who seeks to meet the continuing challenge of understanding the diseases and disorders of the musculoskeletal system.

C. McCollister Evarts, M.D.
Chief Executive Officer
The Milton S. Hershey Medical Center
Senior Vice-President for Health Affairs and Dean
Pennsylvania State University College of Medicine

Preface

Recognizing the proliferation of both specialists and nonspecialists in the field of orthopaedics, we have written a book for those who desire a comprehensive reference to the diseases, disorders, and injuries of the musculoskeletal system. An unfortunate by-product of the profusion of laboratory and radiologic tests available to the physician has been a loss of the sense of satisfaction derived from diagnosis by artful listening and careful examination. In orthopaedics, however, successful practice still relies heavily on clinical findings, which have been emphasized in the text.

Believing that a mind that grasps principles will find appropriate methods, we have stressed fundamental precepts of structure and function. This volume is not a "cookbook," with recipes for casts and braces; rather it is designed for those who, in dealing with musculoskeletal conditions, wish to anchor clinical decision-making in basic pathophysiology.

We have made a particular effort to standardize terminology, style, syntax, and format to avoid the ambiguity inherent in multiply authored texts, and endeavored to illustrate graphically those aspects of conditions for which words alone seemed inadequate.

To produce a book that would guide and inform the management of orthopaedic disorders, we needed and received able assistance from many. To our contributors for their lucid explications; to Jennifer Wilson for her clear and accurate artwork; and to Cathy Wells, for her tireless excellence in preparing the manuscript, we are particularly indebted.

Frank C. Wilson and Patrick P. Lin

General
Orthopaedics

Part *I*

The Musculoskeletal System

Chapter 1

Historical Landmarks

Frank C. Wilson

HISTORY OF MEDICINE: GENERAL DEVELOPMENTS

Anesthesia

Antisepsis

Drugs and Vaccines

X-ray

Materials and Metallurgy

Genetics

HISTORY OF MEDICINE: ORTHOPAEDIC DEVELOPMENTS

Descriptions of Disease
> *Infections; Tumors; Joint Diseases; Neuromuscular Diseases; Vascular and Epiphyseal Disorders; Traumatic Disorders; Metabolic and Endocrine Disorders*

Therapy
> *Splints, Braces, Casts, Traction, and Prosthetics; Operations on Bone; Operations on Joints; Operations on Tendons*

SUMMARY

HISTORY OF MEDICINE: GENERAL DEVELOPMENTS

Many early descriptions of disease were those of Hippocrates, who possessed remarkable powers of observation and common sense. Although believed by his countrymen to be a descendant of Aesculapius, the mythical god of healing, Hippocrates avoided attributing disease to the wrath of the gods; rather, he studied the patient and the resultant findings. His 42 descriptions of clinical cases were almost the only such record for the next 1700 years, and it would be hard to improve on his first aphorism: "Life is short and the Art long; the occasion fleeting; experience fallacious, and judgement difficult."

Orthopaedics as we know it began with Nicholas Andry, who, in 1741, coined the term *orthopaedia* [from the Greek *orthos* (straight) and *pais* (child)]. Its progression, in fits and starts, since that time has resulted from the juxtaposition of discoveries in basic and other clinical fields with advances in orthopaedics itself. The introduction of anesthesia, antisepsis, antibiotics, and blood transfusion, for example, reduced operative morbidity and mortality from a lottery pick to reliability and safety.

The direction of orthopaedic surgery has also been influenced by changes in humans and their environment. As they moved from arboreal to terrestrial means of locomotion, prehension became more important in the upper and less so in the lower limbs. Terrestrial movement led to other and more rapid means of transportation, which introduced musculoskeletal problems that had to be met by innovations in orthopaedic technology; however, before considering developments upon which the modern practice of orthopaedics is based,

we should recall discoveries in other fields that permitted these advances.

Anesthesia

General anesthesia was introduced in America in the 1840s. Active debate has encircled its discoverer: Crawford W. Long began to use ether as a surgical anesthetic in 1842; however, as he did not publish his experience, we cannot assign credit to him for introducing anesthesia to the world at large. In 1846, William T. G. Morton used ether anesthesia at the Massachusetts General Hospital for removal of a superficial vascular tumor on the neck.

In 1847, Sir James Young Simpson, professor of obstetrics at Edinburgh, substituted chloroform for ether in his midwifery practice and was so impressed with its advantages over ether that he published his results a week later. The "death of pain" occasioned by these discoveries led to less haste and more deliberation in surgical procedures, as well as an easier time for both patient and surgeon.

Halsted, after perilous experimentation upon himself, developed the use of cocaine for nerve blocks in 1885. Novocaine, employed by Balfour in 1913, also abolished pain without the systemic effects of general anesthesia or cocaine.

Antisepsis

Primed by the work of Semmelweis in obstetric antisepsis (1840s), Pasteur's work on preventive vaccination (1880), and Koch's postulates for establishing the pathogenic character of a given microorganism (1882), antisepsis found its way into surgery with the work of Lord Lister, who, in 1865, performed his first operation under antiseptic conditions.

In spite of his report to the British Medical Association 2 years later, that he had not had a single case of "pyaemia, hospital gangrene, or erysipelas" in his surgical wards for the preceding 9 months, many years elapsed before the principle of antisepsis was widely adopted in surgical practice. It was Pasteur, too, who discovered the *Staphylococcus,* noting that this organism might cause extensive bone destruction.

Drugs and Vaccines

Antibiotics, antitoxins, nonaddictive analgesics, and vaccines have changed the face of orthopaedic practice. Beyond doubt, the greatest single contribution to surgery in general and orthopaedic surgery in particular was the introduction of the first effective chemotherapeutic agent, sulfonamide, by Domagk in 1935. Fleming followed with penicillin from bread mold in 1941. Antituberculous drugs and wide-spectrum antibiotics came later. Death, which occurred often, and recurrent infection, which was almost the rule, became rare sequelae of acute osteomyelitis after the development of antibiotics. Similarly, tetanus and poliomyelitis have been almost eradicated by vaccination. Tetanus vaccine came into use during the First World War; Salk (and later Sabin) developed polio vaccine in the 1950s.

Nonsteroidal anti-inflammatory drugs (NSAIDs), which reduce the manifestations of inflammation but do not eliminate it, have been developed and used for symptomatic management of various musculoskeletal aches and pains. They derive their effect from the suppression of prostaglandin synthesis. Although the term *nonsteroidal anti-inflammatory drug* was first applied to phenylbutazone, which was introduced in 1949, willow and poplar barks containing salicin have been used since antiquity to treat gout, pain, and fever. The marketing of indomethacin in 1965 stimulated the development of many other drugs to suppress inflammation.

X-ray

In 1895, Wilhelm Conrad Röentgen, professor of physics in Würzburg, discovered "x-rays," which, he noted, would pass through cardboard, wood, and limbs. Within weeks, x-rays were applied to the human body. Many skeletal diseases were subsequently discovered, not in the dissecting room or through the microscope but in radiographs, even though they were used initially to localize metallic foreign bodies.

The introduction of computed tomography (CT) in 1973 revolutionized imaging practices by its capacity to display cross-sectional anatomy. It also discriminates small differences in tissue densities much better than conventional radiography.

Also in 1973, Lauterbur described image formation with nuclear magnetic resonance. First applied to the central nervous system, the process of magnetic resonance imaging (MRI) is now used to study all parts of the body. It finds particular application in orthopaedics for tumor staging and demonstration of intervertebral disk pathology.

Materials and Metallurgy

To Sir William A. Lane of London and Albin Lambotte of Belgium must go the credit for founding modern fracture surgery. During the first decade of the twentieth century, each published books describing the use of steel plates attached to bone by screws for fracture repair.

Unfortunately, technical innovation preceded the development of antibiotics and knowledge of corrosion, which frequently necessitated early removal of these devices. Understanding that the variation in chemical reactivity of different metals produces an electric current generated by destruction of the more reactive metal, Venable and Stuck began to study the problem of corrosion in the 1930s, which led to the development of stainless steel, an iron alloy containing chromium, nickel, and molybdenum. Vitallium, a nonferrous alloy of cobalt, chromium, and molybdenum developed in 1929, was found to be even more inert than stainless steel. Both metals have been used extensively for implant surgery since that time, greatly reducing the need for implant removal.

Nonmetallic materials in current use in orthopaedics include polyethylene, polymethylmethacrylate (bone cement), silicone, and ceramic; these materials have been developed and improved for use as implants during the past 35 years. Polyethylene, used for acetabular cups and tibial trays in joint replacement, has been improved by the development of newer ultrahigh-molecular-weight polyethylene, which has superior wear characteristics. Polymethylmethacrylate, used to cement implants in place, has been made stronger by the addition of carbon fibers, but there are continuing efforts to find prosthetic materials that will bond directly to bone, eliminating the need for a methacrylate interface. Silicone polymers are used for replacement of non-weight-bearing joints, although poor wear properties often lead to synovitis and failure with prolonged use. Ceramics, while brittle and possessing poor crack-resistant characteristics, have high compressive strength, contain inert materials, and bond ionically to bone.

Genetics

In 1865, the Augustinian monk Gregor Johann Mendel announced the results of his experiments on hybridization of peas in the form of a law, which has been applied to the experimental study of heredity. Sir Francis Galton in 1889 published *Natural Inheritance,* which introduced the statistical study of biological variation and inheritance. From experience with the primrose, de Vries in 1901 advanced the hypothesis of *mutation* or spontaneous origin of variations. The effect of these studies was to de-emphasize the role of environmental or external factors in the struggle for existence in favor of internal biochemical forces.

HISTORY OF MEDICINE: ORTHOPAEDIC DEVELOPMENTS

Descriptions of Disease

Like the more general developments listed above, many of the original descriptions of orthopaedic disease were made by people other than orthopaedists, in part because this particular branch of medicine was not recognized as a distinct entity prior to the twentieth century.

Infections

Although there is evidence in early archaeological specimens of bone infections, the term *osteomyelitis* was not coined until the early nineteenth century. Sir Benjamin Collins Brodie of London described a localized chronic abscess of long bones, since known by his name, in 1819; and in 1884, Rodet produced experimental hematogenous osteomyelitis by intravenous injection of staphylococci.

Tuberculosis has also been present for centuries. Perhaps the earliest description was of spinal tuberculosis by Hippocrates in the third century B.C.; he described the gibbus and its association with respiratory difficulty and "unconcocted tubercles in the lungs." Sir Percivall Pott published the first modern account of tuberculous paraplegia in 1779, since which time spinal tuberculosis has been eponymically known as *Pott disease.*

Tumors

Skeletal tumors were also recognized in antiquity; the earliest recorded bone tumor was an *osteochondroma* noted on the femur of the Java man, oldest of subhuman fossils. Differentiation among benign and malignant bone tumors did not begin until the nineteenth century: in 1845, Boyer differentiated and named *bone sarcoma.* In the same year, Lebert described a neoplasm later recognized as *giant-cell tumor.* Dalrymple described *multiple myeloma* in the *Dublin Quarterly* in 1848; and in 1924, Ewing applied the term *endothelial myeloma* to the tumor that later became known as *Ewing sarcoma.*

Joint Diseases

The term *internal derangement of the knee* was coined by William Hey in 1803 to recognize injury to the meniscus and the loss of full extension frequently associated with this condition. In 1941, Brantigan and Voshell published their studies on ligamentous and meniscal functions in the knee, stimulating a bewildering number of like reports since that time.

The history of *rheumatoid arthritis* is ambiguous, perhaps because recognition of the disease evolved very slowly. The earliest writing thought to refer to a patient with rheumatoid arthritis was by Soranus in the first century A.D.; others believe that it became a specific entity only recently. A. B. Garrod, in an 1859 treatise entitled *Gout and Rheumatic Gout,* was the first to employ the term *rheumatoid arthritis;* however, he did not distinguish it from other forms of chronic joint disease. His son A. E. Garrod classified chronic arthritides into osteoarthritis and rheumatoid arthritis, recognizing the first as characterized by bone hypertrophy and the second by atrophy.

Unlike rheumatoid arthritis, *osteoarthritis* has been clearly documented through paleopathologic examination of prehistoric fossils. Thus, it is an ancient disease, the signs of which have been recorded throughout history by art historians as well as physicians.

Anecdotal accounts of what is now presumed to have been *gout* date from the writings of Hippocrates, though the term *gout* was not applied until the thirteenth century by de Vielehardouin.

After seminal observations by McCarty and Hollander in 1961 of non-urate crystals in the joints of two patients with presumed gout, knowledge of articular disorders caused by crystalline calcium deposition expanded rapidly. The original term, *pseudogout syndrome,* was soon replaced by *calcium pyrophosphate deposition disease,* which accented pathophysiology rather than symptomatology.

Jean-Martin Charcot, who became, in 1882, the first professor of nervous diseases in the world, provided the initial description of neuropathic joint disease, now known as *Charcot joints.* His 1868 paper attributed this disorder to "irritative lesions of the spinal cord, especially those which occupy the gray substance."

Neuromuscular Diseases

Cerebral palsy, known in its spastic form as *Little disease,* was first mentioned by William John Little in 1843, although his definitive paper to the English Obstetrical Society was not read until 1862. His life and study were shaped by his own talipes equinovarus deformity, which resulted from poliomyelitis in childhood. Convinced by his own personal experience with Achilles' tenotomy that this treatment for the deformity was correct, he advocated tenotomy of *any* tendon producing deformity and was thus a pioneer in the early treatment as well as the description of this disorder.

Although Smellie (1768) is often credited as the describer of the *brachial plexus injury* that occurs in the newborn and Duchenne reintroduced the subject of "obstetrical palsies" in 1855, eponymic credit went to William H. Erb for the description of birth-related brachial plexus injuries—although of the five cases Erb marshaled to support his argument that such paralyses usually conform to a pattern, only one was in a child. Augusta Klumpke, one of the first female physicians in Paris, distinguished, while a student, the varieties of brachial paralysis that might occur, using animal experimentation to support her concepts. She acknowledged paralysis of the upper roots as *Erb palsy* and the complete plexus palsies of the Duchenne-Erb variety, but went on to describe a third type that involves primarily the forearm and hand *(Klumpke palsy).* She described as constant in all true lower root palsies the "oculo-pupillary phenomenon . . . characterized by miosis, narrowing of the palpebral fissure, and in some cases by the eyeball retracting and becoming smaller."

The first case of *poliomyelitis,* then called "infantile paralysis," was described by Under-wood in his treatise *Diseases of Children* published in 1784; in 1855 Duchenne localized the lesion in this disease to the anterior horn cells of the spinal cord. During the latter half of the nineteenth century, orthopaedic treatment of flaccid paralysis and deformity—more commonly involving lower limbs and trunk than upper limbs—was by crutches and bracing. With the development of surgical approaches to deformity, the twentieth century brought tenotomy, tendon transference, and arthrodesis to the management of these problems.

Although *sciatica* was described in 1764 and disk protrusion noted at necropsy 90 years later, it was another 80 years before the connection between these two observations was fully understood. Goldthwait in a 1911 paper discussed the occurrence of paraplegia after spinal manipulation, opining that disk prolapse, among other things, could cause root compression; but it was not until 1934 that Mixter and Barr established fully the connection between commonly encountered disk protrusions, or "chondromata," and sciatica.

Pseudohypertrophic muscular dystrophy was described by Duchenne in 1868 as another type of progressive palsy, which he thought due to a peripheral lesion involving the musculature itself.

Although compression of the median nerve at the wrist was recognized by Paget in 1853, the first known *carpal tunnel release* was performed by Woltman in 1941. It is now one of the most frequently performed operations on the hand.

Vascular and Epiphyseal Disorders

The first systematic studies of the circulation of blood in bone by Lexer demonstrated the vascular network of the bones; however, the relationship of the vascular pattern to bone survival, i.e., of pathology to anatomy, was demonstrated by Robert W. Johnson in 1927. In 1930, Phemister correlated the microscopic and radiographic changes of *avascular necrosis* and recognized (in agreement with Axhausen) that dead bone was gradually absorbed and replaced by new bone, for which he coined the term *creeping replacement.*

Although the inciting event was often unclear, recognition of the pathologic and radiographic changes in avascular bone led to the description of a number of related bone diseases recognized loosely as the *osteochondritides* and specifically by an eponymous connection to those who described them.

Another vascular disorder of bone was described by Sudeck, who, in 1900, described a painful posttraumatic atrophy of bone *(Sudeck atrophy),* which he considered to be inflammatory, though later studies classified it as a vasomotor disturbance based on dysfunction of the sympathetic nervous system.

The reaction of muscle to ischemia was described in 1881 by Richard von Volkmann. The prompt and permanent paralysis and contracture that follow complete occlusion of the blood supply to muscle *(Volkmann contracture)* occurs most often following supracondylar fracture of the elbow in children.

Traumatic Disorders

The earliest description of shock was by Marshall Hall, who in 1825 recorded the physical effects of blood loss. Reduction of circulating blood volume results in hypotension, which triggers the neuroendocrine response to shock elucidated by Francis Moore and others over a century later.

Little was known about *fracture healing* before the eighteenth century, which embraced the work of John Belchier, who developed a vital stain to study bone formation (1738); Albrecht Haller, who emphasized the role of the blood vessels in callus formation; and John Hunter, who described the morphologic sequence of fracture healing.

The twentieth century saw research in fracture healing tracked beyond morphology to collagen production, mineral uptake, oxygen tension, and other factors, although the triggering mechanisim for bone mineralization has remained an enigma.

A means of quantification of the reaction to injury, known as the trauma score, was developed in 1982 by the American Trauma Society and is used for selection of more precise resuscitative methods and assessment of outcomes following injury.

Metabolic and Endocrine Disorders

As with many categories of illness, knowledge of metabolic and endocrine disorders originated with observations of human disease, followed by written and graphic illustrations, with, in the modern era, greater emphasis on underlying pathophysiology. One of the earliest pictures of *rickets* was provided by Homer in the second *Iliad.* Francis Glissen in 1650 is credited with the most authoritative early study on rickets, and Fletcher in 1911 was the first clearly to demonstrate the coexistence of rachitic deformity and interstitial nephritis, or *renal rickets.*

The parathyroid glands were discovered by Sandstrom in 1881; their importance was defined shortly thereafter by the tetany produced when the parathyroid glands were inadvertently removed during surgery for thyroid disorders. Jaffe in 1931 produced the bone changes of hyperparathyroidism *(osteitis fibrosa cystica)* in rabbits by the injection of parathyroid hormone. In 1962, Kopp et al. reported the discovery of *calcitonin,* a hormone that reduced plasma calcium and inhibited bone resorption.

Therapy

Splints, Braces, Casts, Traction, and Prosthetics

The first use of *splints* dates at least to the time of Hippocrates, who, in his treatise *Fractures,* described broken femurs realigned by traction, with the position maintained by firm bandages to support the part—following which he stated, "The thigh bone is consolidated in 50 days." It was also known to the ancients that "exercise strengthens and inactivity wastes," a principle that has been regularly rediscovered since that time.

Bracemaking, which began in the fifteenth and sixteenth centuries under the direction of Ambroise Paré, progressed through the development of simpler and more ingenious devices by Glissen and Andry in the seventeenth and eighteenth centuries. However, bracemaking attained its apogee toward the end of the nineteenth century, largely from the work of Hugh Owen Thomas of Liverpool, who stressed the importance of rest for injured or diseased joints. The particular value of Thomas's contributions was to deemphasize the mechanical aspects of braces in favor of the physiological principles underlying their use.

Appliances for applying sustained *traction* utilizing weights and pulleys were devised by French surgeons of the fifteenth and sixteenth centuries, especially Ambroise Paré, although his apparatus for reducing dislocated shoulders and hips was similar to those described by Hippocrates. For correction of foot deformities, Paré used plasters and special shoes. His

casts were made from linted bandages impregnated with egg whites, the albumin in which gave support to the covered part.

The *plaster-of-paris* bandage was introduced by Mathijsen in 1852; it reduced dependence on braces and splints, although for many practitioners the brace remained the only means of splintage. Hugh Owen Thomas, in fact, once remarked that "nothing so barbarous as plaster of paris is used any longer." Subsequently, open reduction and external fixation, coupled with early mobilization, reduced the need for external forms of splintage.

In 1907, Fritz Steinmann of Switzerland provided the first description of skeletal traction by means of weights attached to a nail inserted through the distal fragment, which led Böhler to the use of various methods of skeletal traction.

Operations on Bone

The history of operations on bones is essentially the history of fracture treatment: reductions (closed and open), internal fixation, osteotomy, and bone grafting. Early closed reduction consisted merely of passive straightening of the limb by means of manual or mechanical traction. Gradually, manual manipulation of individual fragments was added.

The volume of literature related to the operative treatment of fractures would make a book in itself, beginning perhaps with Guthrie's report crediting La Puyade and Sicre for wire fixation of a fracture in 1775. (Another account of this event has the patient dying 2 days after the operation.)

In 1870, Berenger-Ferand used screws to maintain proper apposition of bone fragments, but he credited Rigaud, a countryman, with having first used screws to internally fix a fracture of the olecranon. Bonnet added metal bars placed externally to the skin, through which screws were implanted in the bone, with the bars serving as an external splint. This device was the forerunner of the external fixators in use today.

Lane (1905) and Lambotte (1907) were the first to use metal plates attached directly to the bone. Since that time, there have been many efforts to improve the type of plate and its manner of fixation to bone. The need for both plate and screws to be made of the same material was emphasized by Venable and Stuck in 1938, after observing the corrosion produced by apposition of dissimilar metals.

John Rhea Barton reported the first corrective *osteotomy* for limb deformity in 1837. Subsequently, many such procedures were done for rickets, a very prevalent condition at that time.

Although performed to fill osseous defects as early as 1682, *bone grafting* did not become safe until the advent of antiseptic surgery. In 1911, Fred Albee of New York, using electrical saws and cortical grafts, popularized grafting operations. The value of cancellous bone grafting was not widely appreciated until the Second World War, when Mowlem, a plastic surgeon, showed its clear superiority for ununited fractures.

Operations on Joints

The first recorded instances of opening a joint cavity, or *arthrotomy*, date from the Renaissance and were performed for the drainage of purulent material. Following Lister's establishment of the principles of surgical antisepsis, surgeons in the 1880s began to accompany arthrotomy with the instillation of various antiseptics; however, failure to control infection was far more frequent than success until the introduction of sulfonamides and penicillin,

which were used parenterally as well as locally.

Until the last half of the eighteenth century, intractable joint infection was managed most often by amputation until, toward the end of the century, Henry Park of Liverpool began the practice of *joint excision* for destructive joint disease, although technical difficulties and absence of anesthesia prevented wide acceptance of this procedure. The support of James Syme, the great Edinburgh surgeon, led to the incorporation of joint excision into general surgical practice in England. In the absence of ensuing arthrodesis, the operation did not reliably control infection and often led to unacceptable instability in the lower limb; however, since joint replacement and fusion began with joint excision, the development of this procedure was not wasted.

John Rhea Barton is credited with the first operation designed to mobilize a stiff joint in 1825. He restored motion to a fused hip by an intertrochanteric osteotomy followed by passive movement, thus creating a false joint, or *pseudarthrosis*. Joint excision, another form of arthroplasty, was confronted, especially in the lower limb, by the problem of achieving an appropriate balance between mobility and stability. If the joint reankylosed, mobility was lost. If not, instability and pain were frequent sequelae. This dilemma began the search for an ideal interpositional material. A variety of materials were tried, ranging from chromicized pig's bladder to cellophane; however, none was successful enough to justify continued use. In 1908 Lexer began his experiments in joint transplantation, but he reported in 1924 that even when the transplanted tissues "took," results were unsatisfactory. In 1925, Smith-Petersen began work with molded interpositional materials, reporting hip arthroplasty with an interposed vitallium cup in 1938, a procedure that found favor for the ensuing 30 years. Complete replacement of joints with metal, polyethylene, or both, spearheaded by the monumental work of John Charnley, began in earnest in the late 1950s, leading to dramatic results in the treatment of disabling joint disease.

Even as arthroplasty was being developed, other surgeons were seeking to induce surgical fusion, or *arthrodesis,* of joints. The procedure, introduced by Albert of Vienna in 1878, was quickly adopted for instability of the knee joint to eliminate the use of braces. Three years later, Albert extended the indications for arthrodesis to the paralytic shoulder, where fusion of the glenohumeral joint increased active scapulothoracic motion in the shoulder girdle. By fusing a tuberculous knee in 1911, Russell Hibbs of New York added infection as a third indication for arthrodesis. In the twentieth century, the decline of poliomyelitis and tuberculosis greatly reduced the need for arthrodesis, so that the most frequent indication for this procedure now is a failed arthroplasty.

In 1877, Volkmann suggested that limited joint excision, or *synovectomy,* might be sufficient for articular tuberculosis in which the disease was limited to the lining and capsular tissues. Even though subsequent experience failed to establish the effectiveness of synovectomy in the eradication of articular tuberculosis, the procedure has been used intermittently for other forms of synovitis, notably rheumatoid arthritis, hemophilia, and synovial metaplasia.

The treatment of internal derangements of the knee focused initially on meniscal injury. Following his description of meniscal tears in 1784, Hey described treatment by manipulation of the joint, followed, if manipulation failed, by a period of immobilization. After Thomas Annandale of Edinburgh reported *The Care of Loose Cartilages Recovered from the Knee Joint by Direct Incision with Antiseptic Precautions,* meniscectomy was gradually adopted worldwide.

Hey-Groves introduced repair of the cruciate ligaments in 1917, passing the lower portion of the iliotibial band through drill holes in the femoral condyles to replace the torn ligament, a procedure surprisingly similar to those used today. Edwards in 1924 proposed a method for repair of the collateral ligaments, both medial and lateral.

Tagaki developed the arthroscope between 1918 and 1920. In 1922, Bircher utilized the end of a Jacobaeus laparoscope for the diagnosis of internal derangements of the knee in 32 patients. In 1925, Kreuscher in the United States described an instrument resembling the cystoscope for examination of the intraarticular space. His work was followed by that of Burman, Mayer, and Finkelstein at the Hospital for Joint Diseases, who developed an arthroscope of their own design. During the 1950s, Watanabe popularized the operation of arthroscopy for diagnosis; its extension to therapy has evolved slowly since that time.

Operations on Tendons

The first name associated with the surgery of tendons is usually that of Isaac Minnius of the Netherlands, who performed a *tenotomy* for torticollis in 1685. Almost 125 years later, Lorenz of Frankfurt made the first attempt to correct a clubfoot deformity by division of the Achilles tendon. General acceptance of the procedure followed the effort and enthusiasm of George F. Stromeyer, whose work beginning in 1831 permanently changed the prognosis for this disorder. After William John

Little underwent Achilles' tenotomy by Stromeyer, he became an enthusiastic advocate for the procedure—leading 2 years later (1837) to his *Treatise on the Nature of Clubfoot and Analogous Distortions.* The technique of tenotomy was quickly extended to other parts of the body, including release of spastic pronator muscles in the forearm by Doubowitski in 1841.

Tendon grafting, which had been attempted repeatedly since Paré's time without success, was restudied as a supplement to tendon lengthening. Rehn's studies, showing that tendon grafts remained viable only if early movement was instituted, led to frequent employment of this procedure for tendon injuries of the hands.

Tendon transference, in which a nearby healthy muscle is used to substitute for a paralytic one, was carried out in 1880 by Nicoladoni of Innsbruck, although the procedure had been performed sporadically in the preceding decade. Codivilla, who recognized the importance of preserving the tendon sheaths in certain locations to prevent peritendinous adhesions, in 1899 reported a technique in which the tendon of the paralyzed muscle was withdrawn from its sheath and the transplanted tendon put in its place. In 1919, Lexer wrote his definitive work on the subject of free autogenous transplants, including tendons and fascia.

Tenodesis, the conversion of tendons to ligaments, was originated by Tilanus in 1898 and used most frequently thereafter for paralytic equinus deformities.

SUMMARY

Third century B.C.		
420–380	Tuberculosis described	Hippocrates
	Gout described anecdotally	Hippocrates
	Splints used for fracture treatment	Hippocrates
	Rickets described	Homer *(The Iliad)*
First century A.D.		
A.D. 50–59	Rheumatoid arthritis described	Soranus of Ephesus
Sixteenth century		
1500–1509	Braces and traction with weights and pulleys used for musculoskeletal disorders	Ambroise Paré
Seventeenth century		
1610–1619	Circulation of the blood described	William Harvey
1640–1649	Term *rickets* coined	Daniel Whistler

| 1670–1679 | Crystals in gouty tophi recognized | van Leeuwenhoek |
| 1680–1689 | Tenotomy for torticollis performed | Isaac Minnius |

Eighteenth century

1740–1749	Term *orthopaedic* used	Nicholas Andry
	Morphologic sequence of fracture healing described	John Hunter
1760–1769	Brachial plexus injury in newborns described	William Smellie
1770–1779	Tuberculous paraplegia described	Sir Percivall Pott
1780–1789	"Infantile paralysis" (poliomyelitis) described	Michael Underwood
	Joint excision for destructive joint disease performed	Henry Park

Nineteenth century

1800–1809	Term *internal derangement of the knee* used	William Hey
	Description of hemophilia	J. C. Otto
1820–1829	Term *osteomyelitis* coined	A. Nélaton
	Shock described	Marshall Hall
	Congenital dislocation of the hip described	G. Dupuytren
	Joint mobilized by creation of a pseudarthrosis	John Rhea Barton
1830–1839	Tenotomy of Achilles tendon performed	William John Little
	Osteotomy performed to correct limb deformity	John Rhea Barton
1840–1849	Antisepsis introduced	I. P. Semmelweis
	Ether anesthesia used	Crawford W. Long
	Bone sarcoma differentiated and named	A. Boyer
	Hyperuricemia of gout described	A. B. Garrod
1850–1859	Plaster-of-paris bandage introduced	Antoninus Mathijsen
	Compression of the median nerve at the wrist (carpal tunnel syndrome) described	Sir James Paget

	Discovery that the lesion in poliomyelitis was localized to the anterior horn cells of the spinal cord	G. B. A. Duchenne
	Term *rheumatoid arthritis* used	A. B. Garrod
1860–1869	Definitive paper on cerebral palsy published	William J. Little
	Surgery performed under antiseptic conditions	Lord S. J. Lister
	Heredity experiments on hybridization carried out	Gregor Mendel
1870–1879	Screws used to maintain apposition of bone fragments	L. J. B. Berenger-Ferand
	Microorganisms causing surgical infection described	Louis Pasteur
	Bandage used to produce a bloodless field in surgery	J. F. A. von Esmarch
1880–1889	Surgical fusion of joints (arthrodesis) performed	Eduard Albert
	Transfer of tendons described	K. Nicoladoni
	Description of muscle reaction to ischemia	Richard von Volkmann
	Differential stain for bacteria developed	H. C. J. Gram
	Parathyroid glands discovered	Ivar Sandstrom
	Neuropathic joint disease described	Jean-Martin Charcot
	Neurofibromatosis described	F. D. von Recklinghausen
	Postulates to establish the pathogenic character of a microorganism listed; tubercle bacillus identified	Robert Koch
	Hematogenous osteomyelitis produced by injection of *Staphylococci*	A. Rodet
	Use of cocaine for nerve blocks described	William Halsted
	Chronic arthritides classified into osteoarthritis and rheumatoid arthritis	A. E. Garrod

	Statistical study of biological variation and inheritance introduced	Sir Francis Galton
	Law on bone transformation in response to stress stated	Julius Wolff
1890–1899	X-ray discovered	Wilhelm Röentgen
	Aspirin introduced	H. Dreser

Twentieth century

1900–1909	Painful posttraumatic bone atrophy described	P. Sudeck
	Urate crystals incriminated as the cause of gouty arthritis	M. Freudweiler
	Osteochondritis dissecans described	J. König
	Era of modern fracture surgery begun; plates used for internal fixation of fractures	Sir William A. Lane; Albin Lambotte
	Apophysitis of the tibial tubercle (Osgood-Schlatter disease) described	R. B. Osgood; Carl Schlatter
	Varieties of brachial paralysis distinguished	Madame Augusta Klumpke
	Novocaine introduced	Alfred Einhorn
	Skeletal traction used with weights attached to a pin passed through the bone	Fritz Steinmann
1910–1919	Legg-Calvé-Perthes disease (coxa plana) described	A. T. Legg; J. Calvé; G. C. Perthes
	Bone grafting operations introduced	Russell A. Hibbs; Fred Albee
	Test for nerve regeneration described	Jules Tinel
	Repair of cruciate ligaments performed	E. W. Hey-Groves
	Treatise on transplantation of autogenous joints, tendons, and fascia published	E. W. Lexer
	Principle of wound debridement established	H. W. M. Gray
	Rickets treated with cod liver oil	E. Mellanby

	"Formication sign" of nerve regeneration described	Jules Tinel
1920–1929	Endoscopic technique for intraarticular examination introduced	E. Bircher
	"Endothelial myeloma" (Ewing sarcoma) described	James Ewing
	Parathormone isolated	J. B. Collip
	Molded interpositional materials used for treatment of joint disease	M. N. Smith-Petersen
	Emboli or thromboses suggested as cause of epiphyseal necroses	G. Axhausen
1930–1939	Microscopic and x-ray changes of avascular necrosis correlated; term *creeping replacement* coined	Dallas Phemister
	Relationship between parathyroid hormone and osteitis fibrosa cystica established	H. L. Jaffe
	Surgical release of carpal tunnel syndrome performed	J. Learmonth
	Connection between disk protrusion and sciatica established	W. J. Mixter; J. S. Barr
	Sulfonamide introduced	G. Domagk
1940–1949	Penicillin discovered	Sir Alexander Fleming
	Ligamentous and meniscal functions in the knee described	O. C. Brantigan; A. F. Voshell
1950–1959	Poliomyelitis vaccine discovered	Jonas Salk
1960–1969	Non-urate crystals in "gouty" patients observed	D. J. McCarty; J. L. Hollander
	Arthroplasty of the hip performed	Sir John Charnley
	Calcitonin discovered	D. H. Copp et al.
1980–1989	Trauma Score developed	American Trauma Society

SUGGESTED READINGS

BICK EM: *Sourcebook of Orthopaedics,* 2d ed. New York, Hafner, 1968.

BICK EM: *Classics of Orthopaedics,* first series. Philadelphia, Lippincott, 1976.

GARRISON FH: *An Introduction to the History of Medicine,* 4th ed. Philadelphia, Saunders, 1929.

HEY W: *Practical Observations in Surgery Illustrated with Cases.* London, James Humphreys, 1805.

KEITH A: *Menders of the Maimed.* Oxford, England, Oxford University Press, 1919.

KELLY WN, HARRIS ED JR, RUDDY S, SLEDGE CB: *Textbook of Rheumatology,* 3d ed, Philadelphia, Saunders, 1989.

MAJOR RH: *Classic Descriptions of Disease.* Baltimore, Charles C Thomas, 1932.

MORTON LT: *A Medical Bibliography,* 4th ed. London, Butler & Tanner, 1983.

RANG M: *Anthology of Orthopaedics.* Edinburgh and London, Livingstone, 1966.

Chapter 2

Formation and Growth

H. Robert Brashear

The tissues of the musculoskeletal system—bone, cartilage, muscle, tendon, and ligament—are highly specialized. Their derivation and the differentiation of their complex cells from one single cell, the fertilized ovum with its 46 chromosomes, is truly one of the remarkable feats of nature. The ovum is fertilized in the outer part of the fallopian tube, and this single cell divides repeatedly as it passes down the tube to the uterus. By the time implantation takes place, about 6 days later, the embryo has become a hollow ball, called a *blastocyst,* consisting of several thousand cells.

During the second week of development, within the wall of the uterus and near the deeper part of the implanted blastocyst, a two-layered plate of cuboidal cells is formed. A part of one of these layers, the *neurectoderm,* is destined to become the outer skin or epidermis, while its midline portion, under the influence of the notochord, will become the central nervous system. The other layer of cells will become the entoderm and give rise to the epithelial lining cells of the viscera. During the third week following fertilization, around day 16, cells invade the plane between these two layers of tissue, forming a third or intermediate layer, the mesoderm. It is from this mesodermal layer that most of the tissues that will ultimately constitute the musculoskeletal system are developed.

The longitudinal midline strip of neurectodermal tissue invaginates to form the neural tube that later becomes the brain and spinal cord. The mesodermal tissue alongside the neural tube proliferates and differentiates to become the *paraxial mesoderm.* This paraxial mesodermal tissue condenses at regular intervals along the long axis of the embryo to form the *somites* (Fig. 2.1). The first pair of somites appears near the end of the third week of gestation. Somite formation continues until the end of the fifth week, when 40 to 42 segments have been formed. The somites ultimately give rise to the vertebrae, ribs, and axial skeletal muscle.

FORMATION OF THE AXIAL SKELETON

Those portions of the somites adjacent to the neural tube and notochord are designated as the *sclerotome* and ultimately will form the vertebral bodies. This mesenchymal tissue undergoes changes such that the mid portion of the somite and its enclosed notochord become the intervertebral disk, and the lower portion of one sclerotome unites with the upper part of the sclerotome below it to form the verterbal bodies (Fig. 2.2). The vertebral bodies are thus intersegmental (between somites) in origin. The mesenchymal tissue surrounds the notochord to form the bodies of the vertebrae and encloses the neural tube to form the neural arch. During the sixth week, chondrification centers appear in this loose mesenchymal tissue on each side of the future vertebral body and on each side of the neural arch. These centers ultimately fuse, and the entire vertebra becomes a cartilaginous model of the future structure (Fig. 2.3).

During the eighth week of development, blood vessels invade the cartilage model, and ossification centers appear in the body and in each neural arch. These centers enlarge and eventually fuse to form the mature bony vertebrae. Failure in the development of the car-

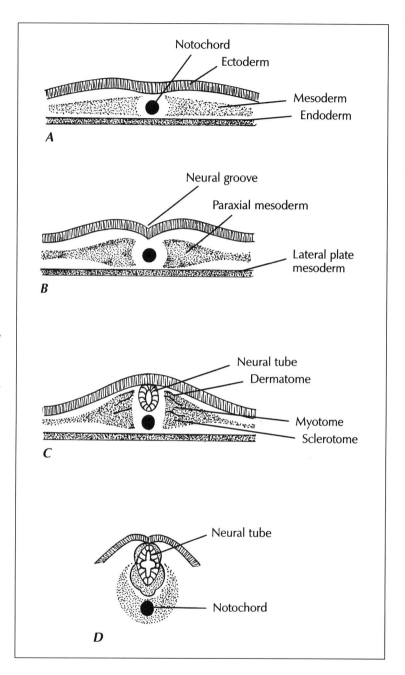

Figure 2.1 Development of the somite. *A.* Initially, the mesoderm exists as a sheet of cells between the ectoderm and the endoderm. *B.* The mesoderm thickens along the notochord to form the paraxial cords of mesenchyme. *C.* The somite is composed of layers—the dermatome, myotome, and sclerotome. *D.* The cells of the sclerotome migrate around the notochord to form the primordium of a vertebra. [Used with permission from Wilson FC (ed): *The Musculoskeletal System: Basic Processes and Disorders,* 2d ed. Philadelphia, Lippincott, 1983, p 7, Chap. 1.]

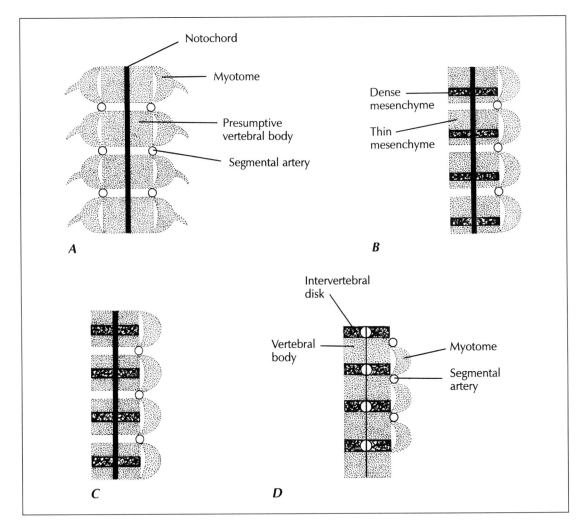

Figure 2.2 Events in the formation of the vertebrae and intervertebral disks. *A.* Early stage: the sclerotome is segmented, and each sclerotomal segment is paralleled by a pair of myotomes: the sclerotomal segments surround the notochord, and a segmental artery courses between the myotomes. *B.* Each sclerotomal segment contains condensed mesenchyme in its caudal portion. *C.* The condensed mesenchyme of the sclerotome migrates cephalad and comes to lie midway between the cranial and caudal borders of the myotome. *D.* The condensed mesenchyme of the sclerotome becomes the intervertebral disk, and the notochord gradually disappears from the vertebral body but enlarges in the intervertebral disk as the nucleus pulposus; the myotome extends from one vertebral body to the next. [Used with permission from Wilson FC (ed): *The Musculoskeletal System: Basic Processes and Disorders,* 2d ed. Philadelphia, Lippincott, 1983, p 7, Chap. 1.]

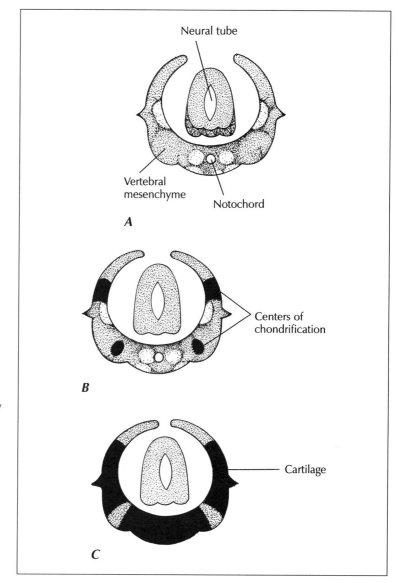

Figure 2.3   Development of a vertebra. *A.* The mesenchymal primordium. *B.* Two centers of chondrification have formed in the body, one on either side of the notochord, and centers have formed laterally in each neural arch. *C.* Extension of the chondrification centers. [Used with permission from Wilson FC (ed): *The Musculoskeletal System: Basic Processes and Disorders,* 2d ed. Philadelphia, Lippincott, 1983, p 8, Chap. 1.]

tilage or bony centers can result in such congenital abnormalities as *spina bifida,* in which the posterior elements of a spinous process do not fuse, or a *hemivertebra,* in which only half a vertebral body forms, resulting in one form of congenital scoliosis.

FORMATION OF THE APPENDICULAR SKELETON

Lateral to the condensations of paraxial mesoderm that become the somites there is a flat layer of mesoderm (middle tissue) called the *lateral plate* (Fig. 2.4). By the twentieth day of gestation, this lateral plate of mesoderm splits into two layers, an outer (parietal) layer and an inner (visceral) layer. The parietal layer of the lateral plate mesoderm is destined to become the connective tissue and muscle of the body wall, while the visceral layer develops into the connective tissue and smooth muscle of the gut and other internal structures. The space between these two layers, the *coelom,* will form the body cavities: peritoneal, pleural, and pericardial.

From the parietal (wall) mesoderm and its overlying ectoderm, limb buds appear at the early part of the fifth week of embryogenesis (Fig. 2.5). The upper limb buds develop lateral to the lower four cervical and first thoracic segments (the region of the future brachial plexus). The buds of the lower limb appear opposite the lower four lumbar and upper three sacral segments (the area of the future lumbosacral plexus) 1 or 2 days later than the upper limb buds. At the time the limb buds appear, the primordia of most of the internal organs have developed, and the musculature of the body wall has already differentiated.

Initially the limb buds consist of a layer of ectoderm covering a mass of mesenchymal tissue. *Mesenchyme* is loose, embryonic connective tissue derived from mesoderm. At the tip of the limb bud, within the ectoderm, is a thickened layer of cells, the *apical ectodermal ridge.* This layer of cells plays an important role in stimulating the growth of mesodermal tissue and the limb bud but has little to do with the cellular differentiation in the developing limb. The bulk of information leading to tissue differentiation and to the development of form apparently lies within the primitive mesenchyme.

A blood supply to the limb bud develops early and well before the ingrowth of nerves. At first this supply consists of a diffuse, fine capillary network arising directly from the primitive aorta. Soon certain channels begin to take preference, and a central artery forms. Around the periphery of the bud, a marginal sinus forms, the remnants of which, in the upper limb, become the basilic and cephalic veins. From the central artery and through a complex series of changes are developed first an interosseous and a median artery and subsequently the radial and ulnar arteries.

During the sixth week of development, the distal portion of the limb bud becomes flattened and paddlelike. Within these paddles, rays that represent the future digits appear. In the proximal part of the limb bud, condensations of the mesenchymal tissue along the central axis of the limb are the first evidence of the skeleton. In the upper limb, the primordia for the scapula and humerus develop first, followed by those for the radius and ulna, and finally those for the bones of the hand. A similar sequence of events takes place in the lower limb, but a day or so later. These condensed mesenchymal cells, designating the future

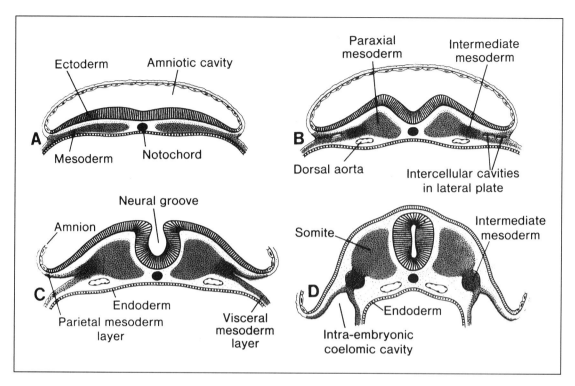

Figure 2.4   Transverse sections showing the development of the
mesodermal germ layer. *A.* Day 17. *B.* Day 19. *C.* Day 20. *D.* Day 24. The
thin mesodermal sheet gives rise to the paraxial mesoderm (the future
somites), the intermediate mesoderm (the future excretory units), and the
lateral plate, which is split into the parietal and visceral mesodermal layers
lining the intraembryonic coelomic cavity. [Reproduced with permission
from Sadler TW (ed): *Langman's Medical Embryology,* 5th ed. Baltimore,
Williams & Wilkins, 1985, Chap. 5, p 64.]

bones, begin to secrete a matrix and become
cartilage. By the seventh week, the cartilaginous model of most of the limb bones is in
place. Gaps between the ends of these cartilaginous segments, where primitive mesenchyme persists, mark the position of the
future joints. Condensations of tissue surrounding these gaps ultimately become fibrous
to form the joint capsules and the ligaments
(Fig. 2.6).

The embryogenesis of limb muscle is complex. In contrast to other connective tissue of
the limb, skeletal muscle is of somitic origin.
Mesenchymal cells split away from the somitic
myotome and migrate into the early limb bud.
At the same time, these cells become elongated
and undergo internal changes to become spindle-shaped myoblasts. By the sixth to seventh
week, as the cartilaginous model of the skeleton begins to appear, the surrounding myo-

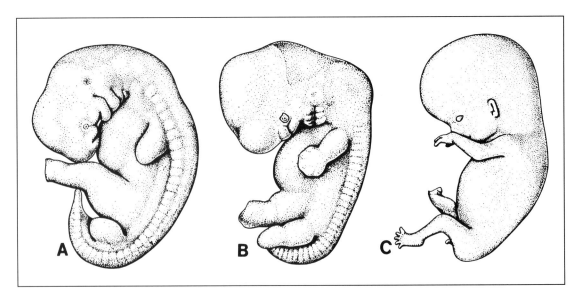

Figure 2.5 Schematic drawings of human embryos to demonstrate the
development of the limb buds: *(A)* at 5 weeks, *(B)* at 6 weeks, *(C)* at 8
weeks. Note that the hindlimb buds are somewhat behind in development
in comparison with those of the forelimbs. [Reproduced with permission
from Sadler TW (ed): *Langman's Medical Embryology,* 5th ed. Baltimore,
Williams & Wilkins, 1985, Chap. 9, p 140.]

blasts begin to fuse, forming elongated multinucleated cells, the myotubes. Within the
myotube there is active synthesis of actin and
myosin, the principal contractile proteins of
muscle. Myofilaments develop, gradually become organized, and, during the third month
of development, typical striated muscle cells
are found. With the increase in volume of
myofilaments, the nuclei of the muscle cells
migrate to the periphery.

On a larger scale, the masses of muscle cells
surrounding the cartilage primordia of the limb
bones split longitudinally, first into large flexor
and extensor masses, then further into bundles
that will form the individual muscles. This
separation begins about the time nerve fibers
start to grow into the muscle masses. The
nerve fibers may influence this process. Tendons arise separately from muscles and only
later join with them. They are derived from
the local mesenchyme and are not of somitic
origin.

As limb development proceeds, creases become evident at the knee, elbow, wrist, and
ankle, and clefts form between digital rays of
the hands and feet. The interdigital clefts form
through programmed self-destruction of the
cells between the rays, a process termed *apop-
tosis.* By the eighth week, at the end of the
embryonic and beginning of the fetal period,
the limb buds have differentiated to a form
similar to that of the adult limb.

Figure 2.6   Major events in the development of a synovial joint. *A.* The cartilaginous models of the two participating bones are surrounded by condensed mesenchyme. Small clefts in the dense mesenchyme between the bones enlarge to form the joint cavity. *B.* Progress in the formation of the joint cavity. *C.* The clefts have coalesced to form the joint cavity; the mesenchyme surrounding the joint has become the joint capsule lined with synovium. Mesenchyme persists over the ends of the two bones. *D.* The mesenchyme over the ends of the two bones is replaced by articular cartilage. [Redrawn with permission from Wilson FC (ed): *The Musculoskeletal System: Basic Processes and Disorders,* 2d ed. Philadelphia, Lippincott, 1983, p 12, Chap. 1.]

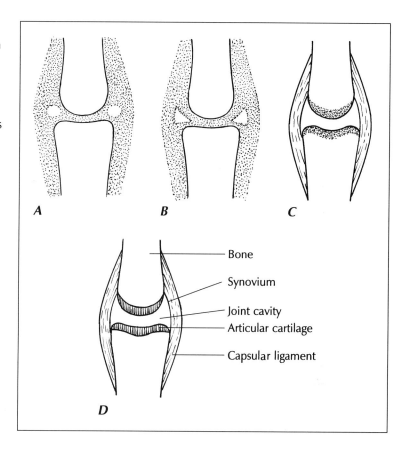

OSSIFICATION OF THE LIMB BONES

With the exception of the clavicle, all of the bones of the trunk and limbs are formed first as cartilage. A portion of the clavicle ossifies directly from mesenchymal tissue *(intramembranous ossification).* The clavicle is also unique in that it is the first bone of the body to ossify. Bone appearing in the clavicle by the end of the fifth week is a good early radiographic marker of fetal development.

Ossification of the cartilaginous model is a matter of replacement of cartilage by bone tissue, not the conversion or metaplasia of cartilage cells into bone-forming cells. This process is called *enchondral* (or *endochondral*) *ossification.* In the long bones, ossification be-

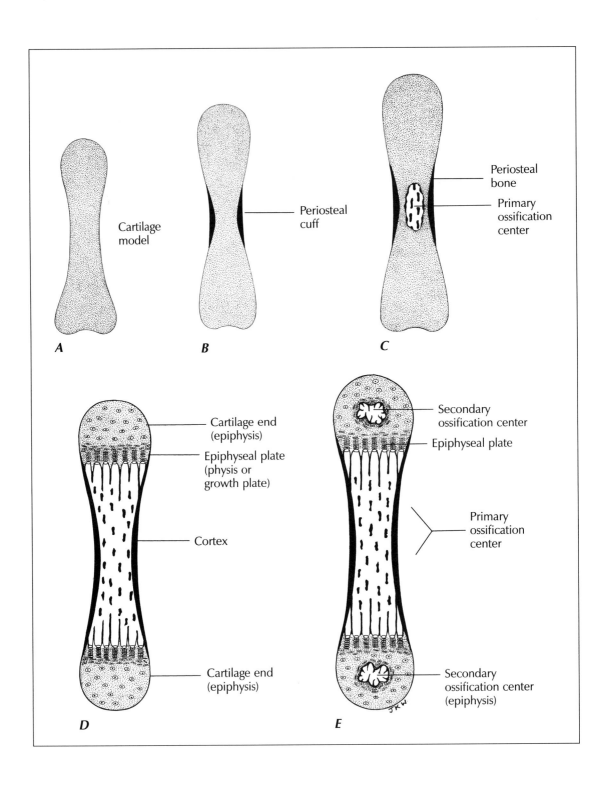

Cartilage
model

Periosteal
cuff

Periosteal
bone

Primary
ossification
center

A

B

C

Cartilage end
(epiphysis)

Epiphyseal plate
(physis or
growth plate)

Cortex

Cartilage end
(epiphysis)

Secondary
ossification center

Epiphyseal plate

Primary
ossification
center

Secondary
ossification center
(epiphysis)

D

E

gins in the middle of the shaft. A condensation of connective tissue cells covers the cartilage model as *perichondrium*. Those cells on the surface of the midportion of the shaft become periosteal osteoblasts and form a cuff of bone around the cartilage model. This periosteal cuff of bone arises directly from the periosteal cells and is thus intramembranous rather than enchondral in origin.

At the same time, the cartilage cells deep in the center of the shaft and beneath the periosteal cuff undergo a series of changes that culminate in their death and destruction. The cells enlarge, their nuclei undergo *chromatolysis*, and the surrounding matrix begins to calcify. Vascular tissue grows in from the periosteal cuff and invades these dead cartilage cells. The cellular elements of the cartilage are destroyed by the invading tissue, leaving only spicules

of matrix. Osteoblasts entering with the vessels deposit bone on these spicules of calcified cartilage matrix. Thus, the extracellular matrix of the cartilage forms a scaffolding upon which the new bone is formed. This is *enchondral ossification*. Although this is first seen in the midshafts of long bones (the *primary ossification centers*), the same type of enchondral ossification is seen later at the epiphyseal plate and within the secondary ossification centers (epiphyses). It is also found in fracture callus and in certain cartilaginous tumors.

Once begun, the primary ossification in the center of the shaft extends rapidly toward the ends of the bone and ultimately occupies the areas that will become the diaphyses and metaphyses. This process begins in the fetal femur around the ninth week and leaves a central

Figure 2.7   The embryogenesis of a long bone. *A.* The cartilage model. As the limb buds are formed, the mesenchyme in their centers condenses, and during the sixth week of development this condensed mesenchyme is replaced by hyaline cartilage that takes the shape of the particular long bone. *B.* The cartilage model continues to grow along with the limb. Cells on its surface differentiate into osteoblasts and form a cuff of periosteal bone around the shaft, which will become the diaphysis. *C.* About the same time vessels grow into the central part of the cartilage model, and a center of endochondral ossification is created. This is the primary ossification center. This center extends at the expense of the hyaline cartilage toward either end of the bone. *D.* At each end of the primary ossification center, cartilage cells become arranged in a linear manner to form the epiphyseal plates, from which future longitudinal growth takes place. Hyaline cartilage covering each end of the bone constitute the epiphyses. This is the condition of most long bones at the time of birth, the exception being the femur, in which the distal epiphysis begins to ossify before birth. *E.* At a later time, which varies with each individual bone, vessels grow into the cartilaginous epiphyses and enchondral ossification results in formation of the bony epiphyses, the secondary centers of ossification.

shaft of bone covered at each end by rounded masses of cartilage (Fig. 2.7). This is the condition of most long bones at the time of birth, the distal femur being an exception.

Within the cartilage masses at the ends of long bones, three separate zones will appear. The cartilage at the periphery of the mass is articular cartilage and has been such since the joints became apparent in the early embryonic period. The cartilage in the center of the mass will undergo the changes described above that precede enchondral ossification: the central portion of this cartilage is invaded by blood vessels and the *secondary centers of ossification,* the *epiphyses,* form. The only secondary center present at the time of birth is that of the distal femur. Other centers appear in specific order during childhood. One of the last major centers to appear is that of the distal ulna, which ossifies during the sixth year. The orderly and sequential appearance of ossification centers, particularly those of the bones of the hand, is used to determine bone age.

The third part of the cartilage mass covering the ends of long bone, that closest to the metaphysis and away from the articular surface, becomes the *epiphyseal plate* or *physis.* The secondary centers of ossification (epiphyses) are separated from the shaft of the bone by the epiphyseal plate as long as the bone continues to grow in length. At varied but again fairly specific times in late childhood and early adult life, epiphyseal plates are obliterated, and the epiphyses and metaphyses are united.

GROWTH OF THE EPIPHYSES (SECONDARY CENTERS)

These secondary centers, the epiphyses and apophyses, begin, as indicated above, as masses of cartilage. At varying times blood vessels grow into the centers of these masses, and a focus of enchondral ossification forms that becomes visible on the radiograph as the epiphysis. At first this center enlarges slowly in all directions and the early bony centers have a roughly spherical shape. This spherical enlargement of the epiphyses continues for several years. However, at a time that varies with each center, growth ceases in that part of the center adjacent to the epiphyseal plate. From that point on, enchondral ossification, and therefore enlargement of the epiphysis, takes place only at those portions of the center adjacent to the articular cartilage. A porous bony plate forms on the side of the epiphysis adjacent to the epiphyseal plate. This subphyseal bone plate functions as a mechanical support for the growth plate, much as subchondral bone supports the articular cartilage. There are numerous perforations in the subphyseal bone plate to permit vessels from the epiphysis to reach the reserve zone and the base of the proliferative zone of cartilage cells of the epiphyseal plate (see below).

Continued enchondral ossification, and therefore growth of the epiphysis beneath the articular cartilage, requires that blood vessels reach the deep surface of the cartilage. The bone of the epiphysis (secondary ossification center) is cancellous (trabecular). As the child grows and weight-bearing and developing muscles put more stress on the articular cartilage, increasing support for the flexible cartilage is required. The cancellous bone just beneath the articular surface begins to align its trabeculae in bars parallel to the joint surface. Because of the need for blood vessels to reach the cartilage for enchondral ossification (and growth) to continue, there are many perforations in this youthful subchondral bone. With maturity, growth of the epiphyses ceases, the perforations in the subchondral bone are filled in, and a solid plate of bone (the subchondral plate) is formed. This is the white line marking the joint margins seen on the radiograph and the solid plate of bone covering the joints of a laboratory skeleton. In the adult the articular cartilage is sealed (bound) to the subchondral bone along a line referred to as the *tide mark*. This basophilic line, often seen as a double line in hematoxylin and eosin (H&E) sections, marks the junction between the end of the bone and the overlying cartilage. Its name comes from its wavy configuration, much like the serpentine line(s) of small beach debris left behind along the shore after high tide.

THE EPIPHYSEAL PLATE (PHYSIS)

Following ossification of the diaphysis and metaphyses (primary center), that part of the cartilage mass covering the ends of long bones nearest the metaphysis becomes the epiphyseal plate, or physis. It is from this plate that growth in length of the long bones takes place. Because bone is a hard tissue, interstitial growth, such as that seen in the liver and other soft organs, cannot occur. Bone growth must take place on a surface. Because the ends of long bones are covered by articular cartilage, a mechanism must be present for the conversion of growing cartilage into bone. Where relatively rapid growth must take place, the highly specialized epiphyseal cartilage plate has evolved. Growth in length can occur directly beneath articular cartilage (see "Growth of the Epiphyses," above), but this process is usually limited and slow. (Consider the length of an epiphysis compared to that of a long bone shaft.)

At the epiphyseal plate, proliferation of cartilage cells is the basis for the longitudinal growth of bone. On the metaphyseal side of the plate, cartilage is exchanged for bone, and this process of enchondral bone formation continues until growth ceases. At the microscopic level, the growth plate is generally considered to consist of four zones or layers (Fig. 2.8). Although these are fairly distinct, one zone merges gradually into the adjacent one. The first zone, that closest to the epiphysis and most distant from the metaphysis, consists of randomly scattered cartilage cells within an abundance of matrix. It is called the *resting* or *reserve zone,* but these names are a bit misleading in that mitotic activity is rarely seen in this area. It is possible that this zone functions as a somewhat flexible base supporting the overlying proliferative zone. Immediately next to the resting zone, toward the metaphysis, the cartilage cells become aligned in regular columns oriented parallel to the long axis of the shaft. This zone is called the *proliferative zone* or *zone of cell columns.* It is at the base of these columns (the end nearest the epiphysis) that mitotic activity is concentrated. Cell division here constantly pushes the epiphysis away from the metaphysis during the growing period.

The height (thickness) of the epiphyseal plate varies with age, rate of growth, and size of the bone. The proliferating zone consists of from ten to twenty cartilage cells and is roughly 100 to 300 μm deep. At the metaphyseal side of this zone, the cartilage cells in the columns begin to enlarge and expand at the expense of the extracellular matrix. This is the third zone or *zone of hypertrophy;* the cellular enlargement here also contributes to growth in length. As the metaphysis is approached, the cartilage matrix alongside the last three or four hypertrophic cells becomes densely calcified,

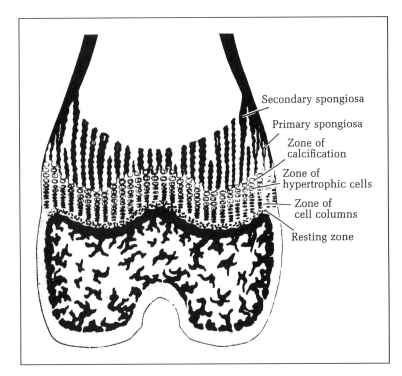

Secondary spongiosa

Primary spongiosa

Zone of calcification

Zone of hypertrophic cells

Zone of cell columns

Resting zone

Figure 2.8   Distal end of the growing femur showing the four layers of the cartilaginous growth plate and the primary and secondary spongiosa of the metaphysis. [Redrawn with permission from Wilson FC (ed): *The Musculoskeletal System: Basic Processes and Disorders,* 2d ed. Philadelphia, Lippincott, 1983, Chap. 6, p 94.]

producing the fourth zone, or *zone of provisional calcification.* Matrix calcification seems to be necessary for the next and final step at the growth plate, the invasion of the last cartilage cell in the column by blood vessels from the metaphysis. This invasion results in the complete obliteration of all intracellular elements of the chondrocyte. If, because of an abnormality in calcium metabolism, calcification of cartilage fails to take place, destruction of the last cartilage cell and vascular invasion do not occur, and hypertrophic cartilage cells continue to pile up. This aberration results in the gross thickening and bulging of the epiphyseal plate characterizing rickets. Normally, with the destruction of the last cartilage cell, all that remains is the calcified cartilage matrix that made up the walls of the former chondrocytes.

In place of columns of cells, spikes of calcified cartilaginous matrix protrude from the growth plate into the metaphysis. This cartilage is more densely calcified than the adjacent bone, for cartilage, being of high water content, can hold more calcium salt than osteoid. It is upon these parallel spikes of calcified cartilaginous matrix that osteoblasts, nourished by capillaries of the metaphysis, lay down a layer of bone that welds the metaphysis to the growth plate. *Enchondral bone,* the microscopic hallmark of enchondral ossification, is a trabecula of bone in which is embedded a segment of acellular, calcified cartilage matrix. This enchondral bone with its core of cartilage persists only a few millimeters into the metaphysis and is called the *primary spongiosa.* Because of its cartilage center, bone of the primary spongiosa is structurally inferior to pure homogeneous bone; presumably for this reason, the primary spongiosa is quickly removed by osteoclasts and replaced by trabeculae of pure bone. This bone, found in the remainder of the metaphysis away from the growth plate, is the *secondary spongiosa.* Persistence of the primary spongiosa and its contained calcified cartilage throughout the metaphysis is a characteristic of the inherited bone disorder of *osteopetrosis* ("marble bones").

GROWTH OF THE LONG BONES

Growth of the long bones takes place in three areas, the epiphysis, the growth plate, and the surface of the shaft (Fig. 2.9). Each of these areas has unique growth features and is considered separately.

The microscopic aspects of epiphyseal growth, as described above, are predominantly those of enchondral ossification from overlying articular cartilage. Although epiphyseal growth is slow, the epiphysis remains proportionate in size to the rest of the bone. The blood supply that furnishes the energy for this growth is from the epiphyseal vessels. Growth of the epiphysis continues until maturity, which is marked histologically by the development of an intact subchondral bone plate (without vascular perforations) and the presence of a tide mark at the junction of the subchondral bone and articular cartilage.

The great majority of growth in length takes place at the epiphyseal plates found at both ends of most long bones but at only one end of some smaller bones, such as the phalanges, metacarpals, and metatarsals. One of the fascinating yet unexplained aspects of physeal

growth is the fairly constant ratio of growth between the proximal and distal ends of bones. For example, growth at the distal end of the femur is about four times as rapid as growth at its proximal end and accounts for about 80 percent of femoral length. The opposite holds for the humerus, as the great part of its elongation takes place at the proximal end. These ratios are retained, with few exceptions, for most mammalian species.

Energy for cell division in the proliferative layer of the growth plate is provided by the epiphyseal vessels. After entering the epiphysis, these vessels ramify and are distributed to the subchondral area to nourish epiphyseal growth. Other branches of these vessels penetrate the openings in the subphyseal plate that supports the growth plate, where they terminate in small capillary tufts at the base of the cell columns. From these tufts, oxygen and other nutrients diffuse through the cartilage matrix to supply the active cells of the epiphyseal plate. Interference with this epiphyseal blood supply, as may occur in epiphyseal avascular necrosis, may seriously interfere with longitudinal bone growth.

As bones grow in length, a proportional increase in the diameter of the shaft occurs. This growth in the width of the diaphysis is produced by osteoblasts in the deep layer of the periosteum. Growth in width of the shaft is thus a matter of membranous bone formation, in contrast to the enchondral ossification of epiphyseal and physeal growth.

Bone on the surface of the diaphysis is added in layers. It is mature or lamellar bone, the lamellae, or layers, being about 8 to 10 μm in width. The parallel collagen fibers of each layer differ in orientation from those in adjacent laminae. For this reason the layers, although visible under ordinary light micros-

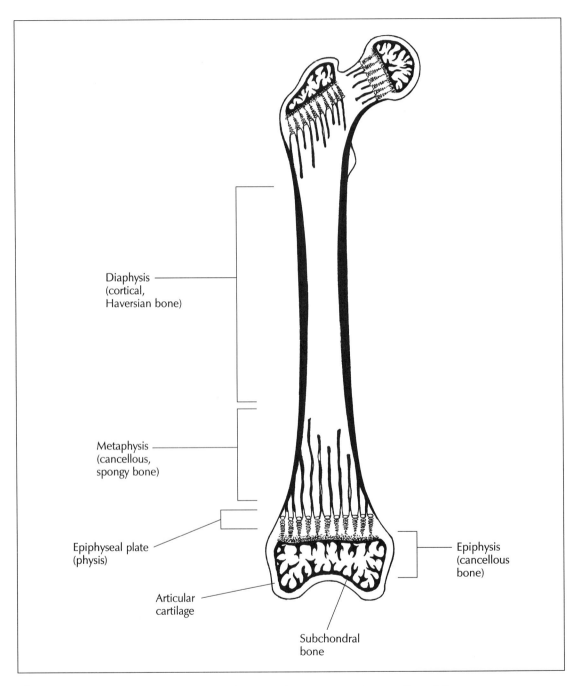

Diaphysis
(cortical,
Haversian bone)

Metaphysis
(cancellous,
spongy bone)

Epiphyseal plate
(physis)

Articular
cartilage

Subchondral
bone

Epiphysis
(cancellous
bone)

Figure 2.9   The immature femur. [Redrawn with permission from Wilson FC
(ed): *The Musculoskeletal System: Basic Processes and Disorders,* 2d ed.
Philadelphia, Lippincott, 1983, Chap. 6, p 90.]

copy, stand out strikingly under polarized light. These layers are laid down concentrically about the shaft as it enlarges. If this were the entire process by which growth in width occurred, the shaft would look very much like the cross section of a tree trunk with its concentric rings and would be a heavy, solid, and inefficient structure. However, as the diameter increases, the bone in the center of the shaft is removed by osteoclasts, producing the familiar tubular shape of bone with its central marrow cavity.

MODELING

If the growth of long bones were merely a matter of enchondral ossification at the epiphyses and membranous bone formation on the surface of the diaphysis, each bone would be of similar shape and would consist of a straight hollow tube in the center, with two inverted cones (apices toward the diaphysis) on each end, and all bones would look alike, which of course is not true. Each radius has a characteristic shape quite different from that of the femur or the tibia. The femoral shaft is round, with a typical anterior bow, while the tibia is triangular in cross section. The process of shaping bones into their adult configuration is called *modeling*. Modeling is the result of a balanced and coordinated action of osteoblasts (bone formation) and osteoclasts (bone resorption).

The epiphyses of most long bones are wider than the metaphyses. Metaphyseal bone formed at the growth plate must be trimmed back and shaped to a reduced diameter. Thus, near the ends of the metaphyses adjacent to the physis, there are osteoclasts rather than osteoblasts beneath the periosteum, which produces a form of modeling of the metaphysis called *funnelization*. Although plastic to a limited degree, bones cannot bend like rubber. The characteristic curves in the radius and the anterior bow of the femur are not a matter of bending but rather of a shift in space brought about by osteoclastic activity on one side and osteoblastic on the other.

It is by these mechanisms that bones attain their distinctive and rather complex adult shape. Though the modeling process may be influenced by stresses on the bone produced by muscle forces and by gravity, most modeling is genetically directed. In a child whose lower limbs have been paralyzed since birth and who has never walked, the femur still has the general shape of a femur.

REMODELING

Secondary change in the shape or structure of a bone as a result of changes in its environment is called *remodeling*. In 1892 a German orthopaedist, Julius Wolff, observed that every change in the form or function of a bone was followed by a corresponding change in its architecture. This is known as *Wolff's law*. If, following fracture, a bone heals with angulation, bone will gradually form along the new lines of stress. This remodeling process continues long after the fracture has healed completely. Bone mass is increased by increased stress, e.g., athletics, and is lost when stress is decreased, as with disuse. The bones of a paralyzed limb are much frailer and contain less osseous tissue than their normal counterparts.

In middle and later life, there is a gradual and progressive loss of bone mass known as *osteoporosis* (see Chap. 16). Some of this loss results from the hormonal changes of aging, but much of it is due to the decreased activity and loss of muscle mass common to later life, which diminish stresses on bone.

SUGGESTED READINGS

SADLER TW: *Langman's Medical Embryology,* 6th ed. Williams & Wilkins, Baltimore, 1990.

WILSON FC: *The Musculoskeletal System,* 2d ed. Lippincott, Philadelphia, 1983.

Chapter 3

Physiology and Biochemistry

Patrick P. Lin and Bruce Caterson

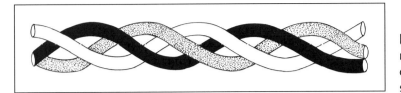

Figure 3.1 Collagen molecules. Note the characteristic triple-helical structure.

The musculoskeletal system may be viewed as an extraordinary feat of engineering. In terms of strength, durability, and efficiency, it is rivaled by few if any structures devised by humans, and attempts to replace parts of the system with metal, ceramic, and plastic have only illustrated the outstanding qualities of nature's original design. The physiologic and biochemical aspects underlying the construction of the musculoskeletal system are the focus of this chapter.

Two types of molecules are ubiquitous in musculoskeletal tissues. *Collagens* are a family of fibrillar proteins that form triple-helical structures (Fig. 3.1). Over eighteen related members of the family have been described; together they are the most abundant proteins in the body, accounting for one-quarter of the total. The amino acid sequence of the proteins is characterized by the occurrence of glycine, the smallest amino acid, in every third position, allowing the molecule to twist into a helical form. Three protocollagen peptides are braided together to form a collagen molecule, which, packed with other molecules, forms a *fibril*. Hydroxylation of proline and lysine enables the strands to be cross-linked for greater strength. The most important structural collagens are types I and II, two similar molecules that form tough, insoluble fibrils. Type I collagen is found in tendon, ligament, and bone, while type II collagen is located primarily in articular cartilage.

Proteoglycans, the other family of musculoskeletal molecules, are characterized by a combination of proteins and *glycosaminoglycans,* which are long chains of repeating disaccharide subunits. The composition of a typical proteoglycan includes a core protein, to which one or more glycosaminoglycans are attached. These glycosaminoglycans possess negatively charged anions, such as sulfate and carboxyl groups, which repel each other and give the proteoglycan the characteristic "bottle-brush" appearance seen in electron micrographs. Numerous proteoglycans have been described, varying in the protein core as well as in the type, size, and number of glycosaminoglycan side chains.

BONES

Structure and Physiology

The primary function of the skeleton is support. Bones create the rigid framework for the body and limbs, and the structure of a given bone varies according to the area it serves. Flat bones create large surfaces for muscle attachment and protect vital organs in the cranium, chest, and pelvis. Cuboidal bones articulate to allow complex motions in the wrist, ankle, and spine. Long bones provide rigid beams to extend limbs and permit actions at a distance.

Each bone is composed of a mixture of *cortical* or surface bone and *cancellous* or trabecular bone. The two types of bone have essentially the same chemical composition but differ in structure and appearance. Cortical bone is much thicker than cancellous bone and has a special vascular system to provide nutrition to the osteocytes (see Chap. 9). The relative amounts of cortical and cancellous bone vary in different regions. In a typical dumbbell-shaped long bone, the *diaphysis* or shaft has a thick cortex with minimal cancellous bone (Fig. 3.2). The diaphysis is similar to a hollow tube in being a light structure with excellent ability to withstand compressive, bending, and torsional forces. The *metaphysis,* which is the flared transition to the end of the bone, is composed mostly of cancellous bone surrounded by a gradually thinning shell of cortical bone. The cancellous bone transfers pressure from the end of a bone to the cortical bone of the diaphysis. The *epiphysis,* or end of the bone, is made up of cancellous bone, which transmits most of the force from the joint to the subchondral bone rather than the cortex. The epiphysis is broadened to increase the surface area and thereby decrease stress on the articular cartilage.

Inorganic Matrix

The essential feature of bone that permits it to serve as a rigid support is *stiffness,* a property imparted by the inorganic constituents of bone. The mineral phase accounts for 65 percent of the dry weight of bone and is composed primarily of calcium and phosphate in hydroxyapatite crystals (Fig. 3.3). Other ions include sodium, potassium, magnesium, fluoride, and carbonate. These substances modify the crystalline structure of hydroxyapatite, but the significance of the alteration is unknown. An amorphous (noncrystalline) mineral phase ac-

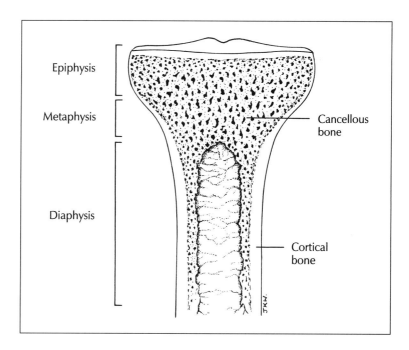

Figure 3.2 Bone structure of proximal tibia. Note the relative amounts of cortical and cancellous bone in different regions.

Epiphysis

Metaphysis

Diaphysis

Cancellous bone

Cortical bone

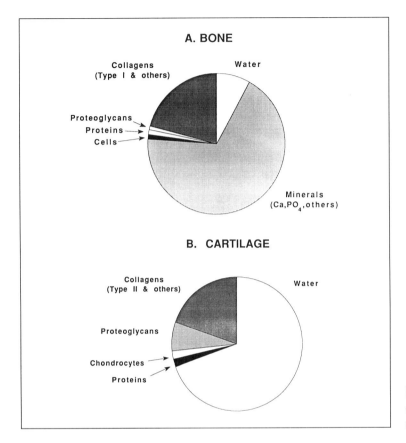

A. BONE

Collagens (Type I & others)

Water

Proteoglycans

Proteins

Cells

Minerals (Ca,PO$_4$,others)

B. CARTILAGE

Collagens (Type II & others)

Water

Proteoglycans

Chondrocytes

Proteins

Figure 3.3 Wet weight compositions of (*A*) bone and (*B*) cartilage.

counts for less than 10 percent of the inorganic phase.

Organic Matrix

The organic matrix, which comprises 35 percent of the dry weight of bone, is nearly all (95 percent) type I collagen. The molecules are staggered by quarter lengths, with "gaps" between the ends of the collagen molecules, where mineralization of the hydroxyapatite occurs (Fig. 3.4). Plates of crystals extend within and between the closely packed fibrils, which take up 80 percent of the available space in bone. The combination of hydroxyapatite and

collagen makes bone analogous to steel-reinforced concrete. Calcium and phosphate, the "concrete," provide hardness and stiffness; collagen fibrils, the "steel rods," afford tensile strength. Bone can be regarded as a two-phase or biphasic composite material, in which the strength of the composite is greater than that of either component alone. If bone lacked mineral, it would not be stiff; conversely, if it were devoid of collagen, it would be brittle, and small cracks would propagate easily. Bone is an *anisotropic* material, since its mechanical properties are not the same in all directions. The orientation of collagen fibrils, which in the cortex parallels the shaft of the bone, helps de-

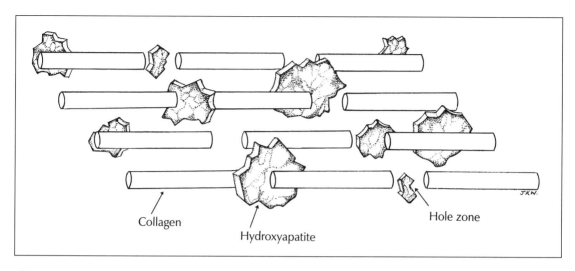

Figure 3.4 Crystallization of hydroxyapatite in the gap regions of collagen fibrils.

termine the direction of greatest tensile strength. The total amount of bone in a given area also affects the strength. According to *Wolff's law* (see Chap. 2), bone formation increases in areas receiving more stress, especially compressive stress. One of the puzzles of bone physiology is how mechanical stress translates into bone formation. One theory is that bone is a piezoelectric material that forms an electrical dipole under strain. Changes in electrical potentials may affect the behavior of osteoblasts.

Other organic molecules in bone include proteoglycans and noncollagenous proteins. The proteoglycans create an amorphous ground substance that surrounds mineralized collagen fibers. Decorin and biglycan are two small proteoglycans that bind to collagen and help regulate the diameter of collagen fibrils. In addition, proteoglycans bind and immobilize other molecules, such as *growth factors*, in the extracellular matrix. The noncollage-

nous proteins include many growth factors; in fact, bone is one of the richest sources of growth factors in the body. Although the specific function of each growth factor in bone is unknown, they can be divided into agents that cause bone resorption and agents that stimulate bone formation. *Interleukin-1* and *tumor necrosis factor alpha* are examples of substances that induce degradation of bone. Their actions may be mediated in part by *prostaglandin E,* which stimulates osteoclastic bone resorption. *Transforming growth factor beta* and *insulin-like growth factor* are examples of proteins that stimulate proliferation of osteoblasts and bone synthesis. *Bone morphogenetic protein (BMP)* is unique because it can induce new cartilage and bone formation and may play an important role in fracture healing.

The biological functions of the other noncollagenous proteins are not well understood. *Osteocalcin,* a glutamic acid–rich protein, chelates or binds to calcium by virtue of multiple carboxyl groups and may be involved in mineralization. *Osteonectin* (also known as SPARC or BM40) is a glycoprotein that also binds calcium and may regulate cell growth. *Bone sialoprotein (BSP)* is a heavily glycosylated protein that promotes calcification. *Osteopontin* is a glycoprotein that specifically binds osteoblasts and prevents crystal growth in vitro. Collectively, these matrix glycoproteins seem to be important regulators of osteoblastic and osteoclastic function.

JOINTS

Classification

There are three categories of joints: *synarthroses,* or immovable joints (e.g., cranial sutures, sternocostal joints); *amphiarthroses,* or slightly movable joints (e.g., symphysis pubis, intervertebral disks); and *diarthrodial* or *synovial* joints, which move freely and contain a synovial cavity. Among the many types of synovial joints, the amount of movement varies greatly. The hinge joint is the most common and allows motion in flexion and extension; examples are the knee, ankle, and interphalangeal joints. The ball-and-socket joint occurs where motion in multiple planes is required, such as the shoulder and hip. Gliding joints are found between the carpal and tarsal bones.

Capsules and Ligaments

Joints are stabilized in three ways. Bony architecture, such as that of the hip socket, imposes rigid constraints. Muscles and tendons provide dynamic stability, which depends on muscular contraction. The joint capsule and ligaments confer static stability, which is independent of muscles. The distinction between capsule and ligament is blurred in some areas, such as the wrist, where the ligaments are simply thickenings in the capsule; however, in other areas such as the knee, the ligaments are discrete structures. Ligaments and capsules are designed primarily to resist tension; they provide almost no resistance to compression and shear. Biochemically, the composition of the two tissues is similar; the chief constituent is parallel-fibered type I collagen molecules, which form 75 to 95 percent of the dry weight (Fig. 3.5). Other components of ligament include proteins and proteoglycans. *Elastin* is a protein that increases elasticity of tissues. The natural tendency of the molecule is to assume a globular form because of the presence of many nonpolar, hydrophobic residues. When incorporated into the extracellular matrix, it elongates like a stretched rubber band. Elastin is a prominent component of certain ligaments, including the spring ligament in the foot, which helps maintain the arch.

Synovium and Synovial Fluid

The synovium is a thin membrane that lines the joint capsule but does not cover the articular cartilage. Two kinds of synovial cells have been described: type A have the appearance of macrophages and are responsible for debridement of the synovial fluid; type B resemble secretory fibroblasts and produce synovial fluid. Lubrication of joints depends on several substances in synovial fluid. *Hyaluronic acid* is a long glycosaminoglycan molecule that imparts a thick, viscous character to synovial fluid. *Lubricin* is a glycoprotein that binds to joint surfaces and provides a slick coating to cartilage. Charged carbohydrate residues on

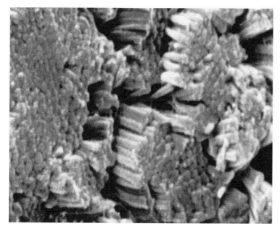

A

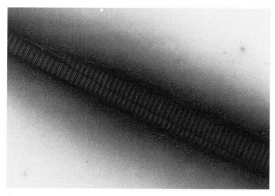

B

Figure 3.5 Type I collagen fibrils in ligament. *A.* Scanning electron micrograph of the cut end of a ligament shows densely packed collagen fibrils. *B.* Transmission electron micrograph of a single collagen fibril demonstrates a light-and-dark banding pattern that reflects the staggered array of collagen molecules. (Courtesy of L. E. Dahners.)

lubricin are responsible for its lubricating properties.

In addition to lubrication, synovial fluid also delivers nutrients to chondrocytes and removes waste products. Synovial fluid is essentially an ultrafiltrate of plasma that contains glucose, amino acids, electrolytes, and growth factors. Articular cartilage is avascular, and chondrocytes depend upon the fluid in the joint for their survival. Movement of molecules across the synovium depends upon their size. Ions and gases diffuse rapidly, while larger entities, such as proteins, migrate slowly. Absorption of waste materials occurs through the cells directly or through spaces between the lining cells. Since it is not composed of epithelium, synovium does not form a continuous basement membrane. During inflammation, clefts appear in the synovial membrane, which ease the passage of large entities such as cells, immunoglobulins, and antibiotics.

Cartilage

Three kinds of cartilage exist in the body: hyaline cartilage, fibrocartilage, and elastic cartilage. Hyaline cartilage and fibrocartilage are important in the musculoskeletal system, but elastic cartilage occurs only in limited areas, such as the outer ear and the epiglottis. Elastic cartilage resembles hyaline cartilage in appearance and composition but is distinguished by the presence of elastic fibers in the matrix.

Hyaline Cartilage
Hyaline cartilage forms the articular surfaces of synovial joints. It is a remarkable material because of its durability, capacity to withstand tremendous compressive forces, and exceptionally low coefficient of friction. The three main components of hyaline cartilage are collagen, proteoglycans, and water (Fig. 3.3). The high concentration of proteoglycans gives articular cartilage a high refractive index and makes the collagen invisible under light microscopy; hence its designation as *hyaline* or

glasslike. Although the appearance of cartilage is amorphous, it has a highly ordered ultrastructure, with the collagen fibers arranged in arcades (Fig. 3.6). At the *surface zone,* or superficial zone, the collagen fibers are parallel to the surface, forming a tight, membranelike sheet that counteracts frictional and tensile forces. Very little proteoglycan is present at the surface. In the *middle zone,* the collagen fibers are more randomly oriented to dissipate shear forces, and the proteoglycan concentration is greater. In the *deep zone,* the collagen fibers become more vertically oriented, allowing firm attachment to the *calcified zone,* but the fibers do not penetrate the underlying subchondral bone, which contains a different type of collagen.

Nearly all of the collagen in hyaline cartilage is composed of type II collagen, making up 60 to 70 percent of the dry weight of cartilage. It is not known why hyaline cartilage contains type II rather than type I collagen, which is much more prevalent in other musculoskeletal tissues. Other collagens, such as types VI, IX, and XI, are present in minute quantities in articular cartilage and have different molecular architectures. These molecules do not form the same large fibrils as type II collagen, and their functions are apparently different. Type XI collagen may be involved in the nucleation of type II collagen fibrils, while type IX collagen may be important for cross-linking and stabilizing the type II collagen network.

Proteoglycans represent approximately 25 to 30 percent of the dry weight of cartilage. The major proteoglycan is *aggrecan,* which is named for its ability to aggregate into giant

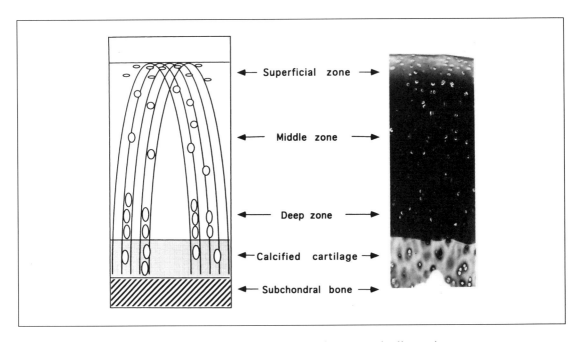

Figure 3.6 Ultrastructure of articular cartilage. Note the Beninghoff arcades of type II collagen fibrils.

macromolecular structures. The proteoglycan clusters exceed molecular weights of 100 million Da and become entrapped in the collagen meshwork. Each macromolecular aggregate consists of a long chain of hyaluronic acid, to which are bound multiple molecules of aggrecan via the G1 globular domain (hyaluronic acid–binding region). This noncovalent interaction is stabilized by the small glycoprotein *link protein,* which binds both to the G1 domain and hyaluronic acid.

The biochemical structure of aggrecan includes a core protein to which are attached approximately 100 chondroitin sulfate chains and 50 keratan sulfate chains (Fig. 3.7). The high charge density of aggrecan accounts for the stiffness of cartilage and its ability to resist compression. Repulsion between negatively charged groups creates an outward, expansile force as the proteoglycans try to spread out. More importantly, however, the charged groups attract water molecules and hold them tightly in the cartilage gel. Almost 75 percent of the total weight of cartilage is water, which is essentially incompressible. When cartilage is loaded, water is squeezed out of the gel, and the concentration of proteoglycan increases, leading to a rise in the charge density and a corresponding increase in stiffness.

Cartilage contains several other species of proteoglycans besides aggrecan, including the small interstitial proteoglycans *decorin* and *biglycan.* Decorin occurs predominantly in the superficial zones of cartilage, whereas biglycan is located in the pericellular matrix around

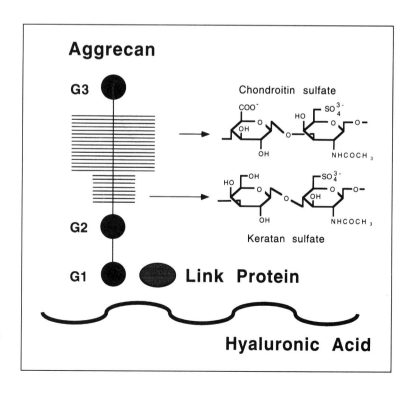

Figure 3.7 Aggrecan (large aggregating proteoglycan). Note the negative charges on chondroitin sulfate and keratan sulfate. The interactions with hyaluronic acid and link protein are noncovalent.

chondrocytes. The structure of these small proteoglycans differs markedly from that of aggrecan. Decorin has only one dermatan sulfate chain attached to the protein core, while biglycan possesses two dermatan sulfate chains. The role of decorin in cartilage is similar to its role in bone. Decorin is believed to be involved in the regulation of collagen fibrillogenesis, and it may also bind to growth factors that affect chondrocyte metabolism. The function of biglycan in cartilage is less certain.

As in bone, where a composite of collagen and hydroxyapatite produces a material structurally superior to the individual components, the composite of proteoglycan and collagen in cartilage creates a more functional substance than either alone. Without collagen to resist expansion, the proteoglycans would swell to five times their volume in cartilage and form a soft gel with little resistance to shear. Conversely, if cartilage were made entirely of collagen, it would be less able to withstand compressive forces.

Like other mechanical systems with moving parts, joints are susceptible to breakdown from constant friction and wear; however, they endure for many years because the materials in the extracellular matrix can be replenished by chondrocytes. The turnover of proteoglycans varies with different molecules, with half-lives ranging from 10 to 80 days. Older reports suggested that the collagen network was inert and did not turn over; more recent work indicates that chondrocytes actively synthesize collagen at a slow rate.

Many agents affect the turnover of cartilage matrix. Certain molecules, such as insulinlike growth factor, increase the production of collagen and proteoglycans, while other molecules, such as interleukin-1 and tumor necrosis factor alpha, induce chondrocytes and synovium to synthesize *metalloproteinases* and other degradative enzymes. Cartilage has an intrinsic ability to resist destruction, since it contains proteins known as *tissue inhibitors of metalloproteinases (TIMPs),* which counteract the proteases. Under normal circumstances there is a surplus of inhibitors, but in disease states, such as osteoarthritis and rheumatoid arthritis, the synthesis of excessive amounts of degradative enzymes enables them to overwhelm the TIMPS.

Fibrocartilage

Fibrocartilage forms numerous specialized structures, including the menisci of the knee, the labrum of the shoulder, and the triangular fibrocartilage of the wrist. Fibrocartilage differs from hyaline cartilage in many respects. The composition is different; fibrocartilage contains more collagen and less proteoglycan than hyaline cartilage. Most cells in fibrocartilage bear a greater resemblance to fibroblasts than to chondrocytes. Fibrocartilage usually arises from fibrous tissue, such as joint capsules, making demarcation between the two tissues difficult to distinguish.

The *meniscus* is probably the best-studied example of fibrocartilage. Type I collagen comprises 75 percent of its dry weight, while type II collagen is present in only trace amounts. The proteoglycan content is less than one-tenth the amount in articular cartilage and accounts for only 1 percent of the dry weight. As a result of these differences, the meniscus is softer than hyaline cartilage but better able to withstand tensile forces. These material properties are well suited to meniscal functions. The knee is an incongruous joint, with nonconforming joint surfaces. The meniscus distributes stresses in the knee more evenly, and its relatively soft material properties allow

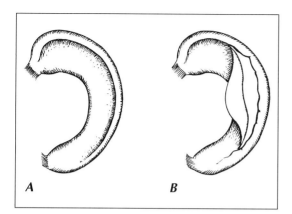

Figure 3.8   *A.* Intact meniscus. *B.* "Bucket-handle" tear, which occurs in line with orientation of collagen fibers.

contact throughout the range of motion. Most of the collagen fibers are arranged circumferentially to resist the large hoop stresses generated by weight-bearing. When the knee is loaded, the meniscus is forced outward and enlarged, causing tension in the meniscus along circumferential lines. The geometry of the collagen fibers accounts for the frequency of "bucket-handle" tears, which occur parallel to the fibers (Fig. 3.8).

MUSCLES

Structure and Physiology

Skeletal muscles are the organs that move the body. Over four hundred skeletal muscles in the human body make up 50 percent of the total body weight. Muscles vary greatly in size and shape (Fig. 3.9). Fusiform muscles (e.g., the biceps) have fibers parallel to the tendon, allowing great excursion. Muscles that require more power have shorter fibers that run obliquely to the tendon. Unipennate muscles have all of their fibers on one side of the tendon, while bipennate muscles, such as the rectus femoris, have fibers on both sides of the tendon. Multipennate muscles, like the deltoid, are composed of multiple small bipennate muscles. All muscles are enclosed by *epimysium,* a sheath of dense connective tissue. Within the muscle, *perimysium* divides the muscle into fascicles, which are further separated by *endomysium* into individual *myofibers,* or muscle cells. The *myotendinous junction* is a specialized structure containing a basement membrane where muscle fibers end and tendon begins. Muscular strains typically occur near this junction because of the change in material properties from inelastic tendon to pliable muscle.

A single axon from a motor neuron may innervate from one to several thousand myofibers. The motor neuron and its muscle fibers constitute a *motor unit.* Muscles that perform fine, delicate movements have small motor units, while muscles used for power have large motor units. Greater strength of contraction is usually achieved by recruitment of more motor units, since muscles contract as an all-or-none response. Muscles rely upon motor neurons not only for stimulation but also for an essential trophic factor. Muscles that lose innervation permanently undergo degeneration and eventual fibrosis.

Biochemistry

Most muscle cells in the body possess the contractile proteins *actin* and *myosin,* which are involved in various processes including movement and cell motility. The unique feature of a muscle cell is the high degree of organization

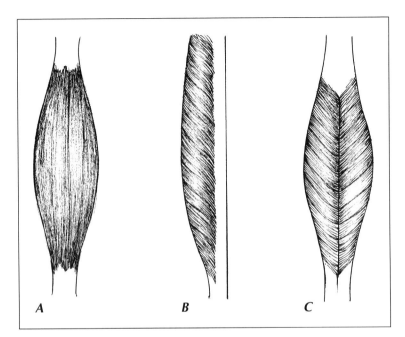

Figure 3.9 Types of muscles: (*A*) fusiform, (*B*) unipennate, and (*C*) bipennate.

of its contractile elements. A mature myofiber is a long, multinucleated cell with multiple *myofibrils* composed of discrete bundles of actin and myosin (Fig. 3.10). Electron microscopy reveals a characteristic light-and-dark banding pattern in the myofibrils. The dark band is composed of thick filaments that contain myosin, while the light band consists of thin filaments that contain actin. The thick and thin filaments interdigitate, and the sliding of the filaments past each other provides the basis of muscular contraction. Each myofibril is divided into multiple, repeating basic units called *sarcomeres,* which include one set of thick filaments and the associated thin filaments (Fig. 3.11). In electron micrographs, the sarcomere can be seen to extend from one Z line, which runs down the middle of the thin filaments, to the next Z line.

Actin is a small 42-kDa protein that forms long filaments by binding together like beads on a chain. Each thin filament consists of two

chains of actin beads that wind around each other (Fig. 3.12). The thick filament is composed of paired myosin molecules, which possess characteristic globular heads projecting outward like oars of a boat. Up to three hundred pairs of "oars" are available on each thick filament for binding actin. In the resting state, actin and myosin are hindered from binding to each other by *tropomyosin,* a protein that winds around the thin filament and blocks the binding sites on actin. When muscles are stimulated, calcium is liberated into the cytoplasm and is bound by the *troponin complex,* which resides on the actin filament. This set of proteins induces a conformational change in tropomyosin and unmasks the binding sites on the actin filament.

Muscle cells are stimulated to contract by electrical input from motor neurons. Electrical excitation, or *depolarization,* occurs throughout the interior of the muscle cell by special involutions of the cell membrane known as *T*

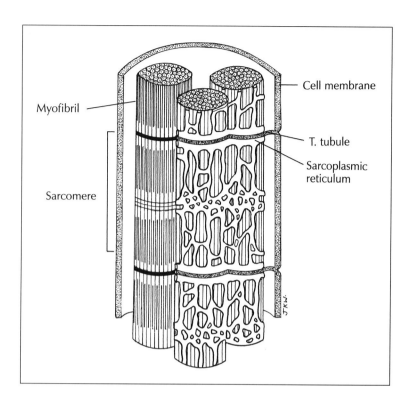

Myofibril

Cell membrane

T. tubule

Sarcoplasmic
reticulum

Sarcomere

Figure 3.10 Internal structure of a myofiber (muscle cell).

tubules. Juxtaposed on either side of each T tubule is the *sarcoplasmic reticulum,* an organelle that stores calcium and releases it into the cytoplasm when the T tubules depolarize. During contraction, the intracellular concentration of calcium rises sharply, but it decreases rapidly as a calcium pump sequesters the ion back into the sarcoplasmic reticulum.

When myosin binds to actin, the myosin head hydrolyzes a high-energy molecule of *adenosine triphosphate* (ATP), resulting in a stable, low-energy "rigor complex." For myosin to be released from actin, it must bind a new ATP molecule. Each cycle of binding results in only 1 percent shortening of the muscle fiber; thus, visible muscle contraction requires many cycles of binding and release. The pool of ATP in muscle is sufficient for only a few seconds of contraction. *Rigor mortis* develops

when there is not enough ATP in the muscle cell to release myosin from actin. Since muscle is capable of expending large quantities of energy in a short period of time, a special system is required to maintain an adequate supply of ATP. *Creatinine phosphate kinase* rapidly replenishes the ATP stores by transferring a high-energy phosphate group from creatinine phosphate to adenosine diphosphate.

Muscle fibers differ in their ability to metabolize energy and have been divided into two types of cells. Type I, or "slow-twitch," fibers utilize aerobic metabolism to obtain energy and are capable of sustained contraction. The fibers are dark in color because they are rich in the cytochromes and enzymes necessary for oxidative phosphorylation. Type II, or "fast-twitch," fibers utilize anaerobic glycolysis and fatigue more rapidly. The fibers are relatively

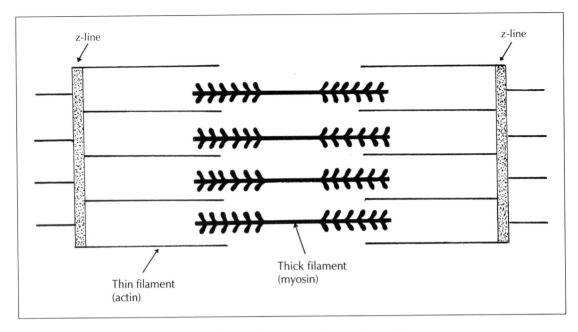

Figure 3.11   Sarcomere. Note the thick filaments with oars (myosin) and thin filaments on both ends (actin and troponin complex).

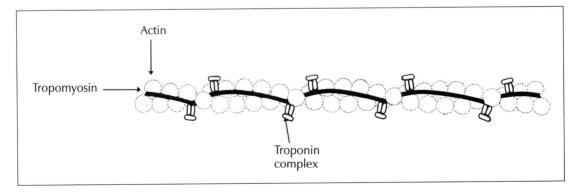

Figure 3.12   Thin filament. Note the double chain of actin molecules.

light in color. Most muscles in the human body contain both type I and type II fibers in varying proportions. Large muscles required for locomotion, such as the quadriceps femoris, contain primarily type I fibers, while muscles engaged in quick, fine movements, like the intrinsic muscles of the hand, contain predominantly type II fibers.

TENDONS

Tendons are the structures that attach muscles to bones and effect specific movements. Like ligaments, tendons are subjected primarily to tensile forces and have similar structures. Approximately 95 percent of the dry weight of the matrix is made of dense, parallel bundles of type I collagen. The remainder is made of types III and V collagen (3 to 5 percent), elastin (1 percent), and proteoglycans (0.5 percent). The collagen fibers of tendons spread and merge with the collagen fibers in bone; the tough bands of tendinous tissue embedded in bone are known as *Sharpey's fibers.* Although the composition of specific tendons and ligaments varies, tendons tend to have more type I collagen and fewer proteoglycans and metabolically active fibroblasts. There may also be differences in the cross links between collagen molecules. The functional significance of the disparities between tendon and ligament is not entirely clear.

Special structures have developed to improve the function of tendons. In areas such as the wrist, *retinacula* prevent bowstringing. In areas of friction, such as the fingers, synovial sheaths surround tendons. The synovial fluid both lubricates and nourishes the tendon. In areas where a tendon is pressed against bone, a *sesamoid bone* often develops within the substance of the tendon, the largest and best-known example being the patella.

SUGGESTED READINGS

ALBRIGHT JA, BRAND RA: *The Scientific Basis of Orthopaedics.* East Norwalk, CT, Appleton and Lange, 1987.

KEUTTNER KE, SCHLEYERBACH R, PEYRON JG, HASCALL VC: *Articular Cartilage and Osteoarthritis.* New York, Raven Press, 1992.

STRYER L: *Biochemistry,* 3d ed. New York, Freeman, 1988.

WEINSTEIN SL, BUCKWALTER JA: *Turek's Orthopaedics: Principles and Their Application,* 5th ed. Philadelphia, Lippincott, 1994.

WOO SL-Y, BUCKWALTER JA: *Injury and Repair of the Musculoskeletal Soft Tissues.* Park Ridge, IL, American Academy of Orthopaedic Surgeons, 1988.

Chapter *4*

Orthopaedic Biomechanics

Douglas R. Dirschl and Frank C. Wilson

Believing that a knowledge of principles facilitates understanding and recall, this chapter explains the responses of musculoskeletal tissues to physical stresses according to the biomechanical principles underlying these behaviors.

Biomechanics examines the action of *forces* on living organisms. Forces are of two basic types: "pushes" or compression and "pulls" or tension. The direction and magnitude of forces are described by *vectors*, usually represented by arrows, with direction indicated by the point and magnitude by the length of the arrow. In addition to producing compression and tension, a force applied to an object may cause it to rotate it about a point. Such forces are called *moments*.

To grasp the effects of forces acting on musculoskeletal tissues, it is necessary to understand the terms *stress, strain,* and *modulus of elasticity. Stress* is force per unit area, which can be tensile, compressive, or shearing. *Strain* measures deformation and may be expressed mathematically as the change in length of an object divided by the original length. A material's *modulus of elasticity* is a measure of

its stiffness or ability to resist permanent deformation; it is determined by dividing stress by strain. While immediate recoil to original shape follows *elastic deformation,* greater stress produces *plastic deformation,* characterized by incomplete recoil and residual deformity. Continued increase in stress levels results in failure of the material. A typical stress/strain relationship for bone or implant materials is shown in Fig. 4.1.

The forces that act on the human body may be internal or external. Study of the effect of forces on bodies at rest, i.e., in equilibrium, is known as *statics. Dynamics* examines bodies in motion and the forces that produce this motion. Dynamics may be subdivided into *kinematics,* the study of motion without reference to cause, i.e., the geometry of motion; *kinetics,* which studies motion in relation to cause; and *kinesiology,* the study of human movement. For a body to be in a static state, the sum of the forces acting on it must be zero, whereas, for an accelerating body, the sum of the forces acting on it is not zero. Kinetic analysis is particularly useful in orthopaedics, because kinetic data can be used to determine the mag-

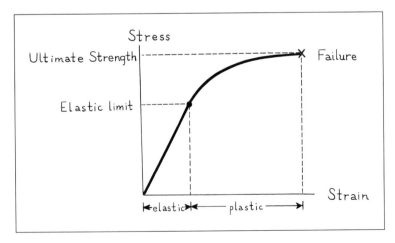

Figure 4.1 Typical stress/strain relationship for bone or implant materials used in orthopaedics. The slope of the linear portion of the stress/strain curve represents the modulus of elasticity of the material. The regions of elastic and plastic deformation are indicated, as well as the failure point of the material.

nitude of forces acting on a joint as a result of muscle contraction, body weight, and externally applied loads.

PRINCIPLES OF BIOMECHANICS

Newton's Laws

Many principles of biomechanics are based on Newton's laws of motion:

Newton's first law, inertia, states that when the sum of all forces and moments acting on an object is zero, the object will remain at rest or move at a constant velocity. This relationship may be stated algebraically by the equation $\Sigma F = 0$. The study of systems in equilibrium is called *static analysis.* If a body is in equilibrium and certain forces acting on it are known, the magnitude of an unknown force may be calculated (Fig. 4.2).

Newton's second law, acceleration, may be stated mathematically as $F = ma$, meaning that the acceleration of a given body is directly proportional to the force applied to it. Acceleration along a straight line is *linear acceleration;* that produced by rotation around an axis is *angular acceleration.* Linear or angular *deceleration* may also occur, as in a person landing on the floor after jumping. Another biological application of this law occurs during extension of the knee: contraction of the quadriceps provides angular acceleration to the lower leg as the knee rotates into extension. Deceleration acts on this system if the accelerating force were countered by the foot striking an object. The greater the quadriceps contraction or resistance of the object struck, the greater the acceleration or deceleration.

Newton's third law, that for every action

there is an equal and opposite reaction, underlies *free body analysis,* by which forces acting on a body part may be identified by the isolation of that part as a free body. The manner in which forces acting on a given joint may be calculated is further considered under "Biomechanics of Joints," below.

BIOMECHANICS OF MUSCULOSKELETAL TISSUES

Bone

Mechanical Properties

The most important mechanical properties of bone are strength and stiffness. Because bone is somewhat pliable, deformation within its elastic and plastic limits does not lead to failure or fracture. When the stress applied to a bone exceeds these limits, permanent deformation and, ultimately, fracture occurs. *Brittleness* and *ductility* are terms that describe the amount of deformation a material may undergo before failure. The bones of the elderly are more brittle, whereas those of children are more ductile.

Cortical bone, being stiffer than cancellous bone, can withstand greater stress but less strain before failure. The strength and stiffness of both are greatest in the direction in which loads are most commonly applied to the bone. Because its mechanical properties differ when it is loaded in different directions, bone is said to be *anisotropic.* (If these properties do *not* vary with changes in loading direction, a material is *isotropic.*) In osteoporosis, a condition of decreased bone mass, the bone is weakened, although the relationship of stress to strain is unchanged. Bony defects resulting from neoplastic or metabolic disorders concentrate

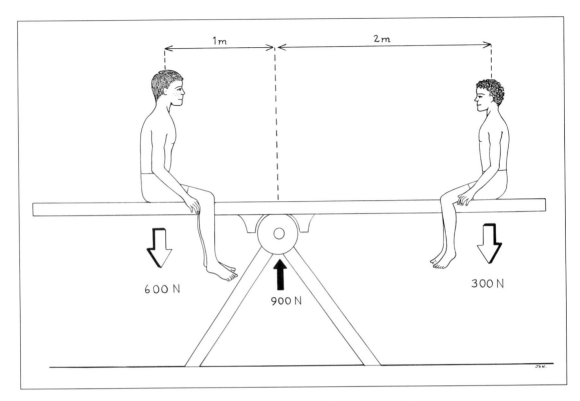

Figure 4.2 An illustration of Newton's first law: since the see-saw is in equilibrium, the sum of the moments and the forces acting at the fulcrum must be zero. In this situation, the sum of the vertical forces (600 N + 300 N − 900 N) is zero. The moment is expressed as the product of the force and the distance over which it acts. One child exerts a moment of (600 N)(1 m), tending to cause counterclockwise rotation about the fulcrum, while the second child exerts a moment of (300 N)(2 m), tending to cause rotation in the opposite direction. The sum of the moments (600 Nm − 600 Nm) is zero, thus satisfying Newton's first law.

forces in a localized area, reducing the amount of force necessary to cause failure.

Bone remodels in response to the mechanical demands placed upon it. This adaptation is expressed in Wolff's law, which observes that bone is added where needed and resorbed where it is not. External callus, for example, provides the rapid increase in strength and stiffness needed during the healing of a fracture, but this cuff of callus is resorbed as the bone remodels and returns to its normal strength.

Biomechanics of Fractures

FRACTURE PATTERNS   Fracture patterns are determined by the mechanism of injury. Bending moments, produced by a fall, blow, or muscular forces, produce tension stresses on the convex side of the bone and compressive stresses on the concave side (Fig. 13.3). Bone subjected to bending fails first in tension, which classically generates a transverse crack extending halfway through the bone. At this point, compressive forces alter the direction of the fracture line, producing an oblique fracture that extends to the cortex being compressed. Thus, tension tends to produce a transverse fracture line and compression an oblique fracture. If the obliquity extends both proximally and distally, an isolated, or "butterfly," fragment will be produced in the cortex subject to compression (Fig. 13.6C). The presence of multiple fragments (comminution) therefore implies a compressive element in the production of a fracture. Bone is also subjected to rotational or torsional forces, which generate a combination of shear, tensile, and compressive stresses that produce a spiral fracture (Fig. 13.3E). Oblique fractures may be distinguished radiographically from spiral fractures by the fact that, in spiral injuries, a fracture line cannot be seen to extend completely across the bone in any one radiographic projection.

Weight-bearing and muscle forces generate significant stresses on bone during activities of daily living. Most fractures occur when excessive force is rapidly applied; however, cyclic or intermittent loading, even with normal forces, may, if repeated long enough, lead to a type of failure known as a *fatigue fracture.* Fatigue fracture begins with microscopic failure of bone and progresses, with continued application of stress, to a point where the bone is weakened sufficiently for normal loading to complete the fracture. Bones with more dense haversian systems have greater fatigue resistance, probably because haversian canals divert extension of the microfracture.

The resistance of bone to fracture is decreased sharply by any defect in its cylindrical structure, such as a hole or notch in the cortex. These *stress risers* reduce the overall strength of the bone greatly. Disuse and *stress shielding* by overlying fixation devices also weaken bone, making it more vulnerable to fracture.

FIXATION OF FRACTURES   Open reduction and internal fixation of fractures is indicated when satisfactory reduction and stability of the fracture cannot be obtained by other means. Fixation devices may be internal or external. Screws, plates, and intramedullary rods are commonly employed for internal fixation. While screws alone do not provide sufficient fixation of fractures in long bones to avoid the need for external immobilization, they are useful where precise reduction is required, as in intraarticular fractures. Plates and intramedullary nails, on the other hand, often provide strong enough fixation to eliminate the need for casting. Plates offer greater resistance to torsional forces than intramedullary devices, whereas the latter more strongly resist bending moments. For this reason, plates are preferred for fixation of forearm fractures to resist the torsional forces of pronation and supination, and intramedullary devices are more useful in weight-bearing bones, such as the femur.

External stabilization of fractures may be obtained through the use of braces, splints, casts, or external fixators. Because of the interposed soft tissue envelope, splints, braces and casts afford less rigid fixation than external fixators, which consist of pins applied first to the fracture fragments, then connected to a rigid external frame. Depending upon the size of the pins and their placement, rigid fixation can be obtained with this device. It also permits wound care for the management of open injuries.

Cartilage

Cartilage is composed of water, which accounts for 70 percent of its wet weight; collagen fibers; and proteoglycans. Collagen, the most abundant protein in the human body, is characterized mechanically by its stiffness and tensile strength. The arrangement of collagen in articular cartilage in three distinct structural zones makes cartilage anisotropic. The proteoglycans, which exist in a gel, have a high affinity for water, most of which can be squeezed out under pressure. The relationship of the collagen fibrils to the proteoglycan gel has been likened to that of twine wrapped around a water-soaked sponge, although the lower permeability of articular cartilage offers much greater resistance to fluid movement under load than exists in a sponge. Under the compressive load of weight-bearing, however, deformation of cartilage further decreases permeability, which causes greater resistance to fluid flow, preventing exudation of the interstitial fluid. With disease and disruption of the cartilage matrix, the permeability of cartilage increases, allowing expression of more of its fluid phase. As a result, the solid or collagenous phase becomes more exposed and susceptible to mechanical abrasion, escalating joint wear.

With *rapid* loading, there is insufficient time for fluid expression, so that cartilage behaves in an elastic manner, with instantaneous deformation and similarly rapid recovery after unloading. Thus, cartilage exhibits material behavior that is dependent on the rate of loading, a property that identifies a material as *viscoelastic.*

Articular cartilage, being relatively acellular, has little capacity for regeneration following injury. Articular cartilage is nourished for the most part by synovial fluid rather than blood vessels, which would collapse under compressive load. Defects in articular cartilage, as result from intraarticular fractures, cause concentration of stresses that may exceed fatigue limits, resulting in cellular degeneration.

Muscle-Tendon

Muscles, which possess the special property of *contractility,* provide the force for active joint movement. Because of long elastic and plastic phases, considerable strain may be tolerated before muscle failure occurs. Although muscle fibers are incapable of active lengthening, contraction is produced by the sliding together of muscle filaments following excitation by electrical signals at the neuromuscular junction.

Muscle is also unique among musculoskeletal tissues in the degree to which it may *hypertrophy.* Repetitive submaximal loading increases both the strength and endurance of muscle. Since muscles assist in stabilizing joints, muscle strengthening is an important aspect of rehabilitation following ligamentous injury. Increased muscular strength, by absorbing more of the stress that accompanies weight-bearing, also reduces compressive forces acting across the joints, which explains the efficacy of strengthening programs for muscles that span arthritic joints.

With aging, the fibrous elements in muscle increase, which reduces its elasticity and increases susceptibility to *muscle strains* (partial tears). This fact accounts for the greater incidence of muscle strains in the aging athlete and suggests the value of stretching before, during, and after vigorous exercise.

Muscles are attached to bone by tendons. The arrangement, in parallel bundles, of dense collagen enables tendons to withstand higher levels of stress than muscle. Where tendons are subjected to high friction forces, e.g., in the wrist and fingers, they are enveloped by a synovial sheath, the cells of which produce synovial fluid to facilitate tendon movement. In other areas, tendons are surrounded by a peritenon of loose connective tissue.

Since the magnitude of force generated by a muscle and transmitted by a tendon is determined by the cross-sectional area of the muscle and tendon, large muscles are usually associated with large tendons. Even though tendon is stronger, its lack of ductility makes it more susceptible to rupture, or partial rupture, than muscle. Tendon rupture is especially common at the myotendinous junction and at its insertion into bone because of the transition in mechanical properties at these junctional sites.

Like ligaments, tendons remodel in response to stress and increase in both strength and stiffness with exercise.

Ligament

Ligaments, along with capsular tissues, stabilize joints, preventing undesirable degrees and directions of movement. Whereas tendons connect muscle to bone, ligaments connect bone to bone. Muscles stabilize joints within their normal arc of motion, and ligaments resist motions at the extremes of normal movement. The collagenous bundles that form ligaments are usually aligned parallel to the direction of the movement to be resisted. Because of this alignment, ligaments resist tensile forces much more effectively than shear forces.

The strength of both bone and ligament under loading is related to the size and shape of the ligament or bone and the speed of loading. The greater the cross-sectional area and speed of loading, the greater the strength. Although both bone and ligament are stronger under more rapid loading conditions, ligaments usually fail first at slow rates of loading; bone fails first at rapid rates.

Ligaments are also similar to bone in having phases of elastic and plastic deformation that precede failure—a fact that has been used to classify ligamentous injury as grade I, II, or III, with I being the elastic phase of deformation, II the plastic phase, and III failure or rupture. Unfortunately, this system does not account for the commonly encountered incomplete rupture of a ligament. In general, joint stability following injury varies directly with the extent of ligamentous rupture. Ligamentous failure through a bony attachment, the so-called *sprain-fracture,* occurs more often with slow rates of loading or when the bone is weakened by a pathologic process, such as osteoporosis.

Another similarity of ligament to bone and tendon is the increased strength and stiffness that results from the mechanical stress of strenuous exercise. Ligaments also atrophy with disuse, as occurs with cast immobilization.

Aging, which is related to disuse, results in a significant loss of strength and stiffness in ligaments. It has not been determined whether vigorous exercise continued into old age prevents or slows these changes.

BIOMECHANICS OF JOINTS

Principles

Friction/Lubrication

The value of lubrication is perhaps best appreciated by the consequences of its absence, in which friction (the force that resists motion between bodies in contact) and joint wear are increased enormously.

Two sources of fluid are responsible for joint lubrication: synovial fluid and the interstitial fluid of cartilage, which is released as a function of the pressure applied to the cartilage.

When a lubricant is placed between moving surfaces, two types of lubrication occur: boundary and fluid lubrication, both of which take place in the human joint. In *boundary lubrication,* each joint surface is coated with a thin layer of fluid molecules that slide on each other, with the lubrication being independent of the physical properties of either the lubricant (e.g., viscosity) or the contacting bodies

(e.g., stiffness). In *fluid lubrication,* the surfaces float on a pressurized layer of fluid, and both the viscosity of the lubricant and the stiffness of the surfaces determine the effectiveness of lubrication. The pressure of the fluid in fluid film lubrication is generated by internal pressure, which may be of squeeze film or elastohydrodynamic type. *Squeeze film lubrication* occurs as the two surfaces moving perpendicularly to each other force fluid out of the gap between them. In *elastohydrodynamic lubrication,* a pressurized wedge is developed as the surfaces slide tangentially over each other. The sliding surfaces (cartilage) are sufficiently soft to be deformed at the trailing edges by pressure in the fluid film. The constriction developed at the trailing edge restricts fluid flow out of the pressure wedge and thus helps maintain it.

Weeping lubrication is also seen in human joints. The compression of cartilage forces interstitial fluid out of the cartilage matrix into the joint space, which increases the fluid film's thickness (Fig. 4.3).

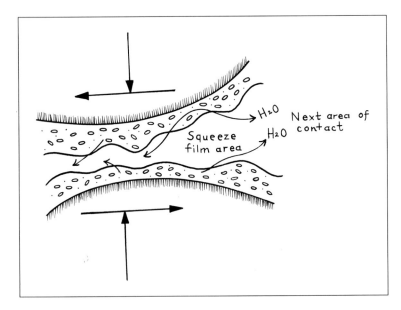

Figure 4.3 Weeping lubrication. As the area of contact between the joint surfaces moves from left to right, increasing contact pressure forces water out of the cartilage matrix into the joint space. This mechanism increases the thickness of the fluid film between the articular surfaces, reduces friction, and improves lubrication. The fluid will return to the cartilage matrix when the contact pressure is decreased.

Other concepts important to an understanding of joint biomechanics are degrees of freedom, coupled force, instant centers of rotation, joint reaction force, and congruence.

Degrees of Freedom

This phrase refers to the six parameters used to define the position of a body. There are three axes for rotation and three for linear motion. To locate the position of the tibial plateau in relation to the femur, for example, one must include its orientation around three axes: vertical (internal or external rotation), sagittal (varus or valgus), and coronal (flexion or extension). Since translation is minimal in most joints, the anteroposterior, mediolateral, and superoinferior locations of the part under study may usually be ignored, which reduces the degrees of freedom from six to three.

Coupled Force

In certain joints, motion around one axis is accompanied by an obligatory motion about another; such motions are said to be coupled. For example, the location and orientation of facet joints in the spine dictate that lateral bending be accompanied by rotation about the vertical axis, as seen in scoliosis.

Instant Centers of Rotation

The center of rotation for a joint is the axis about which the joint rotates. In certain joints, such as the knee, translation of the joint during flexion and extension changes the center of rotation during the arc of motion. Thus, the center of rotation changes from instant to instant—a concept that must be accommodated in the design of prostheses for replacement of the knee or in the reconstruction of torn anterior cruciate ligaments.

Joint Reaction Force

This term refers to the force generated across a joint in response to loading from within or without the body. In general, the higher the joint reaction force, the greater the predisposition to degenerative changes, which may explain the contribution of obesity to the development of osteoarthritis in weight-bearing joints.

Congruence

This term describes the relationship or symmetry of fit between two opposing articular surfaces. When congruence decreases, as in arthritic joints, loading stress in articular cartilage is increased, since weight-bearing forces are distributed over a smaller area of contact.

Biomechanics of Individual Joints: Functional Anatomy, Kinematics, and Kinetics

To analyze the forces acting across a joint, a knowledge of its functional anatomy, kinematics (motion), and kinetics (motion in response to forces) is necessary.

The Spine

The functional unit of motion in the spine consists of two vertebrae and the intervening soft tissues (disks and ligaments). The intervertebral disk is composed of a central colloidal gel, the *nucleus pulposus,* and an outer *annulus fibrosus* of cartilage interlaced with crisscrossed bundles of collagen fibers. This arrangement enables the disk to withstand the large compressive, bending, and torsional forces generated during the activities of daily living. With aging, the disk loses its capacity to retain water; as it becomes inelastic and less able to distribute stresses, it is less capable of resisting loads. Bending produces forces that are mainly tensile and compressive, while rotation produces shear forces. The weight-bearing function of the disk is shared by the facet joints, which, depending upon the spinal segment and forces applied, accommodate up to 30 percent of the load. The particular importance of the facet joints in resisting shear forces is demonstrated by the anterior displacement of the vertebral body in spondylolisthesis, where the facets are detached from the motion segment.

The instant center of spinal motion is located in the disk. Spinal movement is produced by the musculature of the trunk and controlled by the arrangement of the facet joints and ligaments. The motion at each joint is determined by the orientation of the facets; the ribs also limit motion in the thoracic spine. Flexion and extension are greatest in the lower lumbar segments, lateral flexion in the lower thoracic segments, and rotation in the upper thoracic spine. With forward bending, flexion occurs first in the lumbar spine, followed by anterior rotation of the pelvis at the hip joints. With extension, this pattern is reversed: the pelvis is extended first, followed by the lumbar spine.

Since the center of gravity of the body is anterior to the axis of motion in all spinal levels with the body in the erect position, a bending moment is generated in the spine that must be resisted by ligaments and spinal extensor muscles. Bending is also resisted by the kyphotic and lordotic curves of the spine in the anteroposterior plane, which, along with the intervertebral disks and ligaments, confer a springlike structure to the spine, enabling it to withstand greater loads than if it were straight.

Static loading (forces acting on the spine at rest) vary according to spinal position; spinal movement increases loading, which may be described mathematically by an analysis of spinal dynamics. The most heavily loaded spinal segments are those in the lumbar region. In the erect position, pressure in the third lumbar disk is equal to approximately twice the weight of the body above that level because of contributions of intrinsic disk pressure and spanning muscles to the overall intradiscal pressure. Flexion of the spine greatly increases pressure in the lumbar disks, and when torsional loading is added, pressures are further increased. Simultaneous flexion of the hips and knees reduces the forces in the erector spinae muscles needed to balance the flexion moment in the spine and thereby greatly reduces overall spinal loading.

The bending moment of the spine is increased when one lifts or carries objects in front of the body. Holding the object as close to the body as possible reduces the length of the moment arm over which the weight of the object acts and thereby reduces the load applied to the spinal column. Similarly, when a more erect posture is assumed, the bending moment and load on the spine are also reduced.

With normal bone, the vertebral bodies are stiffer than their interposed disks, so that loading failure is more common in the disks. Conditions such as osteoporosis, however, which reduce bone density and stiffness, make the vertebrae more susceptible to compression failure and account for the relatively common vertebral compression fractures of the elderly.

The Shoulder

The shoulder girdle is composed of three bones, four joints, and the muscles and ligaments that bind them together into a functional unit. The clavicle, or "boom" from which the upper limb is suspended, participates in the formation of the sternoclavicular and acromioclavicular joints. The proximal humerus articulates with the scapular glenoid, and the fourth "joint" consists of the movement that occurs between the scapula and the thorax.

Abduction of the shoulder is a smooth, rhythmic, integrated motion in which all shoulder joints participate. This motion was called *scapulohumeral rhythm* by Codman, and it is significant in that asymmetrical movement usually indicates a pathologic disorder of the shoulder girdle (Fig. 5.7).

The glenohumeral joint is a universal joint, permitting a greater range of motion than any other joint in the body. It is shallow, resembling more a grapefruit in a saucer than a ball in a socket. The lack of bony stability and wide range of motion permitted by loose ligamentous and capsular reinforcement account for the fact that the glenohumeral is the most frequently dislocated joint in the body. Loss of the normal capsular laxity, usually associated with disuse of the shoulder, results in limited glenohumeral motion, producing a *frozen shoulder.*

When a weight held in the extended arm is lifted to a right angle in the coronal plane, three forces act across the shoulder joint: the weight held, the force in the deltoid muscle, and the joint reaction force generated against the humeral head by the glenoid fossa. Using free body analysis, it can be determined that the joint reactive force is at least tenfold greater than the weight being lifted. When the unloaded arm is lifted to 90°, the glenohumeral joint reaction forces approach body weight, suggesting that, for at least certain activities, the glenohumeral joint should be considered a weight-bearing joint.

The Elbow

The elbow serves as a positioner of the hand and as a fulcrum for the forearm lever. The articulation between the distal end of the humerus and the radius and ulna provides motions of flexion and extension, and the articulation between the proximal radius and ulna participates in pronation and supination. The flexion arc of motion is from 0 to 140°; the rotational arc is from 90° of supination to 75° of pronation. The flexion-extension axis of the elbow is in the center of the trochlea, while pronation and supination occur about an axis that extends from the capitellum to the distal ulna.

Stability of the elbow results from the bony interlock between the humerus and the ulna, the collateral ligaments (especially the medial), the annular ligament, which maintains the head of the radius against the ulna during rotation, and the interosseous membrane, which unites the shafts of the radius and the ulna.

Extension of the elbow is provided by the triceps and the anconeus. These muscles deliver maximal extensor force with the elbow in 90° of flexion; however, maximal extensor power is only 50 percent of maximal flexor power.

It is difficult to analyze joint reaction force at the elbow because of the multiplicity of joints and motors. Since its motors insert so close to the axis of rotation, the elbow is an inefficient joint. To support the forearm at 90°, for example, the force developed in the biceps must be approximately three times the weight of the arm and any object carried in the hand. Thus, static loads may approach and dynamic loads exceed body weight.

The Wrist and Hand

The proximal row of carpal bones (scaphoid, lunate, and triquetrum) articulates proximally with the radius and distally with the distal row of carpals (trapezium, trapezoid, capitate, and hamate). The eighth carpal bone, the pisiform, belongs to the proximal row but articulates only with the triquetrum.

Wrist movements include dorsi- and volar-flexion (about 80° each) and radial and ulnar deviation (20 and 35°, respectively). Some two-thirds of the flexion and extension occurs at the radiocarpal joint; about one-third results from intercarpal movement. Radial deviation is primarily intercarpal, whereas ulnar deviation relies on movement at both the radiocarpal and intercarpal joints. The instant center of rotation in the wrist is located at the head of the capitate. Although the distal radius normally bears over 80 percent of the load at the radiocarpal joint, changes in radial or ulnar length can increase or decrease the load borne by the distal ulna.

The radius, lunate, and capitate constitute three "links" in a chain of motion, which reduces the amount of movement necessary for each link. Loss of ligamentous or bony support creates local instability, which interferes with this system of linked motion. Carpal collapse, with pain and limited motion, may follow.

Because the scaphoid spans both carpal rows, it has less mobility than the other carpals, which explains its susceptibility to fracture following a fall on the outstretched hand. Being the only carpal bone with a larger volar than dorsal surface, the lunate is the most frequently dislocated carpal bone, displacing volarward with forced dorsiflexion of the wrist. If fracture or displacement of these carpal bones impairs their blood supply, as is often the case, avascular necrosis may result.

The carpal bones are bridged volarly by the transverse carpal ligament, a heavy band of fibers that stretches from the hamate and pisiform medially to the scaphoid and trapezium laterally. Through this fibro-osseous tunnel pass the flexor tendons to the fingers and the median nerve. A decrease in the size of this canal or an increase in the volume of its contents may cause compression of the median nerve, producing *carpal tunnel syndrome* (see Chap. 10).

Finger motion includes 100° of flexion at the metacarpophalangeal (MCP) joints, with slightly more than that amount occurring in the proximal and slightly less in the distal interphalangeal joints. Abduction and adduction enjoy 40 to 50° of freedom at the MCP joints, but this motion is prevented at the interphalangeal joints by their bony and ligamentous configurations.

The most important joint of the hand is the saddle-shaped carpometacarpal (CMC) joint of the thumb. The configuration of this joint permits the circumduction movements of the thumb necessary for its opposition to the fingers in pinch. It is actually a composite motion made up of abduction, flexion, and adduction. The ability to oppose the thumb is one of the traits that distinguishes humans from lower primates.

Gliding of the flexor tendons (flexors digitorum profundus and superficialis and flexor pollicis longus) is assured by their encasement in synovial sheaths. Bowstringing of the flexor tendons is prevented at the wrist by the transverse carpal ligament and in the fingers by encircling retinaculae that bind the tendons to the phalanges.

During pinch, the forces of joint loading are concentrated at the thumb CMC joint. Because this joint has a small surface area over which to distribute the load, it develops the highest contact pressure and is therefore prone to the development of degenerative changes. Occupations requiring repetitive power gripping concentrate forces at the MCP joints; hence, degenerative changes favor the MCP joints in heavy laborers.

The Hip

In contrast to the upper limb, the lower limb has a stable bony connection to the trunk. The hip joint unites the cup-shaped acetabulum and the head of the femur. The acetabulum is the site where the ilium, ischium, and pubis unite to form the innominate bone. The femoral head forms two-thirds of a sphere and is joined to the shaft of the femur by the femoral neck, which makes an angle with the femoral shaft of approximately 125°. When this angle is over 135°, *coxa valga* is said to exist; when it is less

than 120°, *coxa vara* is present (Fig. 4.4). The neck-shaft angle is not parallel to the frontal plane of the body; rather, the neck and head are located anterior to the frontal plane and to the shaft of the femur, i.e., the shaft of the femur is internally rotated with respect to its neck and head. In the adult, this angle *(anteversion)* is between 5 and 15°. When it is greater than 15°, increased femoral anteversion is present; when it is less than 5°, femoral *retroversion* exists (Fig. 4.5). A patient with increased femoral anteversion walks with an in-toeing gait, whereas femoral retroversion produces increased out-toeing.

Motion in the hip joint takes place around

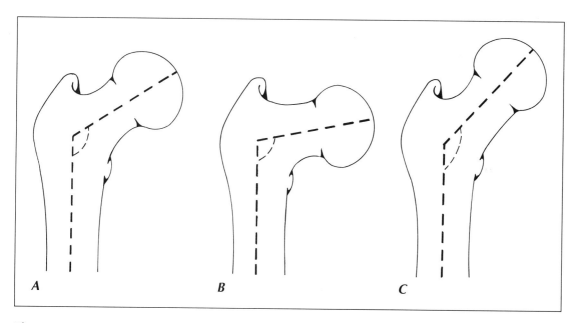

Figure 4.4   The nomenclature describing the relationship between the femoral neck and shaft. *A.* The usual neck-shaft angle is approximately 125°. *B.* When the neck-shaft angle is less than 120°, coxa vara is present. *C.* When the angle is greater than 135°, coxa valga exists. [Redrawn with permission from Wilson FC (ed): *The Musculoskeletal System: Basic Processes and Disorders,* 2d ed. Philadelphia, Lippincott, 1983, Chap. 4, p 56.]

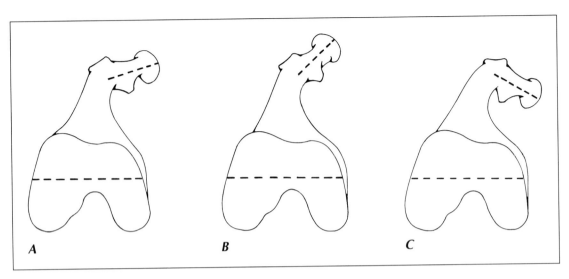

Figure 4.5　The nomenclature describing femoral torsion (version). *A.* Normally, the femoral neck projects anterior to the plane of the femoral condyles, creating femoral *anteversion* of 5 to 15°. *B.* When the angle is greater than 15°, increased femoral anteversion exists. *C.* When the angle is less than 5° or the femoral neck projects posteriorly, it is referred to as femoral *retroversion.* [Redrawn from Wilson FC (ed): *The Musculoskeletal System: Basic Processes and Disorders,* 2d ed. Philadelphia, Lippincott, 1983, Chap. 4, p 57.]

sagittal, frontal, and vertical planes. Since normal use of the hip entails motion in several planes simultaneously, determination of an instant center of rotation is impossible for this joint. Kinematic analysis has shown that for the activities of daily living, at least 120° of flexion (movement in the sagittal plane), 20° of abduction (movement in the frontal plane), and 20° of external rotation (movement in the transverse plane) are necessary.

By kinetic analysis of the hip joint, it has been demonstrated that erect stance can be maintained without muscle contraction, which produces a joint reaction force on the head of each femur of approximately one-half the su-

perincumbent body weight. Subtracting the weight of the legs, each of which is approximately one-sixth of body weight, the true load on each hip joint is approximately one-third of body weight. Contraction of muscles spanning the hip joint increases the forces across the joint. In one-legged stance, tremendous forces must be developed in the abductor muscles of the weight-bearing hip to prevent the force of gravity (acting through the midline of the body) from causing the pelvis to dip downward on the non-weight-bearing side. The forces developed in the abductor muscles and superimposed body weight produce a total joint reaction force in one-legged stance of approximately three times body weight. The abductor muscle forces are further increased in the weight-bearing hip during walking and running; in fact, joint reaction forces of up to seven times body weight may be reached during ambulation. Joint loading is reduced by the use of a cane, especially if it is held in the opposite hand, which increases the distance, or lever arm, over which the weight assumed by the cane acts (Figs. 4.6A and B).

The Knee

The knee joint, the largest and arguably most complex joint in the body, is formed by the femur, tibia, and patella. Since the femurs converge toward the knee and the tibias are vertical, the femur and tibia meet at an angle of 5 to 8° (anatomic axis). If the direction of the distal part of a joint (here, the tibia) is away from the midline of the body, valgus is said to exist, whereas if the distal part angles toward the body's midline, the joint is in varus. Since the tibiofemoral joint is only slightly dished, most of the knee joint's stability is derived from the medial and lateral collateral ligaments, which control abduction and adduction, and from the anterior and posterior cruciate ligaments, which limit anteroposterior translation of the knee. Because of the direction of the collateral ligaments (the medial downward and forward, the lateral downward and backward), they also oppose external rotation of the tibia and internal rotation of the femur. The joint capsule also contributes to static stability of the knee. Further dynamic stability is provided by the powerful quadriceps and hamstring muscles that span the knee anteriorly and posteriorly.

Contributing to the stability of the knee but of most importance in distributing the forces of weight-bearing are the menisci. These fibrocartilaginous, crescentic structures bear from one-third to one-half of body weight; their removal increases tibiofemoral contact stresses up to three times.

Most knee motion takes place in the sagittal plane, which allows a flexion arc of 140°. Little or no rotation occurs with the knee in full extension; however, in flexion, up to 45° of internal and external rotation exists. Similarly, in the frontal plane, little abduction or adduction is possible in the extended knee, whereas in 30° of flexion, several degrees of both adduction and abduction can be obtained. For normal walking, approximately 75° of flexion and 10° of both abduction and adduction and rotation are needed; faster walking requires greater excursion. For other activities of daily living, such as stair climbing or arising from a seated position, 115 to 120° of flexion are necessary.

Because the knee glides in the anteroposterior plane during flexion and extension, the instant center of rotation for the knee varies with the degree of flexion.

The rotational movement of the tibia about the femur during flexion and extension is a function of the medial femoral condyle being about 1.7 cm longer than the lateral. As the weight-bearing knee extends, the femoral condyles rotate internally, a process known as the screw home mechanism.

Kinetic analysis has suggested that joint reaction forces at the tibiofemoral joint during normal walking range from two to four times body weight. Since the contact area of the medial tibial plateau is almost half again as large as that of the lateral plateau, most of the weight-bearing load is borne by the medial compartment.

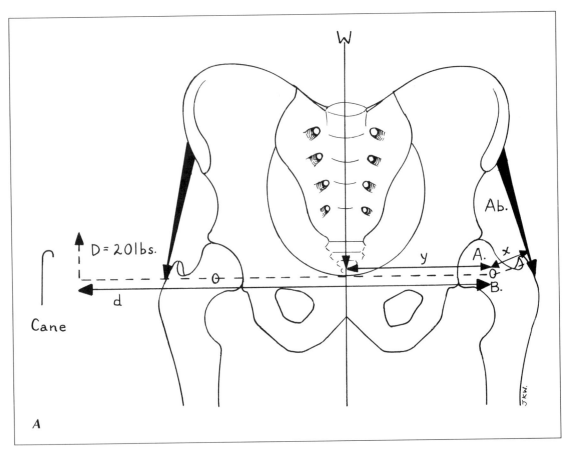

A

Figure 4.6   Vector analysis demonstrating the effect of using a cane on the joint reaction force in the hip joint. The drawings represent a patient in single-leg stance on the left leg (the patient is facing the reader). Point *B* is the center of rotation of the left hip; *W* is the weight of the body above the hips, and *y* is the distance over which the force acts; *Ab* is the force generated by the hip abductors, and *x* is the distance over which this force acts; *D* is the force placed on the cane, and *d* is the distance over which it

As the knee moves from extension to full flexion, the patella slides distally about 7 cm around the femoral condyles. Full contact between the patella and condyles exists between 0 and 90° of flexion; beyond that point, the patella rotates externally. By lengthening the quadriceps lever arm, the patella reduces the force generated by the quadriceps for extension of the knee, which reduces joint loading. In the patellectomized knee, 30 percent more force may be required to extend the knee than with the patella in place. In full flexion, the

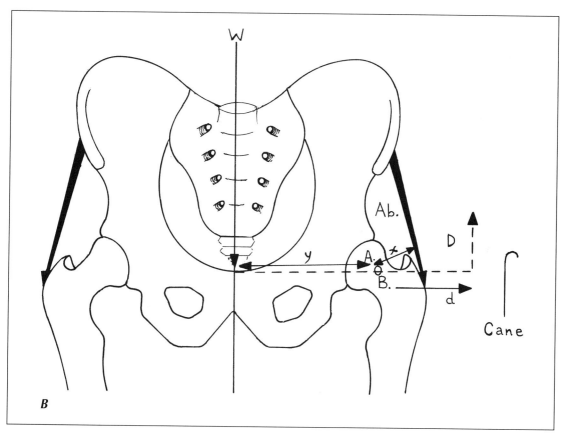

B

acts. Note that distance *d* is much greater (*A*) when the cane is carried in the right (contralateral) hand than (*B*) when it is carried in the left (ipsilateral) hand. As a result of the force acting through this longer lever arm, a much greater moment can be generated; consequently, a more effective reduction of the hip joint reaction force can be achieved by use of the cane in the right (contralateral) hand than in the left (ipsilateral) hand.

patellofemoral moment arm is shortest, so that more quadriceps strength is required to extend the knee from this position. Since muscle strengthening, especially of the quadriceps, is important in the management of many intra-articular disorders, limiting the flexion arc to 30° when quadriceps strengthening exercises are performed reduces the joint compressive force and the pain of exercising.

The Ankle and Foot

At the ankle, the tibial plafond joins the spool-shaped upper surface of the talus, which articulates below with the calcaneus. The ankle is a uniplanar hinge joint of the mortise-and-tenon variety, with the talus as the tenon and the tibial and fibular malleoli forming the medial and lateral walls of the mortise. The tibia and fibula are united distally by the tibiofibular and interosseous ligaments, and the malleoli are anchored to the tarsus medially by the deltoid ligament and laterally by the three fascicles of the lateral ligament. The bones of the ankle mortise and their uniting ligaments form a ring. Since ligaments do not stretch, this ring, like any other "rigid" ring, requires that it be broken in two places for displacement to occur—a concept important in the treatment and prognosis of ankle injuries.

The total range of movement at the ankle joint is about 50°, with 20° being dorsiflexion and 30° plantarflexion. Since the talus is wider anteriorly, the mortise is more completely filled in dorsiflexion, which confers greater stability to the ankle and explains the more frequent occurrence of sprains with the ankle in plantarflexion. The axis of rotation of the ankle joint passes through the talus from the tip of the medial to the tip of the lateral malleolus.

Weight-bearing produces joint reaction forces in the ankle joint at least as great as those transmitted across the hip and knee; however, its larger load-bearing surface (11 to 13 sq cm) creates lower loads per unit of surface area than are encountered in the hip or knee. The highest joint compression forces encountered in normal walking are approximately five times body weight, which occurs at the moment of push-off from stance phase. Shift of the talus in the ankle mortise of only 1 to 2 mm, however, increases joint reaction forces precipitously. Thus, even small degrees of talar displacement must be guarded against

in ankle injuries involving two breaks in the ring, e.g., bimalleolar fractures.

The foot, in addition to its obvious weight-bearing function, serves as a lever or thrust for the body in walking and running. The tarsal and metatarsal bones are so arranged that each foot is half a dome. This arched structure provides strength and resilience for weight-bearing as well as protection of soft tissues in the sole from weight-bearing compression. When the articular surfaces of the tarsal and metatarsal bones are positioned anatomically, two arches are created in the foot, a longitudinal arch, which is higher on its medial aspect, and a transverse arch, which is most apparent at the level of the tarsometatarsal joints. The arch is supported statically by joint configuration, strong plantar ligaments, and plantar fascia. While contraction of the posterior tibial muscle can lift the arch temporarily, neither this nor other muscles can support the arch very long under weight-bearing conditions. Increased height of the medial longitudinal arch is known as *pes cavus;* lowering of this arch results in a flat foot, or *pes planus.*

The *subtalar* joint allows approximately 15° of inversion and 10° of eversion of the foot, although walking uses only 6° of the total arc.

The *transverse tarsal joint,* Chopart's joint, lies at the midfoot between the talus and calcaneus proximally and the cuneiforms and cuboid distally. It has two axes of motion, one that contributes to inversion and eversion of the subtalar joint, and another that permits flexion and extension.

Motion in the intertarsal and tarsometatarsal joints is restricted to a few degrees of dorsiflexion and up to 15° of plantarflexion. Of particular importance is the "keylike" configuration formed by the second tarsometatarsal joint, which makes it the most stable of the tarsometatarsal articulations. This stability is especially important during push-off, since the second metatarsal transmits most of the weight in this maneuver.

The metatarsal "break" occurs along the oblique axis of the metatarsophalangeal (MTP) joints. This joint is particularly important in the hallux, which has a range of motion from 90° extension to 30° flexion. The lateral MTP joints admit up to 50° of flexion.

Each foot bears half of the body weight in the erect position, with the weight on each foot distributed evenly between the heel and metatarsal heads. Since there are two sesamoids beneath the first metatarsal head, this bone bears twice as much weight as the heads of the lateral metatarsals. Most of this load is transmitted across the medial longitudinal arch, which is reinforced by the plantar fascia. This fibrous bowstring of the arch is attached to the tuberosity of the calcaneus proximally and to the proximal phalanges distally. Since it has little ability to lengthen, injury to the plantar fascia is a common attritional change, especially in overweight people who spend a lot of time on their feet. These changes commonly take the form of avulsion of a portion of the plantar fascia from its attachment to the os calcis, producing a condition known as *plantar fasciitis,* which is manifest clinically as tenderness beneath the medial tuberosity of the os calcis.

BIOMECHANICS OF GAIT

The biomechanics of gait, both normal and abnormal, are discussed in Chap. 5.

SUGGESTED READINGS

Miller MD: *Review of Orthopaedics.* Philadelphia, Saunders, 1992.

Simon SR, Riggins RS, Wirth CR, Fox ML: *Orthopaedic Science.* Park Ridge, IL, American Academy of Orthopaedic Surgeons, 1986.

Wilson FC: *The Musculoskeletal System,* 2d ed. Philadelphia, Lippincott, 1983.

Wright V, Radin EL: *Mechanics of Human Joints.* New York, Marcel Dekker, 1993.

Chapter 5

Physical Diagnosis of the Musculoskeletal System

Gary D. Bos and Frank C. Wilson

THE MUSCULOSKELETAL HISTORY

Present Illness
Review of Systems
Past History
Family History
Social History

THE MUSCULOSKELETAL EXAMINATION

General Aspects
Spine
    Cervical Spine; Thoracic Spine; Lumbar Spine
Upper Limb
    Shoulder; Elbow; Forearm; Wrist and Hand
Lower Limb
    Hip; Knee; Ankle; Foot
Gait

Most orthopaedic diagnoses can and should be made on the basis of the history and physical examination. This chapter emphasizes the musculoskeletal examination; findings in pathologic conditions are covered in more detail in the chapters that follow.

THE MUSCULOSKELETAL HISTORY

While every patient with an orthopaedic disorder ideally should have a complete musculoskeletal evaluation, time constraints usually limit the history and examination to affected parts; even so, the practitioner must be aware of and investigate the potential relationships of a specific disorder to other bodily parts and systems.

Present Illness

It is helpful to determine early in the history whether a patient's complaint is related primarily to muscle, joint, or bone. Typical muscular complaints are weakness, fatigue, tremor, spasm, wasting, and soreness. Joint complaints include stiffness, swelling, and pain that are characteristically related to movement and weight-bearing, time of day, and weather. Bone pain tends to be aching, deeply seated, and unrelated to movement or activity. There is obvious overlap in the symptoms manifested by bone, joint, and muscle pathology, but careful attention to historical details will, more often than not, define the primary source of the complaint.

The history of an orthopaedic complaint is investigated by inquiries of how, where, what, and when. "How" describes the onset of the problem, e.g., sudden, gradual, posttraumatic,

and so on. The patient may recall a tearing or snapping sensation at the time of injury. Immediate swelling suggests vascular injury, which stands in contrast to later-developing edema.

The "where" of the complaint includes both localization and radiation. Radiating pain may be of primary neurologic origin or referred from regional musculoskeletal pathology. The practitioner must be mindful of the joints proximal and distal to the site of the pain; for example, the pain of hip pathology may be manifest at the knee because the obturator nerve supplies both areas.

"What" addresses the character of the complaint. Most orthopaedic complaints are activity-related and should be precisely localized by having the patient point to the involved area. Important questions are: Is the pain severe enough to alter daily activities? Is sleep interrupted? What relieves the pain? Pain at rest suggests a neoplastic or metabolic condition. Aggravation by movement and relief by rest points to a musculoskeletal origin. Pain that is more severe upon rising often indicates an arthritic process. The character and distribution of the pain are also important. Throbbing pain should arouse suspicion of an infectious process; radiation suggests neural origin.

"When" includes both time of onset and the temporal relationship of the complaint to other symptoms. Did pain, for example, precede deformity? If so, by how long? Did weakness occur after a sensory disturbance was noted or did both begin simultaneously? Knowledge of temporal sequences often identifies the primary cause of pathology.

Review of Systems

Systems related to the complaint should be explored. Fever and sweats point toward infection. A search must be made for a primary site if osteomyelitis is suspected. Weight loss in an older patient with new back pain, cough, or hematuria suggests metastatic malignancy.

Past History

The general health of the patient is probed by questions relating to recent loss or gain of weight, habits, allergies, medications, and surgeries. A careful occupational history may disclose job-related causes of the complaint. Previous similar complaints should be documented and explored.

Family History

Musculoskeletal conditions often have an hereditary basis, and a quick inquiry with respect to similar conditions in family members may provide both diagnostic and prognostic information.

Social History

Socioeconomic factors frequently compound diagnosis and/or influence treatment. The pro-longed treatment often needed for musculo-skeletal disorders imposes financial hardship and stresses family relationships; also, unique features of a patient's living environment may influence treatment options, particularly for elderly patients.

THE MUSCULOSKELETAL EXAMINATION

General Aspects

Watching a patient move about, walk, or dress when he or she is not aware of being observed often affords valuable information, especially when compared with movement patterns during the physician-patient encounter.

Before specific regions are examined, a cursory examination of the limbs and back, including posture, is carried out. Asymmetry of the shoulders, pelvis, and limbs suggests structural deformity, neuromuscular disease, or neoplasia.

Muscle strength in the affected limb is recorded (Table 5.1). Strength in the affected

Table 5.1 Grading of Muscle Strength

Strength Grade	Findings
0 (Zero)	No contraction
1 (Trace)	Palpable contraction of the tendon; no movement of the joint
2 (Poor)	Complete active range of motion with gravity eliminated
3 (Fair)	Complete active range of motion against gravity
4 (Good)	Complete active range of motion against gravity and partial resistance
5 (Normal)	Complete active range of motion against gravity and full resistance

limb should be compared to that of the normal side if the process is not bilateral.

The length of the lower limbs is measured between the anterosuperior iliac spine and the medial malleolus. The upper limb is measured in the standing position from the C7 spinous process across the shoulder to the tip of the long finger (Fig. 5.1). Inequality in length of the upper limbs is less important than a discrepancy in the lower limbs because of the latter's effect on gait.

Circumferential measurements at comparable levels are also made, recognizing that handedness creates normal differences in the upper limbs, which are absent in the lower limbs. Results are often more useful when reported as a difference between sides rather than actual measurements.

Joint motions and contractures are reported in degrees, with zero being the normal starting point. Important principles for assessing joint motion include measurement of joint angles with a goniometer, determination of both ac-

tive and passive motion, and inclusion of joints above and below an affected part.

The function of the major peripheral nerves is an essential part of the examination. Tests for the motor and sensory functions of the major nerves in the upper and lower limbs are listed in Table 5.2.

Spine

Evaluation of the spine includes observation of the patient's movements throughout the encounter. The entire back should be observed unclothed. Modesty is maintained by a gown that opens in the back. The anteroposterior curves of the spine are examined in both erect and forward bending positions. Viewed from the back, the head should be centered over the gluteal crease and the shoulders and pelvis level. Because the spine is deeply situated in the body, direct examination is difficult and evaluation often relies upon indirect signs,

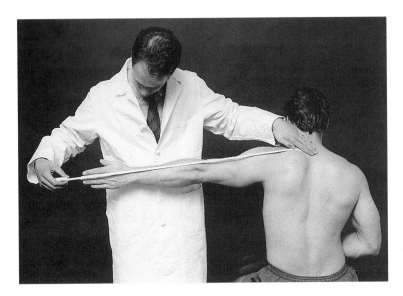

Figure 5.1 Technique for measurement of upper limb length.

Table 5.2   Examination of Major Peripheral Nerves

Nerve	Motor	Sensory
Upper Limb		
Axillary	Abduction of shoulder (deltoid)	Lateral aspect of shoulder
Musculocutaneous	Flexion of elbow (biceps/brachialis)	Radial border of forearm
Radial	Extension of thumb (extensors pollicis longus and brevis)	Dorsal web space between thumb and index finger
	Extension of wrist (extensor carpi radialis, longus and brevis, extensor carpi ulnaris)	
Median	Flexion of fingers (flexor pollicis longus, flexor digitorum superficialis, flexor digitorum profundus to index and long fingers)	Tip of index finger
Ulnar	Abduction of fingers (first dorsal interosseous; abductor digiti minimi)	Tip of small finger
Lower limb		
Femoral	Extension of knee (quadriceps)	Anterior thigh
Obturator	Adduction of hip (adductors magnus, longus, and brevis)	Medial thigh
Sciatic		
Peroneal	Dorsiflexion of ankle (tibialis anterior)	Dorsum of foot
	Dorsiflexion of toes (extensor hallucis longus, extensor digitorum longus)	
Tibial	Plantar flexion of ankle (gastrocnemius, soleus)	Tips of toes, plantar aspect of foot
	Plantar flexion of toes (flexor hallucis longus, flexor digitorum longus)	

such as muscle spasm, weakness, or peripheral nerve dysfunction.

Cervical Spine

The cervical spine may be shortened by vertebral anomaly (e.g., Klippel-Feil syndrome), tilted and rotated by muscle contracture (e.g., torticollis), or flattened by muscle spasm (e.g., disk disease). Other causes of asymmetry include the atrophy of neurologic disease or the swelling produced by a mass.

The spinous processes are palpated for tenderness or malalignment. The C7 spinous process is the most prominent; other spinous processes are partially obscured by the superior nuchal ligament, which extends from the back of the skull to the spinous process of C7. Unless they are in spasm, the paraspinous muscles are soft and pliable. Palpation of the region should extend to the mastoid processes, since paraspinous muscles take origin there. The trapezius, with its extension to the acromion, should be included in the cervical examination. The six motions of the neck—flexion, extension, left and right lateral bending, and left and right rotation—are difficult to measure in degrees and are often reported as a percentage of normal.

A critical portion of the examination entails evaluation of the nerve roots supplying the upper limbs. Sensation, strength, and reflexes should be tested on each side. Normal two-point discrimination is between 5 and 10 mm in the fingers. The dermatomes associated with the cervical roots are illustrated in Fig. 5.2 and the muscles and reflexes in Table 5.3.

Thoracic Spine

The most visible aspect of a disorder of the thoracic spine is deformity. Posteriorly, the spinous processes should be aligned, and the scapulae and shoulders symmetrical and level. In a child, a small, elevated scapula may indicate *Sprengel deformity,* in which the scapula is often tethered to the spine. A sharp increase in the normal kyphosis is called a *gibbus,* usually signifying collapse of a vertebral body from osteoporosis, infection, or metastatic disease. An increase of the normal kyphosis in an adolescent suggests *Scheuermann disease* (Fig. 5.3). *Scoliosis* includes both lateral deviation and rotational deformity of the spine. The rotational deformity produces a rib hump best seen from behind with the patient bent forward, so that the thoracic spine is horizontal (Fig. 8.19B). The rib hump is always on the convex side of the scoliosis.

Palpation of the spinous processes may reveal tenderness or subtle malalignment. The paraspinous, trapezius, and rhomboid muscles should be examined for spasm and pain. Motion in the thoracic spine is more limited than that in the cervical and lumbar areas because of the rib cage. Muscle strength is difficult to assess, but sensory defects in the thoracic dermatomes provide information about nerve root involvement.

Lumbar Spine

The lumbar spine, more flexible than the thoracic spine, reverses its normal lordosis to a kyphotic curve with forward bending. Persistent lordosis during this maneuver may reflect paraspinous muscle spasm from infection or disk disease or joint stiffness from osteoarthritis. Lumbar scoliosis is more difficult to appreciate than thoracic scoliosis because of the lumbar lordosis and the absence of a rib hump, although careful palpation of the spinous processes usually reveals the curve. A lumbar list

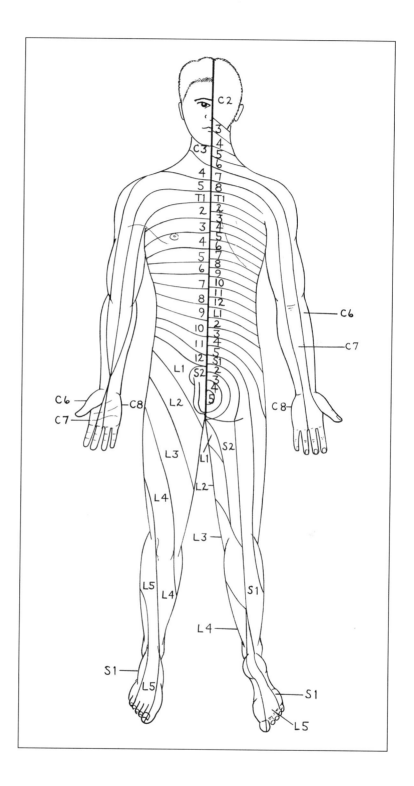

Figure 5.2 Anterior and posterior sensory dermatomes.

Table 5.3   Root Innervations of Muscles and
    Reflexes in the Upper Limb

Root	Muscles	Reflexes
C5	Deltoid	None
C6	Biceps Wrist extensors	Biceps Brachioradialis
C7	Triceps Wrist flexors Finger extensors	Triceps
C8	Interossei Finger flexors	None
T1	Interossei	None

and pain that radiates into a lower limb suggests lumbar disk disease. An abnormal hair patch in the lumbar area, a port wine spot, or a pedunculated soft tissue tumor often signals a congenital anomaly of the spine. *Pelvic tilt* points to leg-length discrepancy, scoliosis, or muscular contracture.

Palpation of the lumbar spine is performed with the patient in both standing and prone positions. Orientation is obtained from the L4-5 interspace, which lies at the level of the posterior iliac crests. With the patient prone, the spinous processes and interspinous intervals are explored. A gap in the process indicates *spina bifida;* a step-off suggests *spondylolisthesis* (anterior displacement of the spine on a subjacent vertebra). Paraspinous muscle spasm is a response to pain, often from protrusion of an intervertebral disk. The sacral spinous processes can be palpated, but the coccyx can be felt adequately only through the rectum. The sacroiliac joints lie 3 or 4 cm deep to the posterior superior iliac spine and cannot be palpated directly.

Motion in the lumbar spine is difficult to quantify because the spine is deeply positioned, and nearby joints, such as the hip, may substitute for lumbar motion. Flexion is measured by having the erect patient with feet together and knees straight reach down as if to touch the floor with the fingers, recording the distance between the fingers and the floor. Extension and lateral bending are estimated from the side and back respectively, with the patient erect and the pelvis steadied. As in the cervical spine, the exiting nerve roots often give the best indication of the level of lumbosacral pathology. Individual dermatomes can be compared by light touch (Fig. 5.2). The subjective localization of numbness is also useful in identifying the site of a spinal disorder. Strength is tested in all muscle groups in the lower limbs, with particular emphasis on those innervated by L5 and S1, since 90 percent of lumbar disk herniations are at the L4-5 or L5-S1 level. Deep tendon reflexes are checked at the knee and at the ankle. The response is recorded as normal, hyporeflexic, or hyperreflexic, and a difference between sides is particularly significant. The muscles and reflexes associated with the most commonly involved lumbar roots are shown in Table 5.4.

Further evidence of irritation of sciatic nerve roots (L4-S3) is provided by special tests. The *straight leg-raising test* (see Chap. 14) is usually performed in the supine position. The examiner lifts the leg at the ankle of the affected limb until the back and/or leg pain is reproduced, noting the angle at which this finding occurs. Hamstring tightness can simulate sciatic pain, so asymmetry and reproduction of the presenting pain are critical for a positive test. If, with the leg elevated just short of reproducing the pain, dorsiflexion of the an-

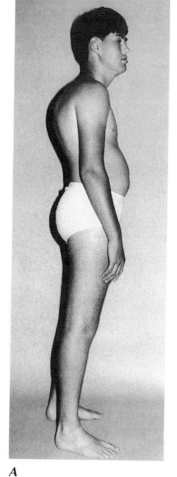

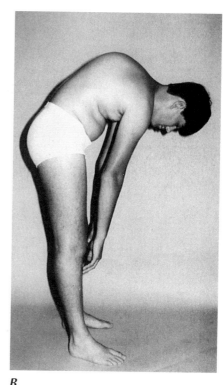

Figure 5.3 Scheuermann disease. Note increased dorsal kyphosis, especially in the flexed spine. (Reprinted with permission from Morcuende JA, Weinstein SL: Physical examination of the pediatric patient, in Clark CR, Bonfiglio M (eds): *Orthopedics: Essentials of Diagnosis and Treatment.* New York, Churchill Livingstone, 1994.)

A

B

kle precipitates the pain (positive *Lasègue sign*), the test is corroborated. If straight leg-raising of the uninvolved leg causes pain in the affected limb (positive *crossed straight leg-raising test*), there is even stronger evidence of root irritation. The sitting *straight leg-raising test* may be used when complaints of sciatic radiation are inconsistent or malingering is suspected. With the patient seated on the edge of the examination table, the knee is straight-

ened under the pretense of a knee examination. Patients with root compression will lean back, extending the hips to reduce sciatic tension.

The sacroiliac joint is examined indirectly by applying posteriorly directed pressure to both anterior iliac crests of the supine patient, which causes pain in the damaged sacroiliac joint; and by the *Gaenslen sign* (Fig. 5.4).

Table 5.4   Root Innervations of Muscles and Reflexes in the Lower Limb

Root	Muscles	Reflexes
L1-2	Iliopsoas	None
L3	Hip adductors	None
	Quadriceps femoris	Patellar tendon
L4	Tibialis anterior	Patellar tendon
	Quadriceps femoris	
L5	Tibialis anterior	None
	Tibialis posterior	Tibialis posterior tendon
	Extensor hallucis longus	None
S1	Gastrocnemius-soleus	Achilles tendon
	Flexor hallucis longus	None

Upper Limb

Shoulder

The shoulder, or shoulder girdle, is composed of three bones, four joints, and the muscles and ligaments that bind them together into a functional unit (Fig. 5.5).

The S-shaped *clavicle* protects the brachial plexus, acts as the "strut" that provides, at the sternoclavicular joint, the only bony connection between the upper limbs and the thorax, and is the "boom" from which the upper limb is suspended. Because of its subcutaneous location, the clavicle is readily visible and palpable. The *scapula,* which serves primarily for muscle attachment and is without bony connection to the thorax, provides two palpable bony landmarks: the *acromion* and the *coracoid process.* The coracoid process projects like a crooked finger from the anterosuperior border of the scapula; its tip is palpable 1 to 2 cm below the outer third of the clavicle. The proximal humerus is difficult to palpate beneath the overlying *deltoid muscle* and coracoacromial arch. Just lateral to the acromion, however, the *greater tuberosity* can be palpated and, medial to it, the *bicipital groove* and *lesser tuberosity. Bicipital tendinitis* is suggested by localized tenderness and by pain in the bicipital groove when the patient attempts to flex the shoulder against resistance with the elbow extended and the forearm supinated (positive *Speed test*) (Fig. 5.6).

The joints of the shoulder are the glenohumeral, acromioclavicular, sternoclavicular, and scapulothoracic.

The *glenohumeral joint,* which lacks strong bony or ligamentous support, allows the greatest range of motion of any joint in the body, at the expense of frequent dislocations. The *acromioclavicular joint* is more exposed, more easily examined, and more subject to injury than its medial counterpart, the *sternoclavicular joint.* Pathology in the acromioclavicular joint is suggested by pain in this area during forced adduction of the shoulder. Shoulder motion also occurs between the scapula and posterior thoracic wall, although this is not a true synovial articulation.

As the arm is abducted 180°, approximately 120° occurs at the glenohumeral joint and 60° in the scapulothoracic articulation, i.e., a ratio of about 2 to 1. During this same 180° arc of abduction, the sternoclavicular joint moves about 40° and the acromioclavicular joint 20°, also a ratio of about 2 to 1. The simultaneous movement in all joints during abduction of the shoulder is called *scapulohumeral rhythm* (Fig. 5.7). The normal arcs of flexion-exten-

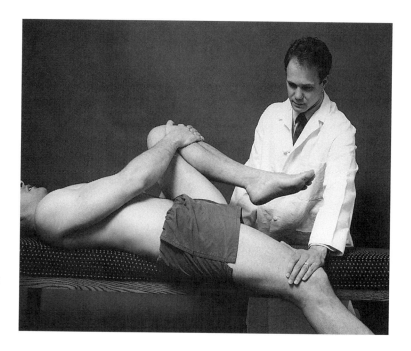

Figure 5.4 Gaenslen sign: pain is produced with disorders of the sacroiliac joint.

sion and internal-external rotation, both of which occur primarily at the glenohumeral joint, are shown in Fig. 5.8.

There are four major muscle groups that move the shoulder articulations: the *rotator* or *musculotendinous cuff* covers the top, front, and back of the humeral head (Fig. 5.9). Because of its location between the humeral head and the overlying coracoacromial arch, these tendons are subject to repeated compression, which may lead to attritional changes, manifest as *calcific tendinitis* ("bursitis"), or *tears of the rotator cuff.* Since the cuff lies beneath the deltoid muscle, it is not directly palpable; however, pathologic changes, which most commonly involve the supraspinatus, are usually manifest by tenderness just below the anterolateral aspect of the acromion. Inflammation of the rotator cuff from repeated compression between the humerus and acro-

mion is suggested by a positive *impingement sign,* in which the internally rotated humerus is passively abducted in slight forward flexion (Fig. 14.18). As the inflamed rotator cuff is thrust upward against the acromion, pain results. These patients also experience a sudden increase in pain at about 90° as the abducted arm is actively lowered from an overhead position—a positive *"drop arm" sign.* Tears of the rotator cuff, especially if large, result in weakness and limited active abduction.

The *trapezius* and *serratus anterior* stabilize the scapular base from which the arm operates. The trapezius also confers the weblike appearance to the neck and functions to rotate and elevate the scapula. Weakness allows the shoulder girdle to sag. The serratus draws the scapula forward in activities such as fencing or boxing; paralysis produces a characteristic prominence of the vertebral border of the scap-

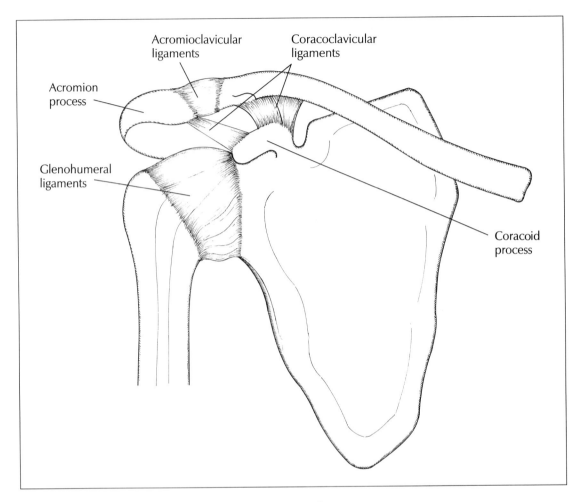

Figure 5.5 Bones and ligaments of the shoulder girdle.

ula ("scapular winging") (Fig. 5.10). The *deltoid,* which abducts the arm after the scapula has been fixed by its stabilizing muscles and the humeral head snugged to the *glenoid* by the rotator cuff, is subject to contusions and strains. Paralysis of the deltoid caused by injury to the axillary nerve results in weakness of all shoulder movements, especially abduction, and visible atrophy.

The major internal rotators (*subscapularis, teres major, latissimus dorsi,* and *pectoralis major*) represent a larger muscle mass than the external rotators (*infraspinatus, teres minor,* and *posterior deltoid*), which explains the greater strength of internal rotation.

The C4, C5, and T1-T4 dermatomes are represented in the shoulder area and should be checked for sensation. The sensory branch of

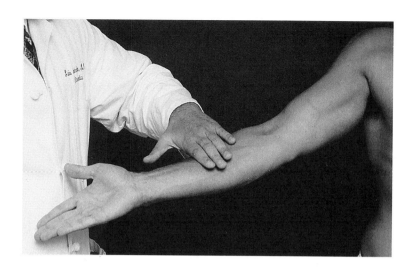

Figure 5.6   Speed test for bicipital tendinitis.

the axillary nerve (C5) supplies the area over the deltoid (Fig. 5.2).

Increased anterior instability of the shoulder, which follows dislocation and leads to its recurrence, is suggested by a positive *apprehension test,* in which the patient's facial expression shows sudden anxiety as the shoulder is passively externally rotated and abducted (Fig. 5.11).

Since shoulder pain is commonly referred from the cervical spine, a history of shoulder pain does not necessarily implicate intrinsic shoulder pathology. Examination of the structures in the shoulder should be followed by thorough evaluation of the cervical spine.

Elbow

The extended elbow lies in 5° valgus, an angle that is slightly greater in females because of their wider pelves. Palpable bony landmarks about the elbow include the medial and lateral epicondyles of the humerus, which serve as origins for the flexor-pronator and extensor-supinator muscles of the forearm and hand, the olecranon, and the radial head. The range of

flexion and extension in the elbow is approximately 0 to 140°, with the most useful arc between 60 and 120°.

Most of the important structures that cross the elbow can be palpated in the antecubital fossa, including, from lateral to medial, the biceps tendon, the brachial artery, and the median nerve. The ulnar nerve is palpable behind the medial epicondyle.

Viewed from behind, the olecranon and two epicondyles form a straight line when the elbow is extended. When the elbow is flexed 90°, they form the corners of an isosceles triangle. The shape of this triangle is unaltered in supracondylar fractures of the humerus (although it may be shifted medially or laterally), but it is distorted by dislocation of the elbow (Fig. 5.12).

Since the elbow is primarily a hinge joint, the most important motors are the flexors (biceps and brachialis) and extensors (triceps), which are tested by resisted flexion and extension of the elbow, respectively. The medial epicondylar muscles and brachioradialis supplement elbow flexion.

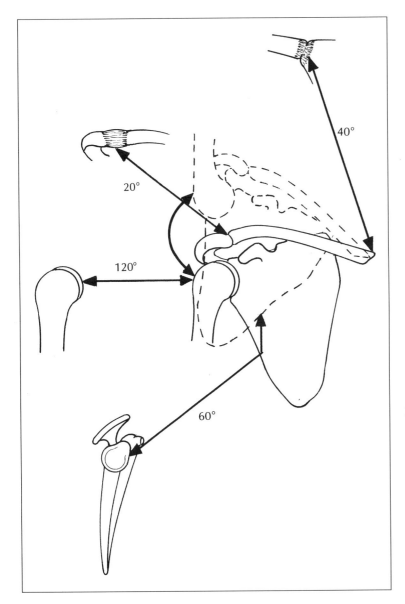

Figure 5.7
Scapulohumeral rhythm illustrating motion in all four shoulder joints during full (180°) abduction of the shoulder. [Redrawn with permission from Wilson FC (ed): *The Musculoskeletal System: Basic Processes and Disorders,* 2d ed. Philadelphia, Lippincott, 1983, Chap. 3, "The Upper Limb," p 41.]

The major nontraumatic conditions that involve the elbow are epicondylitis ("tennis elbow") and *olecranon bursitis. Lateral* (or, less commonly, *medial*) *epicondylitis,* which re-

sults from a partial rupture of the origin of the attached tendons, is associated with pain and epicondylar tenderness that is accentuated by tensing the involved mus-

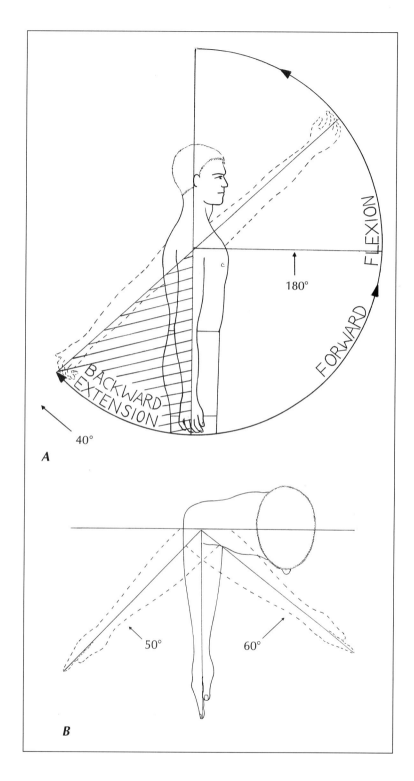

Figure 5.8 Flexion-extension (*A*) and internal-external rotation (*B*) of the shoulder.

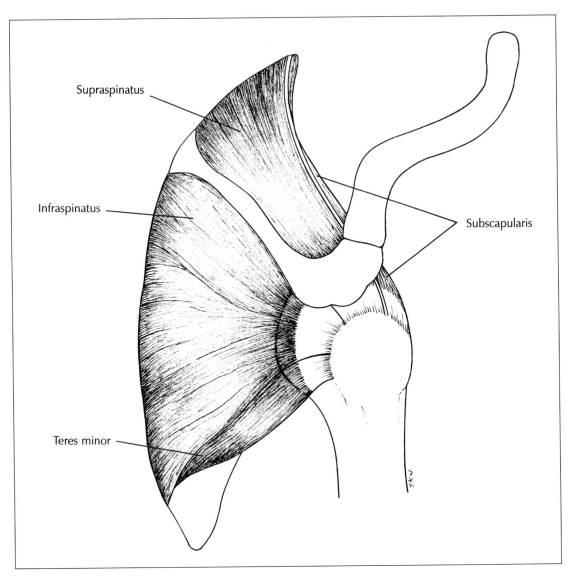

Figure 5.9 Musculotendinous (rotator) cuff.

cles. Olecranon bursitis produces a prominent, fluctuant swelling over the olecranon (Fig. 5.13). If the bursa becomes secondarily infected, the area becomes reddened and tender.

Forearm
The radius and ulna lie parallel to each other in supination. During pronation, the radius crosses the ulna, rotating on an axis that passes

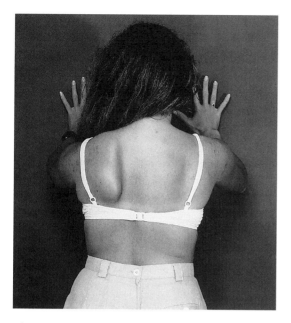

Figure 5.10 Winging of the scapula caused by weakness of the serratus anterior muscle.

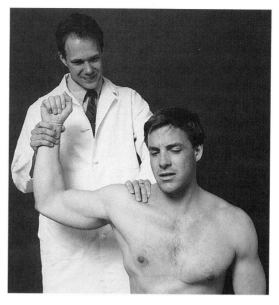

Figure 5.11 Apprehension test for anterior instability of the shoulder.

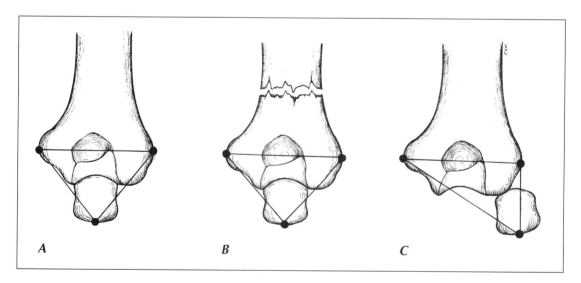

A	*B*	*C*

Figure 5.12 The posterior triangle of the elbow: normal (*A*); supracondylar fracture (no change) (*B*); posterolateral dislocation (*C*).

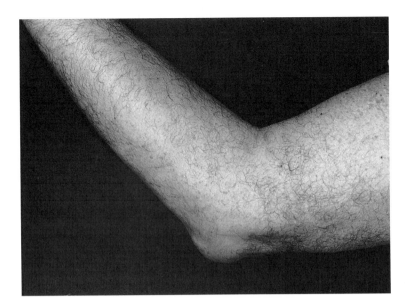

Figure 5.13   Olecranon bursitis.

from the capitellum to the distal end of the ulna. These bones are joined by the proximal and distal *radioulnar joints* and by the *interosseous membrane,* which is directed obliquely downward from the radius to the ulna. Since the ulna does not articulate with the carpus, the direction of this membrane is important for transmission of longitudinal forces from the radius to the ulna. The distal radioulnar joint should be inspected for deformity, and its integrity tested by resisted pronation and supination of the forearm. Fractures of the radius or ulna may result in displacement of the *superior,* or, more commonly, the *inferior radioulnar joint.* If unrecognized and uncorrected, this displacement often leads to a wrist with limited and painful rotation.

The arc of pronation and supination is 150 to 160°, with slightly more supination than pronation.

The forearm is surrounded by tense, unyielding fascia. Bleeding or swelling into the anterior compartment may result in vascular and/or neurologic compromise, producing the devastating syndrome of *Volkmann ischemic contracture.*

Wrist and Hand

The wrist and hand are positioned for use by the elbow and shoulder joints. The functional position of the hand is that of wrist extension with slight flexion of the digits. In this position, both the longitudinal and transverse arches of the hand are visible. Absence of one or both of these arches may signify pathology, such as the flattening of the transverse arch seen with loss of intrinsic muscle function.

Visible landmarks at the wrist are the head of the ulna, the anatomic "snuff box," and the flexion creases. The ulnar head may become displaced and unstable following trauma or rheumatoid arthritis. Scaphoid fractures are characterized by tenderness in the anatomic snuff box. The most distal volar flexion crease marks the proximal edge of the *transverse carpal ligament,* a heavy band of fibers that converts the volar aspect of the carpus into a rigid fibro-osseous tunnel, through which pass the nine flexor tendons to the digits and the median nerve. Compression of the median nerve produces pain, sensory disturbance, and weakness in the distribution of the median nerve (carpal tunnel syndrome).

Palpable landmarks include *Lister's tubercle,* which serves as the pulley for the extensor pollicis longus tendon, and the *radial and ulnar styloid processes.* Normally, the radial styloid projects 1 cm distal to that of the ulna. The pisiform bone is also palpable on the ulnovolar aspect of the wrist and serves to mark the entry, on its lateral aspect, of the ulnar nerve and artery into the hand. Both the ulnar and radial arteries are palpable at this level.

The normal wrist flexes slightly more than it extends, with a total arc of motion from 0 to 160°. Ulnar deviation (30°) exceeds radial deviation (20°).

It is difficult for the examiner to overcome normal dorsiflexion strength at the wrist, and volar flexion is even more powerful. Radial and ulnar deviation are not as strong as flexion and extension.

Special tests for wrist pathology include *Finkelstein's test* (Fig. 14.21) for *de Quervain disease, Tinel's* and *Phalen's tests* for carpal tunnel syndrome, *Allen's test* (Fig. 5.14) for circulation to the hand, and assessment of inferior radioulnar joint stability. The Tinel sign is positive when percussion over the median nerve in the carpal canal produces paresthesias in the distal distribution of the nerve. Phalen's test is performed by maintaining the wrist in maximum volar flexion for 1 min, during which time, if the test is positive, median paresthesias will be noted distally. Allen's test begins with the patient making a tight fist after opening and closing the hand a few times

rapidly; the examiner then occludes both the radial and ulnar arteries by firm pressure. When the patient again opens the hand, the palm is blanched. When either artery alone is released, the hand should flush promptly and completely. Failure to do so from either artery indicates compromised flow from that vessel.

Inspection of the hand should include a search for deformity, discoloration, atrophy, swelling, or masses. Muscle bulk in the thenar and hypothenar eminences should be compared with the opposite side, since thenar atrophy is common in carpal tunnel syndrome. The wrist and hand are also common sites for *ganglia,* which must be distinguished from the synovial and tenosynovial swelling of rheumatoid arthritis. The latter usually occurs more centrally along the extensor tendons; ganglia favor the radial aspect of the wrist. Pale nail beds may signify anemia, while split or pitted nails suggest impaired nutritional status.

Because of their relatively superficial location, the bones and tendons of the distal palm and fingers and their accompanying tendons may be palpated throughout their course, along with intervening joints. Nodules in the flexor tendons frequently accompany rheumatoid arthritis and may lead to snapping or "catching" of the digits during flexion and extension *(trigger finger).* Joint tenderness suggests intrinsic joint disease or recent trauma.

The metacarpophalangeal (MCP) joints have a range of motion from 50 to 60° of extension to 90° of flexion. There is little or no hyperextension of the MCP joints in the thumb. Normal motion in the interphalangeal (IP) joints is 0 to 90°, although 5 to 10° of hyperextension is not uncommon. From a functional perspective, the patient should be able to approximate the fingertips to the palm

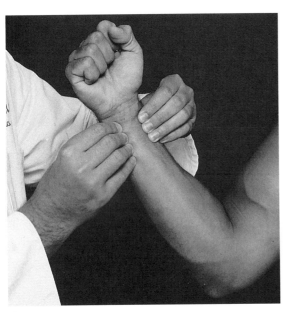

A

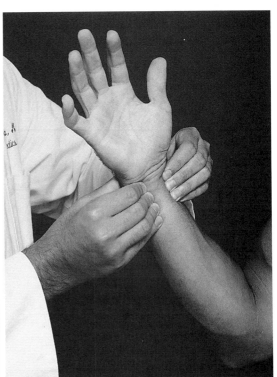

B

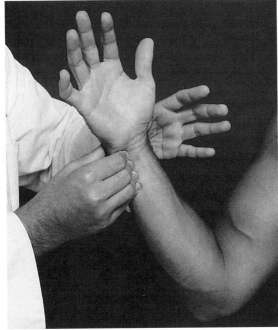

C

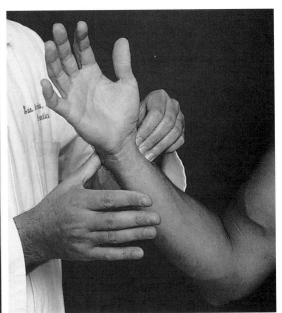

D

and the tip of the thumb to the distal phalanx of the index finger (pinch). If the examiner cannot pull his or her index finger through the patient's pinch mechanism, strength in the first dorsal interosseous muscle is normal.

Function in the flexor digitorum profundus (FDP) tendons is assessed by immobilizing the MCP and PIP joints and noting the power of flexion in the DIP joint. To test the flexor digitorum superficialis (FDS) tendons, the finger to be tested is isolated by securing the MCP and IP joints of the other digits in extension and having the patient flex the PIP joint of the finger being tested. Because the PIP joint may be flexed by the FDP, it must be excluded when the FDS is tested, and since the FDP does not act independently, preventing its action in other digits also excludes its effect on the tested digit (Fig. 5.15).

Abduction of the digits from the long finger is provided by the dorsal interossei; adduction by the volar interossei. The interossei and lumbricales also flex the MCP and extend the IP joints.

Thumb extension (motion away from the second metacarpal in the plane of the palm) is carried out primarily by the extensors pollicis longus and brevis. Thumb abduction (motion in the palmar direction, at right angles to the plane of the palm) is produced by the abductors pollicis longus and brevis. Thumb opposition is a composite motion, requiring abduction, rotation, adduction, and flexion of the thumb.

Sensation in the hand is supplied by the me-dian, ulnar, and radial nerves (Fig. 5.16). Since slight variation in the distribution of these nerves is common, their function should be tested in the autonomous zones, which are, for the median nerve, the volar tip of the index finger; for the ulnar nerve, the volar tip of the little finger; and for the radial nerve, the dorsum of the first web space.

The nerve supply to the muscles of the hand is relatively easy to test if one recalls that the median nerve innervates all volar extrinsic muscles in the hand except the FDP to the ring and little fingers, the thenar muscles except for the adductor pollicis, the deep head of the flexor pollicis brevis, and the third and fourth lumbricales, which are supplied by the ulnar nerve. The remaining volar muscles and all of the interossei are innervated by the ulnar nerve. The dorsal muscles are supplied by the radial nerve.

Deformities of the fingers that are especially common in rheumatoid arthritis are *ulnar drift, swan-neck,* and *boutonnière deformities,* which result primarily from synovitis and imbalance between the intrinsic and extrinsic motors of the digit. The *boutonnière* deformity results from rupture of the central slip of the extensor tendon at its insertion into the base of the middle phalanx, which allows the lateral bands to slip below the axis of rotation of the PIP joint, causing its flexion. Since the bands then pass dorsal to the axis of rotation of the DIP joint, it is commonly hyperextended. A swan-neck deformity follows contracture or

---

Figure 5.14   Allen's test for collateral circulation in the hand. *A.* Exsanguination by making a fist and occluding radial and ulnar arteries. *B.* The palm is blanched when the hand is opened. *C.* Release of the radial artery should lead to flushing. *D.* Steps *A* to *C* are repeated and the ulnar artery is released.

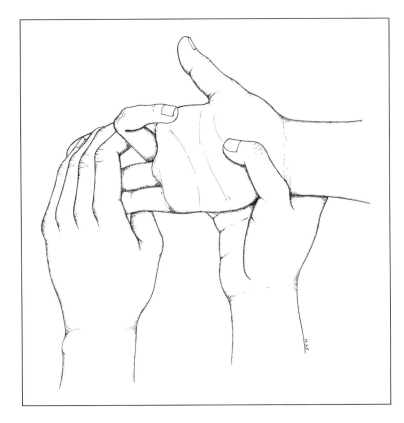

Figure 5.15   Test for function of the FDS. The FDP, which cannot act independently, is blocked from flexing the PIP joint of the long finger by immobilizing the DIP joints of the other fingers.

spasm of the intrinsic muscles, most commonly from rheumatoid arthritis, which causes flexion of the MCP and DIP joints and hyperextension of the PIP joints (Fig. 5.17).

A *claw hand* (or *claw finger*) is characterized by MCP hyperextension and IP flexion (Fig. 5.18). It results from loss of intrinsic muscle function in the presence of continued extrinsic function, such as that resulting from laceration of the median and ulnar nerves at the wrist.

A *mallet finger,* identified by a flexion posture of a distal phalanx, results from rupture of the extensor tendon at its insertion into the base of the distal phalanx. The most common cause of these deformities is trauma.

Lower Limb

Hip

Unlike the upper limb, which is connected to the trunk by the weak sternoclavicular joint, the lower limb has a strong osseous connection through the hip joint. Its ball-and-socket configuration provides great bony stability, which is reinforced by a well-developed capsule and strong ligaments. While direct inspection and palpation of the hip joint is impossible, abnormalities of skin folds, pelvic tilt, muscle atrophy, and asymmetry may provide indirect evidence of pathology in the hip joint.

Palpable bony landmarks about the hip include the anterior and posterior iliac spines,

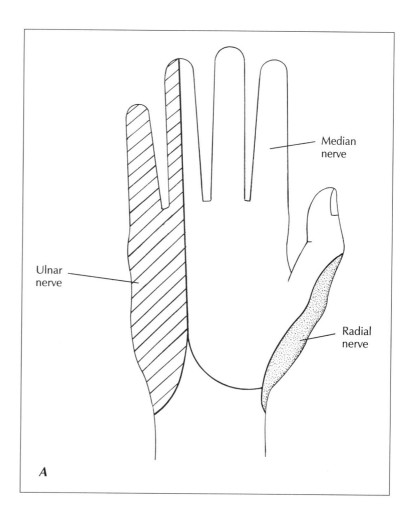

Median
nerve

Ulnar
nerve

Radial
nerve

Figure 5.16   Distribution of sensation in the hand: palmar aspect (*A*); dorsal aspect (*B*).

A

iliac crest, greater trochanter, ischial tuberosity, and sacroiliac joint. Also palpable are the sciatic nerve, which follows a course midway between the ischial tuberosity and the greater trochanter, and the femoral artery, which passes immediately behind the inguinal ligament between the femoral vein medially and the femoral nerve laterally. The artery is useful as a guide to aspiration of the hip joint: a needle inserted 2.5 cm lateral to the artery and 2.5 cm below the inguinal ligament passes directly into the joint cavity.

Motion of the hip joint is tested with the patient supine and the uninvolved hip flexed against the torso to prevent compensatory motion of the lumbar spine. The normal flexion arc is 0 to 125°. Abduction and adduction are 0 to 45° and 0 to 25°, and internal and external rotation are 0 to 25° and 0 to 45°, respectively. Rotational movements are slightly greater when the hips are in 90° flexion. When testing motion of the hip joint, particularly abduction and adduction, one of the examiner's hands should rest on the opposite pelvis to separate

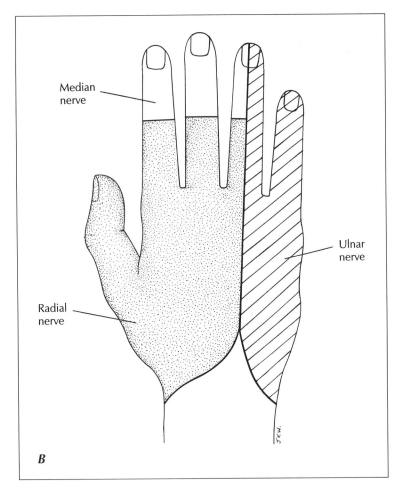

B

Figure 5.16 Continued

motion in the hip from pelvic tilt. Loss of passive movement in the hip suggests articular pathology. With arthritic change, all movements are restricted; however, flexion and extension, being the most frequently used, are preserved longer than rotation and lateral movement. The slipped capital femoral epiphysis of childhood is often associated with striking limitation of internal rotation because of posterior displacement of the femoral head. Increased internal torsion (anteversion) and external torsion (retroversion) of the femur allow increased internal and external rotation of the hip, respectively.

Limited active movement in the presence of full passive motion of the hip indicates a neuromuscular deficiency rather than articular pathology. The muscles about the hip may be tested in functional groups. The *iliopsoas,* innervated by the femoral nerve, is the major flexor of the hip. The chief extensor is the *gluteus maximus,* which is supplied by the *inferior gluteal nerve.* The *hamstring muscles,* innervated by the sciatic nerve, assist in extension.

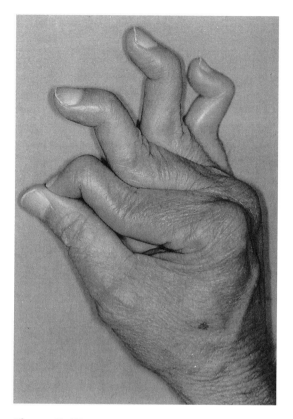

Figure 5.17   Swan-neck deformities caused by rheumatoid arthritis. Note MCP and DIP flexion and PIP extension.

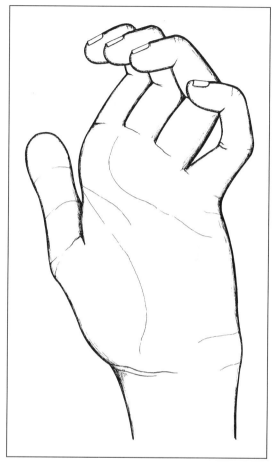

Figure 5.18   Claw hand. Note MCP hyperextension, IP flexion, and flattening of the thenar and hypothenar eminences.

The abductors of the hip are the *gluteus medius* and the *gluteus minimus,* which are supplied by the *superior gluteal nerve.* External rotation of the hip is provided by the gluteus maximus and several small posterior muscles. The gluteus minimus and medius and the *tensor fascia lata* are the principal internal rotators.

Special tests include leg length determinations as well as the *Trendelenburg, Patrick,* and *Thomas tests.* Leg lengths are measured between the anterosuperior iliac spine and the medial malleolus. The Trendelenburg test assesses strength in the hip abductors (Fig. 5.19).

The Patrick test is primarily an indicator of sacroiliac joint pathology (Fig. 5.20). The Thomas test stabilizes the lumbar spine to allow more accurate assessment of a flexion contracture in the hip (Fig. 5.21).

Knee

The knee is primarily a hinge joint, although both rotation and gliding occur during flex-

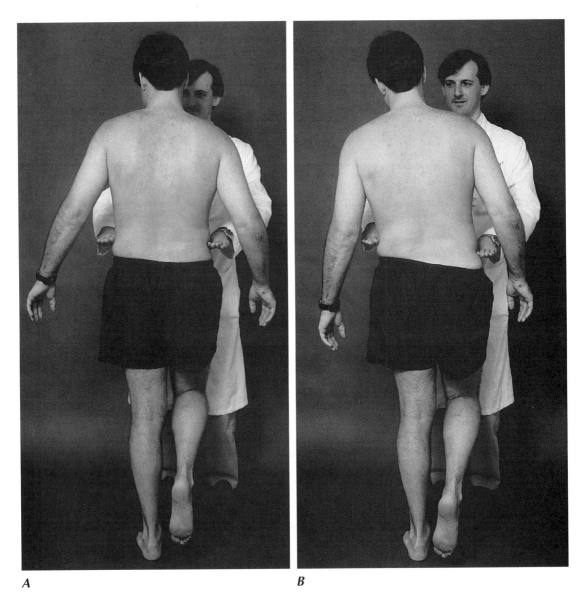

A   *B*

Figure 5.19   Normal single limb stance (*A*), positive Trendelenburg test (*B*),
      weakness of the left gluteus medius muscle.

ion and extension. As a weight-bearing joint that exists at the ends of the two longest lever arms in the body, it is subject to great angular and compressive stresses. Stabil-ity, necessary in the coronal plane, must not interfere with freedom of movement in the sagittal plane. Since the tibias are nearly ver-tical and the femurs converge from the pelvis

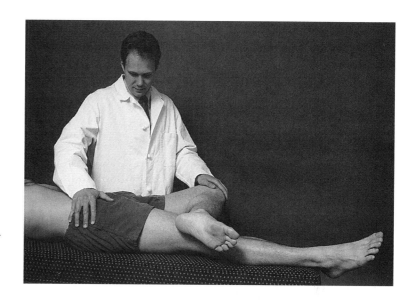

Figure 5.20   Patrick's test. Pain with abduction and external rotation suggests pathology of the hip joint.

to the knees, the femur and tibia meet in the adult at an angle of 5 to 8°. A greater angle results in *genu valgum* (knock-knee), a lesser angle in *genu varum* (bowleg). Physiologic increases in varus are common between birth and 2 years of age and in valgus from ages 2 to 8.

Inspection of the knee should include comparison with the opposite side. Normally visible bony landmarks may be obscured by ef-

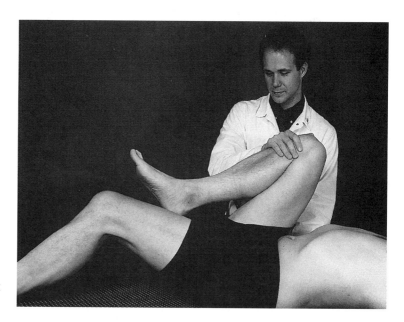

Figure 5.21   Positive Thomas test, indicating a flexion contracture of the left hip joint.

fusion. Undue prominence of the tibial tubercle is seen in *Osgood-Schlatter disease.* Abnormal position of the patella usually results from congenital or traumatic disorders. The patella should track smoothly between the femoral condyles during flexion and extension; lateral displacement during the terminal arc of extension is seen in patients with recurrent displacement of the patella. The most common masses encountered at the knee represent accumulation of fluid in one of the many bursae that surround the knee. Enlargement of the popliteal bursae *(Baker cyst)* usually reflects intraarticular pathology, such as arthritis or a torn meniscus.

Palpable bony landmarks at the knee include the tibial plateaus, femoral condyles, fibular head, patella, tibial tubercle, and joint lines. Careful palpation of the joint lines is particularly important, since meniscal pathology produces tenderness localized to these areas. (The tenderness associated with collateral ligament sprains is vertical, usually extending above and below the joint line, whereas meniscal tenderness is horizontal.) In the swollen or obese knee, the joint lines may not be directly palpable; however, their level is marked by the inferior pole of the patella, which lies at or just above the joint lines when the knee is fully extended.

The intraarticular cruciate ligaments are designed to prevent abnormal anterior or posterior displacement of the knee. Mediolateral (varus-valgus) stability is provided by the straplike medial collateral and the cordlike lateral collateral ligaments. Tests for the integrity of the ligaments of the knee are discussed in Chap. 13. Patellar stability is provided by the tendinous retinaculae. Dislocation of the patella, which is usually lateral, requires tearing of the medial patellar retinaculum. Thus, tenderness following lateral dis-

location of the patella is medial rather than lateral.

The arc of motion in the normal knee is from 0 to 135°, although the amount of flexion varies with the thickness of the soft tissue envelope in the thigh. Hyperextension, determined by lifting the heel of the supine patient and noting posterior sag at the knee joint, often indicates disruption of the posterior cruciate ligament. Lack of full passive extension or flexion suggests meniscal pathology or a loose body. Hamstring spasm, which often accompanies intraarticular pathology, may also limit extension.

Under normal circumstances, it is difficult or impossible for the examiner to overcome the quadriceps or hamstring muscles. The ability to do so may reflect either weakness in these muscles or pain associated with their testing. The rapid atrophy of the quadriceps muscle that follows injury to the knee is most easily quantified by circumferential measurements of both thighs at least 5 cm above the superior pole of the patellas. If measured lower, effusion may mask atrophy. The ability to extend the knee with full strength denotes integrity of the entire quadriceps muscle, including the patella, from the hip to the tibial tubercle.

Special tests used in examining the knee include the *McMurray test* for meniscal pathology, the *drawer, Lachman,* and *pivot shift tests* for cruciate pathology (see Chap. 13), the *apprehension test* for patellar instability, and patellar ballottement for effusion. The apprehension test, usually positive in patients with recurrent lateral displacement of the patella, is performed by allowing the knee to flex passively while the examiner's thumbs displace the patella laterally. A positive response is indicated by a sudden facial grimace as the patella returns from its displaced position over the lateral condyle to its normal position between the femoral condyles. *Patellar ballottement* is performed by compressing the suprapatellar pouch with one hand while, with the other, the patella is tapped downward toward the femoral condyles. If an effusion is present, the patella will be felt to click against the condyles.

Palpable soft tissue structures include the quadriceps and patellar tendons, often the site of partial or complete ruptures, the former producing *tendinitis*, the latter associated with a palpable defect and inability to extend the knee with normal strength. The iliotibial band, appreciable just posterior to the lateral border of the patella, may be subject to painful irritation when passing over the femoral condyle during flexion and extension of the knee, producing the *iliotibial band syndrome*. Tenderness on the anteromedial face of the proximal tibia, particularly if associated with swelling, suggests *pes anserinus bursitis*, an inflammation of the bursa lying deep to the three tendons (sartorius, gracilis, and semitendinosus) that insert in this area. Other bursae about the knee are described in Chap. 14. If the patient is not obese, the popliteal artery should be palpable in the popliteal space. The common peroneal nerve (L4-S2), vulnerable to stretch or compression injury, becomes subcutaneous behind the head of the fibula and can be rolled beneath the finger as it wraps around the neck of the fibula. Loss of function in this nerve results in diminished sensation on the dorsum of the foot and paralysis of the dorsiflexors and evertors of the ankle and foot.

Ankle

At the ankle, the weight-bearing tibia articulates with the spool-like upper surface of the talus, which articulates below with the calcaneus. The ankle is a hinge joint of the mortise-and-tenon variety, in which the talus is the tenon and the distal tibia and malleoli constitute the mortise. The malleoli also serve as pulleys for tendons that reach from the posterior and lateral compartments of the leg to the foot. Further medial stability is provided by the heavy deltoid ligament that fans out from the medial malleolus to the talus, navicular bone, and calcaneus below. Laterally, three smaller ligaments: the *anterior* and *posterior talofibular ligaments* and the *calcaneofibular ligament* (which lies between the talofibular ligaments) provide stability.

Visible bony landmarks are the medial and lateral malleoli. The tip of the lateral malleolus extends 1 cm distal to that of the medial malleolus and rests 15 to 20° posterior to it. If this angle exceeds 20° after puberty, *external tibial torsion* exists; if it is less than 15°, *internal tibial torsion* is present. This relationship of the malleoli is tested with the knee flexed, the tibial tubercle pointing anteriorly, and a finger on each malleolus (see also Chap. 17).

In addition to inspection of visible landmarks, examination of the ankle includes palpation of the anterior ankle and distal tibiofibular joints, the tendons that cross the ankle (anterior and posterior tibials, toe extensors, Achilles tendon, and peroneals), and the deltoid and lateral collateral ligaments. Palpation of these structures may be precluded by edema, which most commonly follows injury but also results (usually bilaterally) from varicosities and systemic conditions, such as cardiac failure.

Although recent injury may make interpretation difficult, stability of the ankle in both anteroposterior and mediolateral planes should be tested. With an intact mortise, neither inversion nor eversion of the foot should produce appreciable tilting of the talus; however, the presence and degree of talar tilt is best assessed by stress radiographs. Anteroposterior stability is tested by the *anterior drawer test,* in which, with the ankle slightly plantar flexed, an attempt is made to pull the foot forward on the fixed tibia (Fig. 5.22). Abnormal anterior displacement of the foot compared to the opposite side suggests rupture of the anterior talofibular ligament.

Motion of the ankle, recorded as the angle between the anterior tibia and dorsum of the foot, is normally from about 15° of dorsiflexion to 45° of plantar flexion. Dorsiflexion is produced by the anterior tibial muscle and, to a lesser extent, by the toe extensors; plantar flexion is produced primarily by the gastrocnemius-soleus complex, with reinforcement from the posterior tibial and toe flexors medially and the peroneal muscles laterally.

Also important at the ankle are the Achilles and posterior tibial reflexes. Reduction or loss of the Achilles reflex may signify a lesion of the S1 root; an absent posterior tibial reflex, obtained by tapping the posterior tibial tendon between the medial malleolus and the navicular, indicates compromise of the L5 nerve root only if present on the opposite side, since it is difficult to elicit this reflex under normal conditions.

Special tests to elucidate local pathology include *Homan's sign,* in which passive dorsiflexion of the foot produces calf pain in the presence of thrombophlebitis; the anterior drawer test (described above) for lateral ligamentous deficiency; and the *Thompson test* for rupture of the Achilles tendon (Fig. 13.45).

Foot

In addition to being a weight-bearing structure, the foot serves as a lever to raise the body and to convey thrust in walking and running. Its arched structure provides strength and resilience for the large forces involved as well as protection of plantar structures from compression. The bones are arranged so that each foot forms half a dome that is sustained in the normal weight-bearing state by the plantar fascia and ligaments. Inadequate ligamentous support results in collapse of the longitudinal arch when weight is borne (pes planus). The opposite deformity (pes cavus) may be a normal variant or associated with neurologic disorders, such as *Charcot-Marie-Tooth disease* or *Friedreich ataxia.*

Inspection of the foot should include examination of the weight-bearing arches, nails, hair, and a search for deformity, masses, calluses, corns, and warts. Deformity often indicates muscular imbalance; the absence of hair on the dorsum of the toes (along with decreased arterial pulsations) suggests vascular deficiency; plantar calluses and dorsal or in-

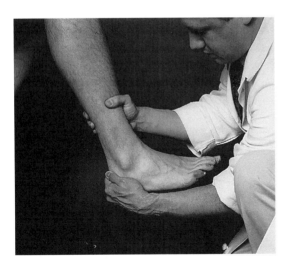

Figure 5.22 Anterior drawer test. Anterior displacement of the slightly plantar flexed ankle indicates rupture of the anterior fibulotalar ligament.

terdigital corns indicate abnormal weight-bearing or shoe pressure and are commonly associated with deformity. *Calluses* beneath the metatarsal heads can usually be distinguished from *plantar warts* by lateral compression, which produces pain if the lesion is a wart.

Palpation should include further assessment of deformity, with particular reference to whether it is fixed or flexible. Deformities due simply to muscular imbalance are usually correctable passively, even when spasticity is present, whereas bony deformity or ligamentous contracture, such as that seen in clubfoot, produces fixed deformities. In the presence of heel complaints, the os calcis must be carefully examined. The two most common causes of heel pain in adults are *plantar fasciitis,* manifest by tenderness beneath the os calcis where the plantar fascia has been partially torn from the medial tuberosity, and bursitis of the Achilles tendon, in which a bursa deep or superficial to the insertion of the Achilles tendon becomes inflamed, swollen, and tender *(Haglund disease).*

Motions of the foot are primarily those of inversion and eversion. Inversion may be broken down into supination (forefoot) and varus (heel); eversion may be subdivided into pronation (forefoot) and valgus (heel). Inversion is usually limited to 15°, eversion to 10°. The major inverters of the foot are the calf and posterior tibial muscles; eversion is produced primarily by the peroneal muscles. Active motion of the toes is limited primarily to dorsiflexion and plantar flexion, with the roles played by the intrinsic and extrinsic muscles similar to those in the hand.

Weakness in the muscles of the foot is commonly the result of injury to a nerve root, as occurs in intervertebral disk disease, or a peripheral nerve, which is most commonly caused by trauma. Determination of the root involved (and hence the level of intervertebral disk pathology) may be determined by careful motor and sensory dermatomal mapping (Fig. 5.2, Table 5.4; see also Chap. 14).

Restricted motion at the metatarsophalangeal (MTP) joint of the large toe, termed *hallux rigidus,* is commonly the result of arthritic changes in that joint. *Hallux valgus,* lateral deviation of the great toe at the MTP joint, is more common in patients with flat feet and in women, among whom footwear with pointed toe boxes is a major contributor. Hallux valgus is associated with increased medial prominence of the first metatarsal head. Continued shoe pressure over this prominence leads to the formation of a medial exostosis with an overlying bursa, which may become inflamed and tender, a constellation of deformities recognized as a *bunion.*

The most common deformities affecting the lateral toes are *claw toe, hammer toe,* and *mallet toe,* which are discussed in Chap. 17. When these deformities place the toe in abnormal contact with the shoe or other toes, painful corns or calluses are likely to develop.

Gait

Normal gait consists of two phases: *stance phase,* which makes up 60 percent of the gait cycle, begins with heel strike and ends with toe-off; *swing phase,* 40 percent of the cycle, begins with toe-off and ends with heel strike. Throughout the gait cycle, the muscles of the lower limb function alternately to accelerate or decelerate joint movement, e.g., the anterior tibial muscle dorsiflexes the foot during the swing phase of gait so that the toes may clear the ground; with heel strike, this muscle decelerates the plantarflexion moment of the ankle, thereby preventing foot slap. Normal stride length, which varies with length of limb and rate of walking, averages about 37 cm. Synchronous action in the joints of the lower limb confers symmetry, rhythm, and smoothness to normal gait. A limp is usually a consequence of pain, weakness, or difference in the lengths of the limbs.

Pain is the most common cause of limp. It produces an *antalgic gait,* which is characterized by a shortened stance phase on the affected side. Pain in the hip *(coxalgia)* causes a lurch of the trunk toward the painful side during stance phase.

A weak gluteus medius muscle allows the opposite side of the pelvis to tip downward during stance phase on the weakened side. To compensate, the trunk leans toward the weakened side during stance to reduce the force required of the abductors to maintain a level pelvis (abductor or *gluteus medius limp*).

When the gluteus maximus is weak, the trunk lurches backward at heel strike on the weakened side to restrict forward motion of the trunk because the gluteus maximus is unable to carry out this function.

With a deficient quadriceps muscle, walking on level ground may appear entirely normal. Such a patient, however, is unable to run and may have difficulty walking on rough or inclined surfaces and climbing stairs. When full extension is not obtained under these conditions of increased stress, the knee tends to buckle into flexion.

Weakness or paralysis of the anterior tibial muscle produces a *steppage gait:* the ankle drops into equinus during swing phase, which is compensated by increased knee and hip flexion to permit the foot to clear the floor.

Laceration of the Achilles' tendon or paralysis of the calf muscles result in inability to push off in a normal manner, producing a "peg-leg" gait.

Difference in the lengths of the limbs is termed *anisomelia.* Compensation for a short leg occurs through downward tilt of the pelvis on the short side, increased knee flexion on the normal side, and/or increased plantarflexion in the ankle of the affected limb. With marked shortening, the normal heel-toe pattern of gait may be reversed to a toe-heel pattern or a toe-toe pattern, in which the heel never touches the ground.

The use of a cane to improve the biomechanics of gait and minimize the limp associated with pathology of the hip joint is discussed in Chap. 4.

SUGGESTED READINGS

HOPPENFELD S: *Physical Examination of the Spine and Extremities.* East Norwalk, CT, Appleton-Century Crofts, 1976.

POST M: *Physical Examination of the Musculoskeletal System.* Chicago, Year Book, 1987.

Chapter 6

Diagnostic Modalities: Imaging, Joint Aspiration, and Arthroscopy

Jordan B. Renner and Frank C. Wilson

IMAGING

Conventional Radiography
Computed Tomography
Magnetic Resonance Imaging
Nuclear Medicine
Ultrasound
Summary

JOINT ASPIRATION

Technique
Glucocorticoid Injections

ARTHROSCOPY

IMAGING

The diagnostic evaluation of the orthopaedic patient is a puzzle often easily solved; in other instances it requires integration of information from disparate sources. The history and physical examination remain the most important means for the evaluation of the patient with musculoskeletal complaints. While other tools, such as clinical laboratory testing, neurophysiologic studies, and invasive diagnostic procedures are often helpful, diagnostic imaging is second in importance to the history and physical examination.

Imaging the orthopaedic patient may require conventional radiography, computed tomography (CT), magnetic resonance imaging (MRI), nuclear medicine, ultrasonography, and occasionally angiography. Conventional radiography is often sufficient to establish a diagnosis, but each imaging modality has distinct sensitivity and specificity, which help the clinician tailor the imaging evaluation to the patient's needs in an efficient and cost-effective manner.

Conventional Radiography

Conventional or plain-film radiography is the cornerstone of imaging for musculoskeletal problems. Radiographic facilities for these studies are relatively inexpensive, easily located in clinical settings, and require less equipment than CT or MRI. Conversely, conventional radiography is the most difficult radiologic procedure to perform well. High-quality radiography requires carefully calibrated and maintained equipment, correct selection of film/screen systems, proper processing, and well-trained technical personnel. Appropriately trained personnel are especially important, since proper selection of radio-

graphic technique and accurate positioning are vital for optimal results with conventional radiography. Restated, it may be easy to do plain film radiography, but it is difficult to do it well.

In many cases conventional radiography alone is sufficient for the orthopaedic patient. It must be remembered, however, that plain films are necessary even when further imaging is anticipated. Seldom can the physician interpret the results of a CT, MRI, or nuclear medicine study optimally without correlative information from plain films.

The sensitivity and specificity of plain film studies vary widely, depending upon the clinical problem. Conventional radiographs are highly sensitive and specific for the diagnosis of a fracture but are often less valuable in the assessment of a patient with low back pain. Plain films can be very specific for arthritis but insensitive for metastatic malignancy. The relative diagnostic strengths of different modalities are emphasized in the discussion that follows.

Plain films are indispensable for the evaluation of musculoskeletal trauma, both to assess the initial injury and to confirm the progress and quality of fracture healing. They are also unsurpassed for characterizing arthritic conditions, offering important information as to the type, distribution, and extent of the arthritic process. Such features may not be apparent clinically but may be diagnostically, therapeutically, and prognostically important. In the evaluation of musculoskeletal neoplasms, particularly primary tumors, conventional radiographs offer information about the lesion's margins, matrix calcification pattern, size, position, and association with new bone formation, all of which may, coupled with the clinical features, lead to a high degree of diagnostic accuracy (Fig. 6.1).

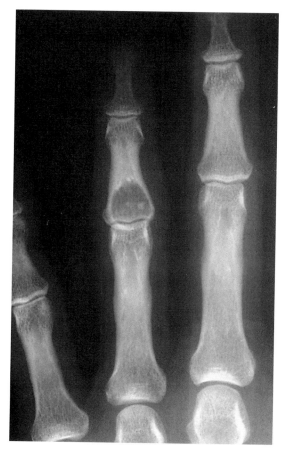

Figure 6.1 Enchondroma. Note the well-demarcated lytic lesion in the proximal end of the middle phalanx, which contains calcification of the chondroid matrix.

Evaluation by conventional radiographs is limited when overlying structures obscure the area of interest or when internal structures cannot be visualized. A refinement of conventional radiography, conventional tomography, either linear or pluridirectional, allows visualization of structures otherwise obscured by overlying anatomy. The extent of spinal trauma and degree of consolidation following fusion are better evaluated by tomography than

by any other modality, including reformatted CT (Fig. 6.2). Conventional tomography is also helpful in the evaluation of complex joint problems, such as fractures of the ankle or tibial plateau, although CT may provide comparable information (Fig. 6.3). As compared with conventional radiographs, tomography requires specialized equipment, is more time-consuming and costly, and exposes the patient to more radiation.

Arthrography allows radiographic visualization of structures within a joint following injection of radiopaque contrast material and/or radiolucent gas, usually air. Arthrography of the knee, which demonstrates the internal architecture of the joint, has been largely replaced by arthroscopy and MRI; but arthrography of other joints, including the shoulder, wrist, elbow, and hip, remains useful, especially in pediatric patients with unossified or partially ossified epiphyses (Fig. 6.4). The wrist in particular is more easily evaluated by arthrography than by MRI. The risks of arthrography include adverse reactions to contrast media and infection, but these complications are rare.

Computed Tomography

With its introduction in 1973, CT revolutionized imaging practices. Although neuroimaging profited most from early advances with CT, other areas of medicine, including orthopaedics, have since embraced its use. Restricted initially to scanning in the axial plane, CT scanners now offer imaging in other planes, limited only by the gantry size, the size of the body part to be studied, and the patient's flexibility. Direct coronal and sagittal scans of limbs, the head, and portions of the pelvis are possible.

The design of scanners for CT has evolved

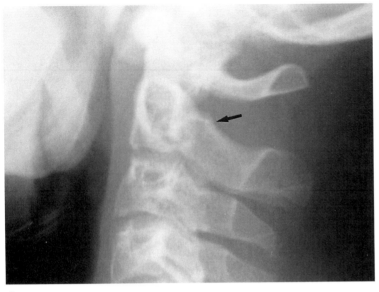

A

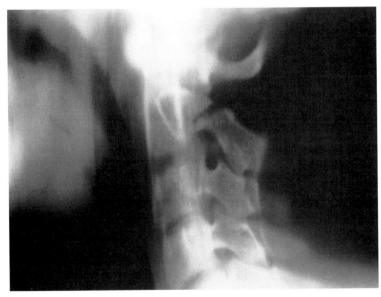

B

Figure 6.2 *A.* A lateral view of the cervical spine demonstrates a possible fracture of the posterior arch of the C2 vertebral body *(arrow). B.* Lateral tomogram clearly shows the fracture of the C2 pedicle.

through several generations, resulting in a reduction in scan times from 3 to 5 min to less than 1 s with current scanners. Regardless of the generation, CT uses an x-ray tube as its radiation source. The tube moves in the gantry around the patient, and x-ray photons passing through the patient are detected by an array of detectors opposite the tube. The information

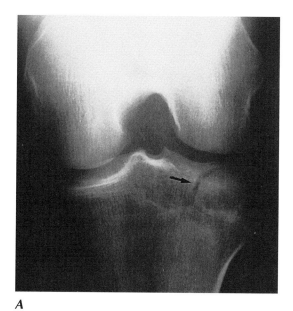

A

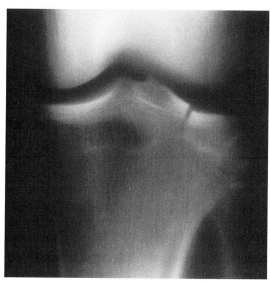

B

Figure 6.3   *A.* An intercondylar notch view of the knee shows a fracture of the lateral tibial plateau *(arrow). B.* An anteroposterior tomogram of the knee demonstrates the fracture and shows slight depression of the articular surface of the tibia, which is not detectable on the conventional film.

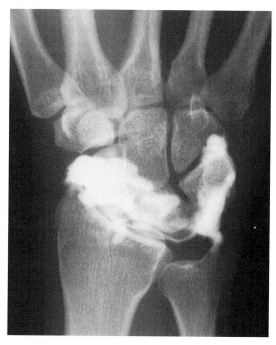

Figure 6.4   A frontal view of the wrist following injection of contrast shows contrast confined to the radiocarpal joint, indicating intact proximal row intercarpal ligaments and an intact triangular fibrocartilage complex.

from the detectors is mathematically processed to produce the CT image.

Computed tomography differs from conventional radiography in several additional ways. The primary advantage afforded by CT is its capacity to display cross-sectional anatomy. Another improvement provided by CT is in contrast resolution; its ability to discriminate small differences in tissue densities is much greater than that of conventional radiography. Its spatial resolution, however, is less than that achieved with plain film. With purchasing costs ranging from hundreds of thousands to more than $1.5 million, CT machines are much more expensive than conventional radiographic units, and radiation exposure is considerably higher from CT than from conventional radiography. Finally, CT images are susceptible to marked degradation when very dense structures, such as contrast medium, implants, and fixation devices, are included in the scan. In such patients, plain films obtained before CT can define scan planes to avoid metallic structures and minimize image degradation.

Because of its display of cross-sectional anatomy, CT is excellent for defining complex articular injuries, detecting subtle fractures, and evaluating spinal column injuries. In the wrist, for example, CT, with proper positioning, can be used to evaluate fractures of carpal bones that may be difficult to interpret on plain films. CT can be used to study an immobilized limb without underlying skeletal structures being obscured by the cast or splint (Fig. 6.5).

In the evaluation of spinal disorders, CT is useful for detection of herniated disks, including laterally directed protrusions, without administration of intrathecal contrast material (Fig. 6.6). Computed tomography is less helpful in the study of the postoperative spine because of image degradation by implants. In the postoperative patient with recurrent low back pain, CT following administration of intrathecal or intravenous contrast is used to distinguish scarring from residual disk material.

Both CT and MRI are used to evaluate musculoskeletal neoplasms. Although MRI is often performed in such cases, CT depicts subtle areas of cortical bone destruction and tumor calcification better than MRI. Computed tomography also characterizes soft tissue masses more accurately than plain films, but, as noted above, cannot equal conventional radiographic

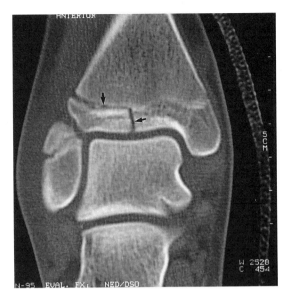

Figure 6.5 A coronal computed tomogram of the distal tibia reveals a fracture of the distal tibial epiphysis and widening of the lateral aspect of the distal tibial physis *(arrows)*. Although the limb is immobilized in a cast, the cast material does not preclude CT scanning.

analysis in the assessment of primary osseous lesions (Fig. 6.7).

Refinements of CT have led to improved image display and to imaging in planes that cannot be scanned directly. Three-dimensional (3D) reformatting of CT slices is helpful in assessing articular trauma and spinal disorders and in designing customized endoprostheses (Fig. 6.8). Planar reformatting allows display in any plane, even along a curved surface, but image resolution is usually less than can be obtained by direct scanning in the plane of interest. Congenital and developmental abnormalities, including developmental dysplasia of the hips, femoral anteversion, tibial tor-

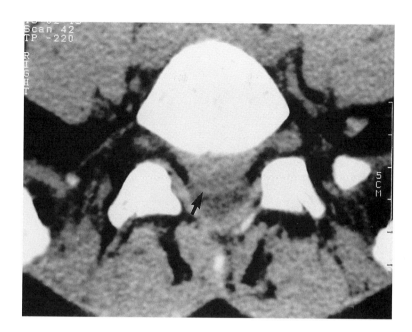

Figure 6.6   A transverse computed tomogram of the L5-S1 intervertebral disk. Note central herniation of the disk *(arrow)*.

sion, and hindfoot coalitions, are easily studied with CT.

Magnetic Resonance Imaging

Nuclear magnetic resonance (NMR) was a commonly used tool in chemistry long before Lauterbur described image formation with the technique in 1973. Since that time, NMR imaging, now termed MRI, has developed into a standard imaging tool. As was the case with CT, MRI was first applied to the central nervous system but now is used to study all parts of the body.

The physical basis of MRI is complex. In brief, the body part to be studied is placed into a uniform high-strength magnetic field, called B_0, causing the body's protons to align along the direction of this magnetic field. A second magnetic field, the gradient field, is applied perpendicularly to B_0. The gradient field varies linearly along its axis and helps provide anatomic localization. A radiofrequency (RF) coil is aligned perpendicularly to B_0 and to the gradient field. When a current pulse at a particular frequency is applied to the RF coil, the coil emits a magnetic field, known as B_1, the RF magnetic field. This emitted field causes the protons to absorb energy and to tip away from the axis of B_0; the degree to which the protons flip off axis depends on the amplitude of the RF pulse and on the length of time the RF coil is energized. As the protons flip away from B_0, they come partially into the axis of B_1. After the RF coil current is turned off, the protons return to alignment with B_0, releasing their absorbed energy. This released energy is detected and forms the basis for the MRI image.

The MRI signal of a particular tissue is determined by the strength of the magnet, the RF coil frequency, the local proton density, T1, and T2. T1 and T2 are intrinsic tissue charac-

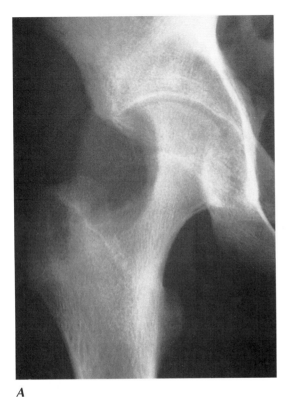

A

Figure 6.7   *A.* The conventional film demonstrates a focal destructive lesion in the femoral neck, containing faint calcifications.
B. A transverse computed tomogram through the femoral neck shows a well-demarcated lytic lesion as well as an effusion in the hip joint *(open arrow)* and fluid levels within the lytic lesion *(arrow),* typical for an aneurysmal bone cyst.

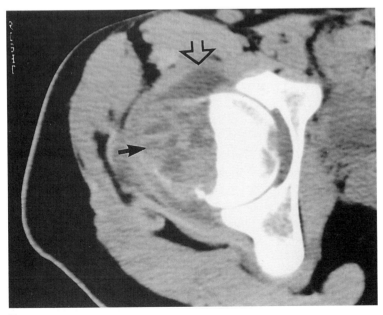

B

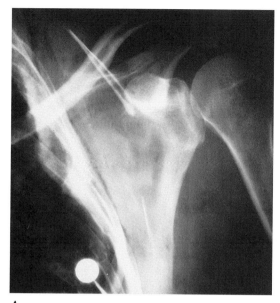

A

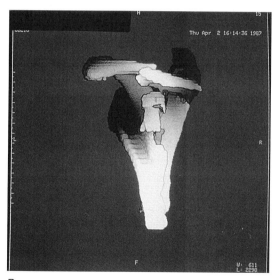

B

Figure 6.8 *A.* A standard anteroposterior radiograph of the shoulder demonstrates a comminuted fracture of the scapula. *B.* A three-dimensional reconstruction of a CT scan of the shoulder shows the scapular fracture, with overriding of the fracture fragments.

teristics and indicate the time required for the protons to release their absorbed energy. By manipulating the MRI scanning parameters, primarily the duration and timing of the RF pulses, differences in T1, T2, and the proton density are detected and comprise the MR image. In standard spin echo MR sequences, scan parameters may be selected to emphasize differences in T1, T2, or proton density, hence the terms T1-weighted and T2-weighted images. Although their appearances vary depending on scan parameters, with standard spin echo sequences bone is dark (no signal) on both T1- and T2-weighted images, fat is relatively bright on standard sequences, and fluid is bright on T2-weighted images and dark on T1-weighted images. Muscle is gray on T1- and T2-weighted images, and cartilage is fairly dark on T1- and T2-weighted sequences. Many other scanning strategies are available; some will display cartilage as a bright structure. Others can suppress the signal from the fat, rendering it dark on the resulting images.

Aside from being complex, MRI scanners are costly to purchase, install, and maintain. Tissue contrast with MRI is higher than that of CT, although MRI scanning is more time-consuming than CT. Unlike CT, MRI can scan in any desired plane, but like CT, plain film correlation is vital for the interpretation of MRI. Magnetic resonance imaging is safe and has no known lasting biological hazard. Complications from MRI are infrequent; they include claustrophobic reactions to the physical confines of the scanner and very rare reactions to gadolinium, the contrast agent used in MRI scanning. Patients with pacemakers, certain aneurysm clips, and prosthetic cardiac valves cannot undergo MRI scanning safely. Orthopaedic fixation devices do not preclude MRI scanning, but they may produce marked local degradation of the image.

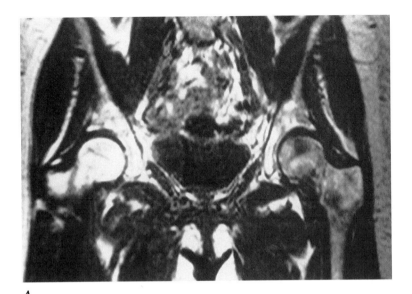

A

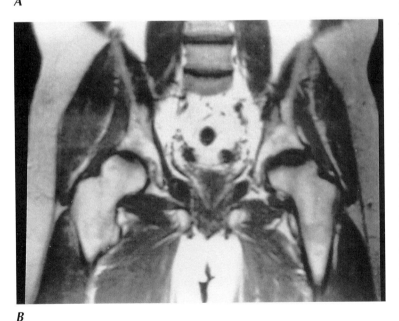

B

Figure 6.9 *A.* A T1-weighted MRI scan (TR 300 ms/TE 20 ms) of the proximal femora shows mottled replacement of the normal fat signal throughout the femoral head and proximal metaphysis of the left femur, typical for transient osteoporosis. *B.* A T1-weighted MRI scan (TR 500 ms/TE 25 ms) of the hips in another patient shows loss of the bright fat signal confined to the superior aspect of the femoral heads bilaterally, typical for avascular necrosis of the femoral heads.

Although bone itself is dark on all currently available MRI sequences, fat-containing bone marrow is easily seen. Processes replacing normal marrow, such as neoplasms, osteonecrosis, and infection, are well demonstrated by MRI. Magnetic resonance imaging can differentiate among causes of an abnormal marrow signal, e.g., between osteonecrosis and transient osteoporosis of the hip, both of which may be associated with pain and minimal findings on standard radiographs (Fig. 6.9).

For the evaluation and staging of musculoskeletal tumors, MRI is excellent and has largely replaced CT. As most tumors are associated with adjacent fluid, they usually appear as bright structures on T2-weighted images. The extent of a lesion within the marrow cavity, soft tissue invasion, skip lesions within bone, and involvement of adjacent neurovascular structures are readily assessed by MRI (Fig. 6.10). The advantage of MRI in this setting is in staging the tumor, but plain films offer more important clues about the histology of a musculoskeletal tumor and must not be

omitted. The use of gadolinium in MRI evaluation of neoplasms is controversial, but it may be helpful in guiding biopsies.

In the spine, MRI demonstrates disk pathology very accurately and reveals intracanalicular and intraosseous pathology better than CT (Fig. 6.11).

In many cases MRI has replaced arthrography for articular imaging, particularly in the knee (Fig. 6.12). Some investigators report excellent results in imaging the shoulder, although imaging of the wrist, ankle, and elbow is less well developed. Regardless of the joint, appropriate surface coils must be available if MRI is to be effective.

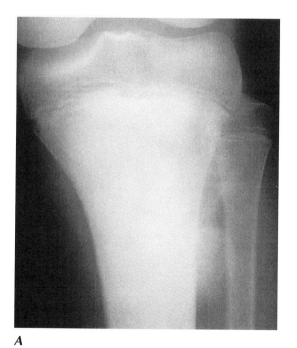
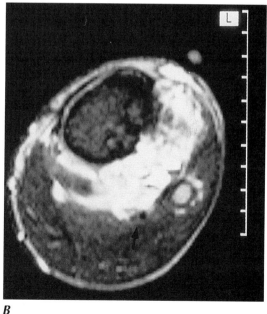

A   *B*

Figure 6.10   *A.* A sclerotic lesion in the proximal tibial metaphysis contains dense osteoid matrix calcification, typical for an intramedullary osteosarcoma. *B.* A T2-weighted axial MR scan (TR 3000 ms/TE 80 ms) shows intraosseous and extraosseous tumor and displacement of the neurovascular bundle *(arrow).*

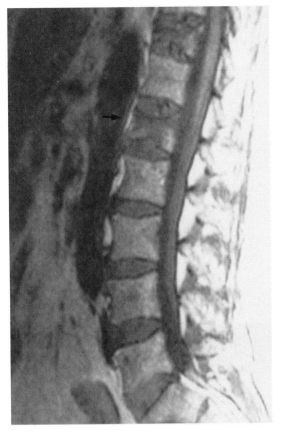

Figure 6.11 A T1-weighted sagittal MRI scan (TR 419 ms/TE 17 ms) reveals a diffusely decreased marrow signal and a compression fracture of L1 *(arrow)* in a patient with multiple myeloma.

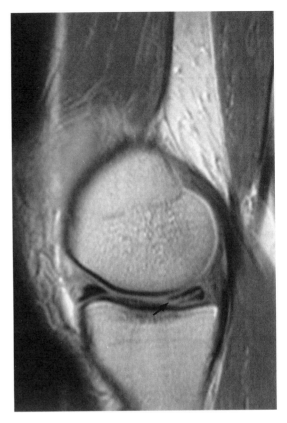

Figure 6.12 A sagittal MRI scan of the knee (TR 1939 ms/TE 29 ms) demonstrates a horizontal tear *(arrow)* in the posterior horn of the medial meniscus. The tear communicates with the articular surface of the meniscus.

Nuclear Medicine

Nuclear medicine (NM) continues to have an important role in musculoskeletal imaging, although its importance has been diminished by the advent of MRI. Bone scanning with strontium 85 was reported in 1961, but technetium 99m (^{99m}Tc) is most often used today. This isotope has a short half-life and a single gamma emission at 140 keV, making it ideally suited for imaging with available gamma cameras. Technetium 99m can be easily bound to a number of organ-specific compounds; ^{99m}Tc phosphates and ^{99m}Tc phosphonates are most frequently used for bone scanning. Gallium 67 citrate and white blood cells labeled with indium 111 are useful adjuncts to ^{99m}Tc phosphonates when scanning is performed to evaluate the possibility of bone infection. Bone scanning agents are safe; ^{99m}Tc-containing compounds in particular deliver very low radiation doses, and adverse reactions to the phosphonates are extremely rare.

Bone scanning with ^{99m}Tc phosphonates is often used to exclude osseous neoplastic and metastatic disease. These areas are generally characterized as regions of increased bone turnover. More of the radiopharmaceutical agent accumulates in neoplastic deposits than in normal bone (assuming an intact blood supply to the bone in question), which appear as areas of increased activity, or "hot spots" (Fig. 6.13). Bone scanning in this arena is very sensitive and can detect metastatic deposits before they become apparent on plain films. Bone scanning is, however, nonspecific. Any area of increased bone turnover will produce a hot spot, and differentiation of metastatic disease from other causes of accentuated bone turnover often requires correlation with another imaging modality, especially plain films.

Bone scanning is also useful in the diagnosis of occult trauma and stress fractures. Stress fractures in particular may be difficult to appreciate initially on plain films but are usually quite obvious on bone scans (Fig. 6.14).

Nuclear medicine studies are frequently used to evaluate bone infection. Osteomyelitis is notoriously difficult to detect on conventional radiographs, particularly early in the disease. Three- or four-phase ^{99m}Tc phosphonate bone scans may be useful in the diagnosis of osteomyelitis, even with normal plain films. Gallium 67 and indium 111–labeled leukocyte scanning are useful adjuncts, but in most cases they are less specific than three- or four-phase ^{99m}Tc phosphonate scanning.

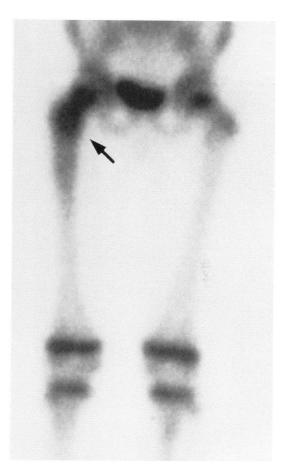

Figure 6.13   A bone scan with increased uptake in the right proximal femur *(arrow)* indicating metastatic disease in this patient with a neuroblastoma. Note the normal, symmetrical uptake in the physes.

Ultrasound

Although most discussions concerning ultrasound (US) focus on its abdominal and obstetric applications, US can be helpful in evaluating musculoskeletal disease. State-of-the-art musculoskeletal US uses real-time, linear array, high-frequency (7.5 to 10 MHz)

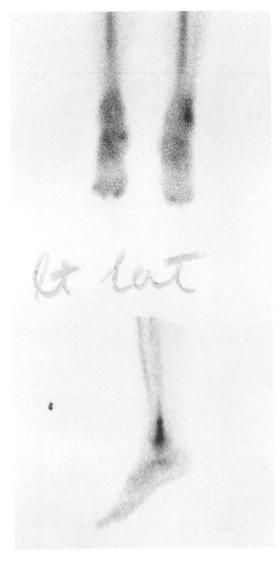

Figure 6.14 Stress fracture. Note the characteristic accumulation of the tracer in the distal fibula. This fracture was later visible on conventional films.

transducers and is well suited for the evaluation of superficial structures. Like MRI, it is associated with no known biological hazards, but it is much less expensive than MRI or CT.

Ultrasound is very operator-dependent; the ultrasonographer must be well trained in anatomy, pathology, and ultrasound if optimal use of this modality is to be achieved.

Generation of an US image depends upon the reflection of sound waves. As the high-frequency sound waves leave the transducer and enter the body, they are reflected at tissue interfaces. Whenever the acoustic impedance (sound transmissibility) of adjacent tissues differs, sound is reflected from their interfaces, and an ultrasound echo results. The collection of these echoes makes up the ultrasonic image. A structure that is free of tissue interfaces (a fluid-filled cyst, for example) generates no echoes and is shown as a homogeneous structure. Such structures also enhance sound wave transmission to deeper structures; posterior acoustic enhancement is a common feature associated with the ultrasonic appearance of fluid-filled structures. Because sound waves cannot penetrate air or bone, air-filled and bony structures cannot be evaluated with US.

Ultrasound is well suited to the identification of fluid-filled structures. Popliteal cysts can be seen with US and can be differentiated from other masses in the popliteal fossa, including tumors and abnormalities of the popliteal artery (Fig. 6.15). Ruptured popliteal cysts, however, may not be detectable with US. Other fluid collections such as abscesses, seromas, and lymphoceles are easily evaluated with US.

Tendon abnormalities have also been studied with US. Patellar tendon lesions such as jumper's knee and patellar tendinitis can be seen, and the Achilles tendon is well suited to ultrasonic evaluation (Fig. 6.16). Pediatric hip disorders, particularly developmental dysplasia, and adult shoulder lesions, such as rotator cuff tears, can be analyzed with US. Again,

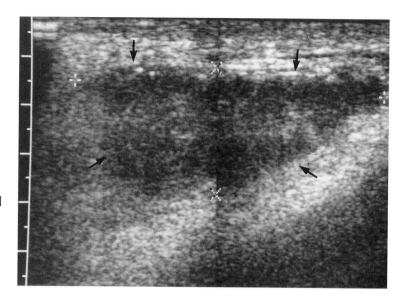

Figure 6.15 A longitudinal ultrasound scan of the popliteal fossa demonstrates a hypoechoic, fluid-filled mass *(arrows)*, indicating a popliteal cyst.

however, imaging is limited by the proficiency of the operator.

Summary

Studying the patient with musculoskeletal disease requires a carefully planned approach to imaging. Most conditions can be defined by conventional radiography, which is also needed if further imaging is required. Computed tomography, MRI, NM, and US may contribute diagnostic information, but their use should be tailored to the clinical question.

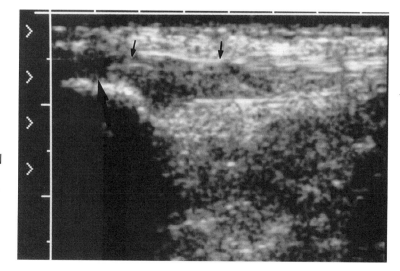

Figure 6.16 A longitudinal ultrasound scan of the knee shows rupture of the patellar tendon *(arrows)*, with accumulation of fluid at the torn margin of the tendon *(large arrow)*.

JOINT ASPIRATION

Joint aspiration, or *arthrocentesis*, is often useful for the diagnosis and/or treatment of joint disorders, especially when pyogenic or crystalline arthritides are suspected.

Technique

After explaining the procedure to the patient, checking for hypersensitivity to local anesthetics, and obtaining written consent for the procedure, the patient is arranged comfortably on the examining table, usually in the recumbent position. Observing sterile techniques, 3 to 5 mL of 2% lidocaine is used for local anesthesia. The fluid removed is sent for cytology, culture, a mucin test, crystal search, protein determinations, and other desired tests. If a glucose determination is necessary, part of the fluid must be put into a tube containing sodium fluoride and potassium oxalate and

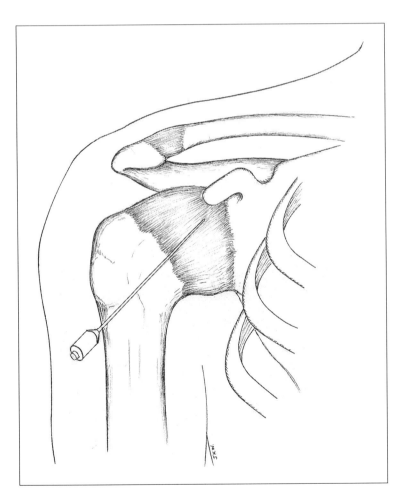

Figure 6.17 Aspiration/ injection of the glenohumeral joint. The needle is inserted approximately 1 cm lateral to the tip of the coracoid process, which is palpable as a slightly tender bony prominence 1 to 2 cm below the outer clavicle.

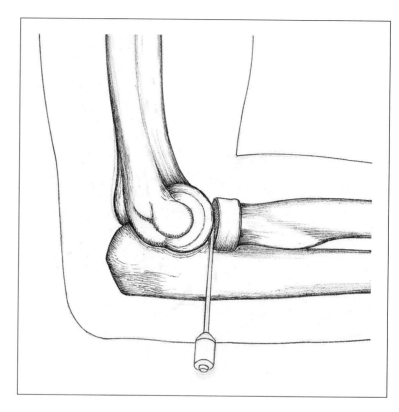

Figure 6.18 Aspiration/ injection of the elbow joint. The interval between the head of the radius and the capitellum is determined by palpating the radial head as the forearm is pronated and supinated. Since the adjacent capitellum is stationary, the interval is easily defined.

blood drawn for a simultaneous serum glucose level. If the glucose level in the joint fluid is more than 50 mg/dL below the serum level, bacterial infection is suggested. Although aspiration of the hip may require fluoroscopic control, all peripheral joints can usually be reached by the experienced clinician (Figs. 6.17 through 6.21).

If the initial fluid aspirated contains blood, a *hemarthrosis* is present; if the fluid is initially yellow but then becomes bloody, bleeding has been produced by the tap. Most hemarthroses result from trauma, which may be so slight as to be unremembered by patients on anticoagulants or with bleeding disorders. The white cell count and search for crystals are particularly important tests that are better performed by an experienced rheumatologist than hospital laboratory personnel. After examining the slide for crystals under a polarizing microscope, smears should be made for a Gram stain and a Wright stain for the differential leukocyte count. Normal synovial fluid is sufficiently clear to read print through it, and, since clotting factors are absent, it does not clot. Because of its hyaluronate content, the fluid is extremely viscous; when a drop is placed between two gloved fingers, they may be separated by 5–7 cm before the string of fluid breaks. The viscosity of synovial fluid is reduced in most infections.

Because the results of culture are often delayed, the leukocyte and differential counts in synovial fluid are particularly important in the

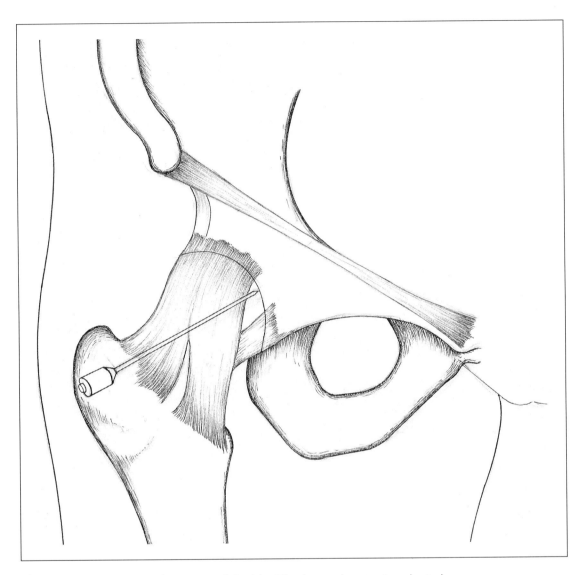

Figure 6.19   Aspiration/injection of the hip. The femoral artery is palpated
as it crosses the inguinal ligament; the needle is then introduced 2.5 cm
lateral and 2.5 cm distal to this point and advanced proximally and
medially along the femoral neck into the joint.

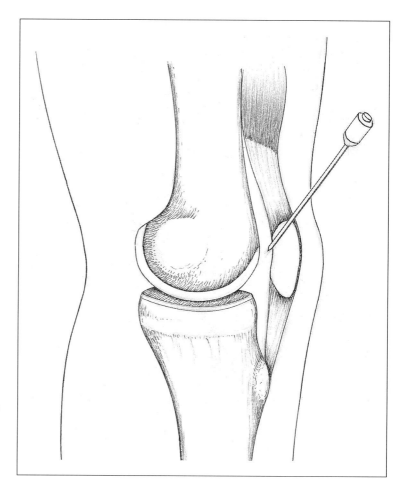

Figure 6.20 Aspiration/ injection of the knee. Viewing the patella as the face of a clock, the needle is inserted just behind the patella at either 10 or 2 o'clock (i.e., laterally or medially).

diagnosis of inflammatory joint conditions. Gram stains, even when carefully performed, are subject to artifactual interpretive errors that may lead to false-positive or false-negative results.

Although they have great diagnostic specificity when found, both gout, with monosodium urate (MSU) crystals, and crystal deposition disease, with calcium pyrophosphate dihydrate (CPPD) crystals, are relatively uncommon.

Synovial fluid may be classified by its leukocyte count into noninflammatory fluids [white blood cells (WBC) less than 2500/mm^3], inflammatory fluids (WBC 2500 to 25,000/mm^3), and infectious fluids (WBC over 50,000/mm^3). As the total count rises, so does the number of neutrophils, while the mucin test degenerates. Normal synovial fluid contains only 60 to 70 cells per mm^3, with few neutrophils. Since there is considerable overlap in leukocyte count between in-

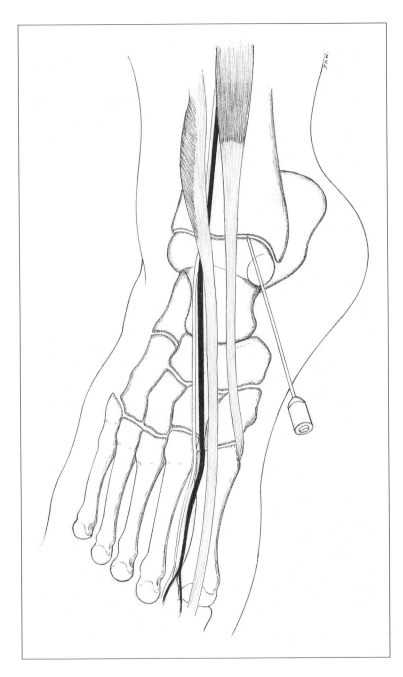

Figure 6.21 Aspiration/ injection of the ankle. The location of the joint is determined by palpation as the patient dorsiflexes and plantarflexes the ankle. To avoid neurovascular or tendinous structures, the needle is introduced at either the medial (shown here) or lateral corner of the joint.

fected and uninfected fluids, a positive culture is required to confirm the diagnosis of infection.

Glucocorticoid Injections

Indications for intraarticular glucocorticoid injections include rheumatoid arthritis, crystalline arthritis, osteoarthritis, and, occasionally, acute traumatic "arthritis." Injection of a glucocorticoid into a septic or unstable joint is contraindicated, since it may increase the morbidity of these conditions. The other contraindications are overlying cellulitis and a bleeding diathesis, such as hemophilia. The former objection can often be circumvented by locating an aspiration site not overlain by cellulitis and the latter by factor replacement before the joint is aspirated. Failure to respond to previous injections of glucocorticoids is a relative contraindication, since multiple injections may increase cartilage breakdown ("steroid arthropathy") and potentiate infection. The length of symptomatic improvement following corticosteroid injection is related to the preparation used: hydrocortisone acetate usually lasts only a few days to a week, whereas triamcinolone hexacetonide relieves inflammatory symptoms for longer periods of time. The joint injected may also bear on the results obtained; for example, improvement is usually more dramatic and long-lasting following injection of the first carpometacarpal joint of the thumb than that after injection of the hip. The amount of glucocorticoid injected ranges from 1 to 2 mL for large joints down to 0.1 to 0.5 mL for small joints. Mixing the corticosteroid with a local anesthetic is helpful in preventing an early postinjection "inflammatory flare."

ARTHROSCOPY

Since the application of cystoscopic principles to the knee joint by Takagi in 1918, continuing improvements in technique and instrumentation have enabled surgeons to expand the role of arthroscopy both for diagnosis and therapy of joint disorders. Reduction of the risks from anesthesia and infection, along with more rapid and comfortable rehabilitation, have all but eliminated the need for wide exposure to treat meniscal tears and disruptions of the anterior cruciate ligament. As with all technical advances, however, the potential for overuse is great, since the existence of a particular technology may become an indication for its use. Indeed, the allure of increased diagnostic accuracy and immediate therapeutic intervention has too often led practitioners to bypass the careful history taking and examination by which other procedures may frequently be avoided; however, a clinician who has the ability to use arthroscopy as an adjunct to clinical findings and judgment will be a more effective practitioner than one who does not have this technique available.

Imaging techniques such as MRI have also become highly reliable in the diagnosis of intraarticular pathology, but diagnosis must often be followed by arthroscopic treatment; thus, clinical findings that strongly suggest a mechanical disorder should usually be followed by arthroscopy rather than MRI, so that the diagnosis may be confirmed and treatment implemented in the most cost-effective manner.

Arthroscopy is indicated as a diagnostic tool (1) when clinical and radiographic studies have not led to a clear diagnosis and (2) prior to operative treatment to detect additional, unanticipated pathology that may be present.

The major contraindication to arthroscopy is infection in the skin or subcutaneous tissues overlying anticipated portals of entry. Abrasions, pustules, and rashes should be allowed to heal before arthroscopy is undertaken.

Because of the reduction in size of the arthroscope from Takagi's 7.3-mm instrument to scopes less than 2 mm in diameter, it has become possible to examine small as well as large joints, although most arthroscopies today are done with rigid telescopes that are about the size of an ordinary pencil. The arthroscope is attached to a small television camera that permits viewing on an operating room monitor, and a videotape record of the operation is preserved for physician and patient instruction and follow-up evaluations.

Operations that are now being performed endoscopically include suturing of torn menisci, reconstruction of torn anterior cruciate ligaments, stabilization of unstable shoulders, acromioplasty, debridement, biopsy, synovectomy, and reduction of intraarticular fractures.

Since more of the knee joint can be visualized arthroscopically than through a standard arthrotomy, arthroscopy is particularly valuable for this joint. The synovium, suprapatellar pouch, patellofemoral joint, femoral and tibial condyles, menisci, and anterior cruciate ligament can be inspected through the arthroscope once orientation techniques and the distortion of normal structures by magnification are understood. Redundant synovial folds, scarring from previous surgeries, joint debris, and enlargement of the fat pad may limit visualization; even under optimal conditions, there are "blind spots" in the joint. For these reasons, it is important that arthroscopy be carried out by an experienced surgeon. At least fifty supervised examinations are needed for an operator to acquire the skills necessary to visualize, interpret, and correct intraarticular lesions.

While arthroscopy can be performed as either an outpatient or inpatient procedure and under local or general anesthesia, a majority of arthroscopies are now performed as outpatient procedures. The choice of anesthesia depends upon such patient-related factors as age and temperament and upon the skill and experience of the surgeon. Children and anxious patients are often better served by general anesthesia. Shoulder arthroscopy usually requires general anesthesia because of the difficulty in achieving adequate analgesia with regional or local blocks. Additional advantages of general anesthesia include muscular relaxation and the ability to stress joints more fully for better viewing.

Undoubtedly, further developments in instrumentation and procedural technology will expand the horizons of arthroscopy. Better optics, lighting, and instruments and perhaps other forms of energy will play major roles in improving the management of intraarticular disease.

SUGGESTED READINGS

Imaging

CURRY TS, DOWDEY JE, MURRY RC: *Christensen's Physics of Diagnostic Radiology,* 4th ed. Philadelphia, Lea & Febiger, 1990.

BERQUIST TH: Magnetic resonance imaging of primary skeletal neoplasms. *Radiol Clin North Am* 31:411, 1993.

RUBIN SJ, FELDMAN F, DICK HM, ET AL: Heterogeneous *in vivo* MR images of soft tissue tumors: Guide to gross specimen sampling. *Magn Res Imaging* 10:351, 1992.

THRALL JH: Technetium-99m labeled agents for skeletal imaging. *CRC Crit Rev Clin Radiol Nucl Med* 8:1, 1976.

RESNICK D: *Diagnosis of Bone and Joint Disorders,* 3d ed. Philadelphia, Saunders, 1995.

HUDSON TM: *Radiologic-Pathologic Correlation of Musculoskeletal Lesions.* Baltimore, Williams & Wilkins, 1987.

Joint Aspiration

KRAY PR, BRANDT KD: *An Analysis of Synovial Fluid.* Summit, NJ, Ciba-Geigy Corporation, 1992.

Arthroscopy

O CONNOR RL (ED): *Arthroscopy.* Kalamazoo, MI, The Upjohn Company, 1977.

Chapter 7

Principles and Techniques of Rehabilitation

Walter B. Greene

Rehabilitation is the key to maximal recovery following injury. It should be recognized as an integral part of therapy and planned from the outset rather than as a separate and distinct process after "definitive" care is rendered. The goal is a return to optimal function as quickly as possible, which, because of the time required for the healing of musculoskeletal injuries, often demands more time and skill than other parts of the treatment algorithm. For most injuries, however, rehabilitation does not require complicated equipment, extensive therapy sessions, or detailed knowledge of physiatry or physiotherapy. For these patients, a physician who understands the basic principles can usually prescribe and monitor an effective program. On the other hand, patients with such conditions as paraplegia, chronic arthritis, amputations, multisystem trauma, and intractable low back pain are often best rehabilitated through the coordinated efforts and expertise of various physicians and allied health specialists.

It is important to realize that regaining *maximal* function does not necessarily mean *full* restoration, which is impossible for some conditions or injuries. Successful rehabilitation means that the patient has been provided with the physical and psychological means to function independently when recovery is complete and therapy curtailed.

Although this chapter focuses on nonoperative methods of rehabilitation, surgical procedures are often an integral part of the rehabilitative process. Tendon transfers in the upper limb, for example, may greatly enhance the function and independence of a patient who is tetraplegic as the result of an injury to the cervical spine.

MEASURING AND RESTORING MOTION

Immobilization, whether by cast or self-imposed by the pain and swelling of injury, results in muscle weakness and joint stiffness. As a general principle, regaining a functional arc of motion should be accomplished prior to embarking on vigorous strengthening exercises.

Restricted motion after immobilization is caused by contracture of the involved ligaments, joint capsules, and musculotendinous units. Restoring movement requires stretching of these contracted soft tissues. Regaining motion is more difficult when (1) the injury was intraarticular, (2) immobilization was prolonged, (3) the joint was arthritic, or (4) a combination of these factors was present. Fortunately, most sprains, strains, and simple fractures do not involve these factors and the physician can personally outline a home rehabilitation program. The therapeutic modalities discussed later in this chapter are helpful adjuncts for more complicated injuries.

Exercises to regain joint motion can be classified as active, active-assisted, and passive. *Active exercises* are voluntary movements under the direct control of the patient and are, therefore, less likely to exceed an injury threshold. With more difficult rehabilitation problems or with reluctant patients, assistance is required to regain mobility. *Passive exercises* are performed by having a therapist, family member, or the patient himself move the joint. For example, passive stretching of a stiff wrist and fingers can easily be performed with the uninvolved hand. Passive exercises are also used to prevent contractures that follow paralytic disorders. Reinjury may result from passive exercises if the manipulation force exceeds the strength of healing tissues, but this complication is uncommon if the force of passive stretch is increased gradually.

Active assisted exercises combine voluntary muscle contraction with assistance or passive manipulation. Assistance may be provided throughout the arc of motion and passive stretch applied at the termination of movement. This type of exercise both strengthens muscles and stretches periarticular tissues. Therefore, active assisted exercises are particularly useful in the early phase of rehabilitation when there is limited motion and the muscles are too weak to move the joint through a full arc of motion.

Measuring joint motion provides a simple, objective assessment of progress in a rehabilitation program. Range of motion also is an important determinant of when an athlete may return to competition or when a factory worker can rejoin the assembly line, and disability ratings for disorders of the limbs and spine are based largely on impairment of joint motion.

Standardization of the starting, or zero, position is critical for effective communication among physicians and therapists. For most joints, the zero starting position is the extended "anatomic position" of the limb. To avoid confusion, this position is described as 0° rather than 180°. Although joint motion can be estimated visually, a goniometer enhances accuracy of measurement, is inexpensive, and is easily applied to the measurement of motion in the elbow, wrist, finger, knee, ankle, and great toe, where bony landmarks allow reproducible alignment of the goniometer (Fig. 7.1).

Motion in an affected limb should be compared with that in the normal limb, since joint

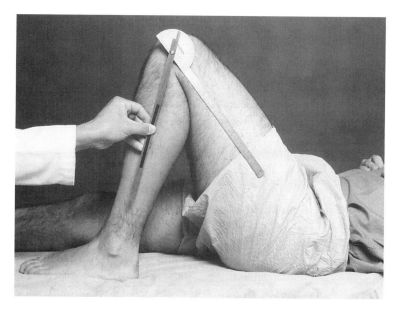

Figure 7.1 Goniometric measurement of joint motion allows more reproducible and precise assessment of joint mobility. The limbs of the goniometer should be in line with the shafts of the long bones, and the center of rotation of the goiniometer should coincide with that of the joint.

mobility in healthy subjects is equivalent on both sides.

MEASURING AND RESTORING STRENGTH

The primary function of skeletal muscle is to generate movement. At a microscopic level, this function is characterized by tensioning of the myofibril as myosin filaments slide over actin filaments and cross links couple these filaments. Tension in a muscle may develop by concentric, isometric, or eccentric means. During *concentric contraction,* a muscle shortens. Muscle function is typically described in the concentric mode, such as extension of the knee by the quadriceps muscle. However, in daily activities, *isometric contraction,* with no change in external length, and *eccentric contraction,* in which muscle tension is maintained as the muscle lengthens, are frequent. Eccentric contractions are important for controlled movement of joints and for absorbing the impact of weight-bearing or other loading activities. Muscles can sustain greater tension during eccentric contraction and therefore are more vulnerable to rupture when performing work in this mode.

Manual testing of muscles is often important and can be easily performed without special equipment, but its limitations should be understood. Strength is commonly graded on a 0-to-5 scale (Table 5.1), but two facts should be remembered. First, the full range of motion is the *passive* arc of motion. Second, to achieve fair or grade 3 strength, the muscle must be able to move the joint through that range of motion against gravity. For example, if a pa-

tient has a 20° knee flexion contracture but active extension against gravity is only 30°, quadriceps strength is, by definition, less than grade 3.

When testing a muscle, other muscles that can produce the same movement should be eliminated. For example, when the tibialis anterior is being tested, the patient should be instructed to keep the toes flexed. This maneuver inhibits activity of the extensor hallucis longus and extensor digitorum longus muscles, which also dorsiflex the ankle. In addition, the patient should be instructed to pull the foot into dorsiflexion and inversion. This maneuver inhibits firing of the peroneus tertius.

Manual muscle-testing is subjective, and its accuracy depends on the experience of the observer, the ability and willingness of the patient to cooperate, and the availability of an uninjured side for comparison. Furthermore, the manual classification system does not correlate in a linear fashion with actual strength. In a study of children with poliomyelitis who were compared to a group of normal children, Beasley found that grade 4 strength was only 40 percent of that in the normal group; grade 3 was 15 percent, and grade 2 was 5 percent.

Instrumented muscle testing is a new technique, the clinical usefulness of which has not been ascertained. Certainly isokinetic dynamometers provide objective data on muscle torque and allow strength to be measured in either concentric or eccentric fashion. Isokinetic testing also provides a more objective analysis of a patient's progress during rehabilitation, but it is not clear that these data justify the added cost of testing.

Muscles are used for and therefore can be strengthened by isometric, isotonic, and isokinetic exercises. *Isometric exercise* involves contraction of the myofibrils without change in length of the musculotendinous unit. This type of exercise program is particularly useful in the early postoperative period, when joint motion is both painful and limited. For example, isometric strengthening or "quadriceps setting" exercises are the first strengthening exercises instituted after knee replacement.

With *isotonic exercises,* the load placed on the muscle does not change. An example is lifting standard bar bells. However, because the efficiency of a muscle is related to its length, the changing position of the joint and lever arms alters muscular resistance continuously during isotonic exercise.

With *isokinetic exercises,* the limbs move at a constant velocity, and resistance is accommodated to maintain maximal muscular tension throughout the full arc of motion. Isokinetic strengthening requires special equipment that incorporates a hydraulic system to maintain constant velocity against resistance. Since the muscle can contract maximally through its arc of motion, isokinetic exercises should be the most efficient method of conditioning, and many studies have shown that isokinetic strengthening programs do achieve greater strength more rapidly. Because the ultimate strength achieved by either isotonic or isokinetic exercises is similar, it is less clear whether the early difference observed with isokinetic strengthening is enough to offset the cost of the special equipment. As a general principle, eager and well-motivated patients should start with isometric and low-resistance, isotonic exercises, since aggressive use of isokinetic machines may aggravate articular pain and swelling during the early stages of rehabilitation.

THERAPEUTIC MODALITIES

Physical modalities such as heat, cold, water, and electrical therapies are age-old rehabilitation aids. Because these modalities frequently produce comforting sensations, their psychological effect may be difficult to separate from physiologic benefit. Certainly motion and strengthening exercises should be the primary foci of rehabilitation, but physical modalities may enhance the process by decreasing pain and permitting the exercise program to proceed more quickly. Obviously, these modalities are most useful in the early phases of rehabilitation.

Cryotherapy

Cryotherapy, the use of cold as a treatment modality, has traditionally been employed to reduce swelling during the acute phase of injury; however, in recent years, it has been utilized increasingly during the later phases of rehabilitation. Cooling does decrease pain, possibly by acting as a counterirritant (the "gate theory" of pain perception). Spasticity also may be decreased by the application of cold, thereby allowing a more vigorous rehabilitation program.

Techniques of cryotherapy include cold packs, cold compression units, ice massage, cold hydrotherapy, and evaporative, cooling sprays. Cold packs and cold compression units are most beneficial immediately after injury or surgery. Ice massage is most frequently used following exercise to minimize the effects of musculotendinous damage. Cold hydrotherapy, with water temperatures ranging from 13 to 18°C for 1 to 20 min, has been used to reduce spasticity before specific therapy for patients with upper motor neuron disorders, such as cerebral palsy and stroke. In using cryotherapy, care must be taken to prevent damage to the skin or underlying muscles. Rheumatologic conditions exacerbated by cold are contraindications to cryotherapy.

Heat

Therapeutic heat is analgesic, but its mechanism of action, like that for cold therapy, remains unclear. Possibilities include a direct effect on peripheral nerves or an indirect effect as a counterirritant at the level of the spinal cord. The application of local heat increases blood flow to subjacent tissues. This effect is obvious and dramatic in the skin and subcutaneous tissue; however, penetration of heat to deeper, muscular tissues is not only more difficult to obtain but less reliable, as control of blood flow to muscle is more dependent on local metabolic factors. Therapeutic heat may also lengthen collagen fibers in tendons and ligaments, which, if delivered before exercise, facilitates stretching of stiff joints.

Hydrocollator packs and paraffin baths deliver therapeutic heat by conduction. Hydrocollator packs are warmed to approximately 75°C and wrapped in towels to protect the skin from thermal injury. The packs are applied for approximately 15 to 20 min. Deeper tissues are not affected. Paraffin baths are utilized primarily to transfer heat to arthritic digits.

Convection transfers heat by circulating a heated substance over a body part. Convection therapy may be administered by means of moist-air cabinets, contrast baths, hydrotherapy, and fluidotherapy. Of these, *hydrotherapy* is the most frequently used modality and can

be carried out in Hubbard tanks, hot tubs, and whirlpool baths. Indeed, for rehabilitation of minor injuries at home, a warm bath is an excellent place to initiate range-of-motion exercises. In rehabilitation centers, hydrotherapy is most effective when the tank is large enough for the affected body part to be exercised while immersed in warm (39 to 45°C), agitated water. Large tanks allow ambulation, which reduces impact loading and permits endurance training.

Fluidotherapy heats and massages tissue by placing the injured part in circulating, heated air that contains suspended particulate matter (cellulose beads). Sensory stimulation from these beads provides additional sedative and analgesic effects. By alternating heat and cold therapy, contrast baths seek the therapeutic benefits of vasoconstriction and vasodilatation. This therapeutic modality is most often used for painful conditions characterized by marked swelling, such as Sudeck's atrophy.

Radiant energy therapy with infrared and visible-light lamps is rarely used in rehabilitative programs. These techniques heat only superficial tissues, and their energy output or heat dose at the tissue level is difficult to calculate. Diathermy heats deeper tissues preferentially by passing energy through overlying, resistive layers. If the subcutaneous fat layer is thin, microwave diathermy may elongate musculotendinous tissues and can be used to rehabilitate muscular contractures and chronic tenosynovitis. Short-wave diathermy offers the deepest penetration of fat and muscle and has its maximal effect when used in a parallel setup (electromagnetic transfer). Unfortunately, this modality does not provide warning signs of impending thermal injury and must therefore be used with caution.

Ultrasound

Ultrasound, another modality for applying deep heat, uses high-frequency sound waves to penetrate subcutaneous fat and reach deeper layers. Tissues high in collagen content, such as ligaments and tendons, preferentially absorb higher levels of ultrasonic energy. As temperature increases in these structures, the collagen elongates, allowing stretching of contracted tissues. In muscles, ultrasound also has an indirect effect by increasing blood flow. Blood flow may be adversely affected if the ultrasound damages vessels.

Since the energy of ultrasound attenuates rapidly in air, a gel is used between the machine and the skin. Continuous movement of the transducer is recommended to prevent uneven distribution. *Phonophoresis,* an ultrasonic modality that delivers topical medications, such as corticosteroids, to deeper structures, theoretically works by increasing the permeability of soft tissues. Although ultrasound is used for a great variety of conditions, documentation of its effectiveness is lacking. It is contraindicated for use in the groin or near the spinal cord following laminectomy. Other relative contraindications include diabetes, cardiac problems, thrombophlebitis, acute trauma (where bleeding may be exacerbated), and injuries near osseous growth plates in children.

ELECTRICAL MODALITIES

Electrical potentials are widespread in biological tissues and exist in all cells and organs. It is therefore not surprising that electrical therapy has been prescribed to enhance soft tissue healing and reduce pain. Whether electrical therapy has a significant influence on the healing of soft tissues is inconclusive, but electrical stimulation does seem to be a helpful adjunct in the control of chronic pain. Whether its effect is at the spinal cord or at a more central level is unknown.

The use of electrical stimulation for rehabilitation of muscles is probably not justified when voluntary contractions can be generated. However, when immobilization has been prolonged or when voluntary muscle contraction is profoundly inhibited, electrical stimulation is helpful during the initial phases of rehabilitation.

ORTHOTIC DEVICES

The indications for use of an *orthosis* include (1) protection or immobilization of an injured part, (2) improvement of function, (3) prevention of deformity, and (4) correction of deformity. The latter two indications find application primarily in pediatric orthopaedic conditions. For example, owing to muscular imbalance and growth, equinus contractures frequently develop in children with cerebral palsy. The risk or severity of this deformity is reduced by use of an ankle-foot orthosis. Correction of a deformity by an orthosis is illustrated by the use of an abduction splint to reduce and stabilize a neonatal dislocation of the hip (Fig. 8.35).

The most common indication for an orthosis is protection of an injured part. An orthosis typically does not provide as much stability for an injured limb as a circular cast, but it has the advantage of being removable, thereby allowing not only bathing of the affected area but

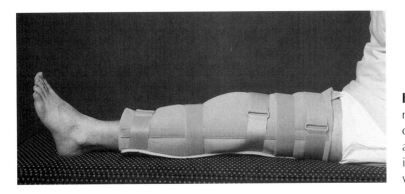

Figure 7.2 A sprain of the medial collateral ligament can be treated initially with a commercial knee immobilizer, which may be worn over clothes.

also, more importantly, early institution of motion. Obviously, the decision to use an orthosis must be individualized, but even immediately after injury, most strains and sprains can be effectively immobilized by an orthotic device (Fig. 7.2).

An orthosis may improve function in weak or paralyzed muscles; for example, a drop-foot gait caused by peroneal nerve dysfunction may be significantly improved by a below-knee brace made of lightweight, thermoplastic material, which decreases the weight of the orthosis and improves its appearance. A below-knee brace made of this material can be worn inside a conventional shoe almost unnoticeably (Fig. 7.3).

CANES, CRUTCHES, AND WALKERS

Canes, crutches, and walkers (in that order) increase balance and stability in the lower limbs. These devices also permit the upper limbs to reduce weight-bearing stresses on the lower limbs.

Crutches offer more support and potential to unload joints in the lower limb, but canes

are lighter, cause less wear and tear on clothes, are more easily stored, and are cosmetically appealing to patients. A cane can be particularly helpful in augmenting the balance and stability of the unsteady geriatric patient who is at increased risk for fracture of the hip. Especially when used in the contralateral hand, a cane significantly decreases stress on an arthritic hip. A "quad cane" has four prongs at its base. This device is more cumbersome than a single-tipped cane but confers a wider base of support and can be quite useful for a patient who, following a stroke, has only one functional upper limb.

Despite frequent use, many physicians do not know how to adjust the length of a cane. A cane that is too long causes excessive flexion of the elbow and increases the demand on the triceps muscle. A cane that is too short requires complete elbow extension, provides inadequate support during stance phase, and compromises stair climbing. For a person of average height, the optimal length of a cane will position the elbow in 20° of flexion when the tip of the cane is placed approximately 6 in. in front of and 6 in. lateral to the fifth toe (Fig. 7.4).

Crutches are intermediate between canes and walkers in support and convenience. For

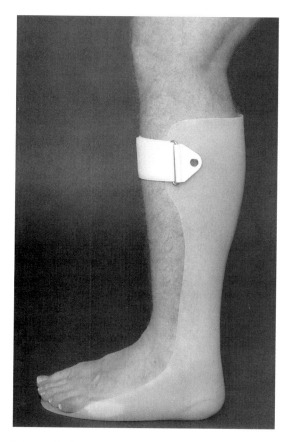

Figure 7.3   A thermoplastic drop-foot brace
is used to prevent equinus contractures,
which can occur with peroneal nerve palsy
or other neuromuscular disorders. The brace
should be in neutral dorsiflexion and may
be worn inside the shoe.

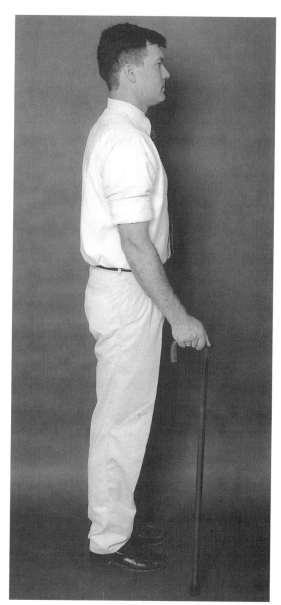

Figure 7.4   The proper length of a cane is
determined by placing the tip 6 in. forward
and 6 in. lateral to the foot. The elbow
should be flexed about 20°.

short-term use, axillary wooden crutches are
satisfactory and more economical. Aluminum
crutches are more durable but cost more and
are therefore prescribed for chronic conditions.
Forearm crutches, usually made of aluminum,
are less bulky and are used for patients with
chronic disorders, but they require better balance and upper limb strength. Platform
crutches allow forces to be transmitted through
the forearm and are useful when patients have

arthritic or traumatic conditions of the wrist and hand.

The length of an axillary crutch is determined with the patient standing. To prevent undue pressure on the axillary neurovascular structures, the top of the crutch should be two finger breadths below the axilla when the tip is positioned approximately 6 in. lateral to the base of the fifth toe. In that position, the hand grips should be adjusted to place the elbow in 20° of flexion.

The gait patterns used with crutches or walkers are listed in Table 7.1. Following injury to a lower limb, the technique most commonly prescribed is a non-weight-bearing, swing-through gait. Walking on level ground by this method is easy to teach, since it involves simply advancing both crutches, followed by the sound leg. Going up and down steps is more difficult, but the key is to advance the crutches first when going down stairs and the sound leg first when going up.

Table 7.1   Gait Patterns Used with Crutches or Walkers

Type	Characteristics
Swing-to	Advance both crutches. Lift the body to advance both feet on line with the crutches.
Swing-through	Advance both crutches. Lift the body to advance both feet beyond the crutches.
Non-weight-bearing, swing-through	Advance both crutches. Shift weight and advance the sound leg.
Four-point	Move one crutch forward, then advance the opposite foot, followed by the ipsilateral crutch, then the contralateral foot. (Three points of contact are always maintained.)
Alternating two-point	Advance one crutch and the contralateral foot at the same time. Shift weight and advance the other foot and crutch. (A progression of the four-point gait.)

A training session with a physical therapist is often helpful.

Through their four points of contact, walkers provide the greatest support . The bulkiness of a walker is its major disadvantage. Some walkers fold down, making storage on public transportation easier, but these models are more likely to break. Walkers with wheels on the front legs are not often used for adults but are commonly prescribed for children with cerebral palsy. The same principles apply for adjusting the length of a walker as for crutches, i.e., the hand grip should be at a height to allow a 20° flexion angle at the elbow when the walker is positioned approximately 6 in. in front of the foot.

Given the prevalence of musculoskeletal disorders in an aging population, it is likely that society's need for rehabilitation will increase. If carefully planned from the outset of treatment, with the essentiality of the patient's role in mind, rehabilitation will be a critical and cost-effective part of the return to maximal function.

SUGGESTED READINGS

ALMEKINDERS LC, OMAN J: Isokinetic muscle testing: Is it clinically useful? *J Am Acad Orthop Surg* 2:221–225, 1994.

BEASLEY WC: Quantitative muscle testing: Principles and applications to research and clinical services. *Arch Phy Med* 42:398–425, 1961.

BURGESS EM, ALEXANDER AG: Canes, crutches, and walkers, in American Academy of Orthopaedic Surgeons: *Atlas of Orthotics: Biomechanical Principles and Application.* St Louis, Mosby, 1975, pp 421–430.

CARY JM, LUSSKIN R, THOMPSON RG: Prescription principles, in American Academy of Orthopaedic Surgeons: *Atlas of Orthotics: Biomechanical Principles and Application.* St Louis, Mosby, 1975, pp 235–244.

WOJTYS EM, CARPENTER JE, KUHN JE: Therapeutic modalities in sports medicine, in Griffin LY (ed): *Orthopaedic Knowledge Update: Sports Medicine.* Rosemont, IL, American Academy of Orthopaedic Surgeons, 1994, pp 73–92.

Musculoskeletal Diseases and Disorders

Chapter *8*

Genetic and Congenital Disorders

Richard C. Henderson and Edmund R. Campion

GENERALIZED DISORDERS

Skeletal Dysplasias
Achondroplasia; Multiple Epiphyseal Dysplasia; Spondyloepiphyseal Dysplasia; Cleidocranial Dysplasia

Down Syndrome (Trisomy 21, or Mongolism)

Mucopolysaccharidoses
Hurler Syndrome; Hunter Syndrome; San Filippo Syndrome; Morquio Syndrome; Scheie Syndrome; Maroteaux-Lamy Syndrome

Arthrogryposis Multiplex Congenita

Neurofibromatosis

Acrocephalosyndactylism (Apert Syndrome)

Fetal Alcohol Syndrome

CONNECTIVE TISSUE DISORDERS

Ehlers-Danlos Syndrome

Marfan Syndrome

Osteogenesis Imperfecta

DISORDERS OF THE HEMATOPOIETIC SYSTEM

Hemophilia

Sickle Cell Disease

Gaucher Disease

REGIONAL DISORDERS

Spine
Os Odontoideum; Klippel-Feil Syndrome; Congenital Muscular Torticollis; Syringomyelia; Congenital Spinal Deformities; Idiopathic Scoliosis; Spondylolisthesis

Upper Limb
Sprengel Deformity; Congenital Pseudarthrosis of the Clavicle; Congenital Dislocation of the Radial Head; Congenital Radioulnar Synostosis; Madelung Deformity; Trigger Digits; Hypoplastic Thumb; Congenital Clasped Thumb; Camptodactyly; Clinodactyly; Polydactyly; Syndactyly; Congenital Constriction Bands

Lower Limb
Developmental Dysplasia of the Hip; Congenital Displacement of the Knee; Deficiencies of the Limbs; Congenital Pseudarthrosis of the Tibia; Clubfoot (Congenital Talipes Equinovarus); Congenital Vertical Talus (Congenital Convex Pes Valgus); Congenital Metatarsus Varus (Metatarsus Adductus); Calcaneovalgus Foot; Polydactyly; Syndactyly; Macrodactyly; Congenital Curly Toe; Congenital Overriding of the Fifth Toe (Digitus Minimus Varus)

Congenital and genetic disorders of the musculoskeletal system include a broad spectrum of abnormalities. Some are *localized* anatomic deformities that are apparent at birth, such as failure of a part to form normally or duplication of a part. Other focal abnormalities, such as dislocation of the radial head and radioulnar synostosis, are commonly overlooked, often for several years, because of more subtle manifestations. Still other congenital disorders, e.g., Madelung deformity and osteochondroma become evident only after abnormal growth.

Among congenital disorders that affect *multiple* bones, joints, or muscles, some again are apparent at birth, such as achondroplasia; others are present at birth but not recognized until later, such as some forms of osteogenesis imperfecta; and conditions like multiple epiphyseal dysplasia become apparent only with growth. Generalized disorders may also involve other bodily systems, with consequences of greater clinical significance, as in Down syndrome, neurofibromatosis, and the mucopolysaccharidoses.

The complex process of human development from a single fertilized ovum is orchestrated by information encoded in the 46 chromosomes. Abnormalities may result from a defect in the original 46 chromosomes or a spontaneous mutation occurring during subsequent cellular multiplication. Disorders also occur from environmental factors that affect genetic expression; for example, the teratogenic effects of thalidomide, radiation exposure, and maternal rubella infection. Mechanical environmental factors contribute to such congenital conditions as dislocation of the hip, constriction bands, and muscular torticollis.

While environmental factors clearly play a role in some disorders, most congenital malformations have a genetic background, which may range from a relatively gross distortion of the normal complement of 46 chromosomes to an isolated defect in a single gene. Down syndrome (trisomy 21), Klinefelter syndrome (45/XXY), and Turner syndrome (45/XO) are examples of the former. Duchenne muscular dystrophy and sickle cell disease are disorders in which specific genetic defects have been identified, and many more undoubtedly will be elucidated as mapping of human chromosomes continues.

Simple Mendelian genetics applies to certain congenital disorders. Achondroplasia, multiple epiphyseal dysplasia, and multiple osteochondromatosis are conditions inherited in an autosomal dominant pattern. In these conditions the affected parent passes the abnormal dominant gene to 50 percent of the offspring. In autosomal recessive conditions, such as Morquio syndrome and some cases of osteogenesis imperfecta, neither parent is clinically affected. One-fourth of their offspring, however, receive the abnormal recessive gene from both parents and will manifest the condition. Sex-linked dominant conditions, such as hypophosphatemic rickets, are transmitted to one-half of all offspring if the mother is the carrier and to all daughters but no sons if the father is the carrier. Variable expressivity or penetrance of the affected gene is common and results in differing severity among members of a pedigree. In some instances, neither parent carries the affected gene, and the condition results from a mutation. These factors may obscure the inheritance pattern.

Many congenital disorders do not conform to simple Mendelian inheritance patterns. When the familial incidence of a congenital disorder is significantly higher than that expected by chance, the condition may have been determined by multiple genes. Variable penetrance, modulation by other genes, and environmental factors add further to the complexity. Congenital dislocation of the hip is a multifactorial disorder, in which siblings of affected children are at 10 to 50 times greater risk for the same condition than siblings of unaffected children. The concordance rate is 43 percent in monozygotic twins but only 3 percent in dizygotic twins.

GENERALIZED DISORDERS

Knowledge of the musculoskeletal manifestations of a generalized genetic or congenital disorder allows one to anticipate problems. For example, once a diagnosis of Down syndrome has been made, knowledge of potential neck, hip, and knee problems is integral to management of the patient and family.

Skeletal Dysplasias

Certain generalized disorders are defined primarily by their musculoskeletal manifestations, a principle clearly illustrated by the skeletal dysplasias. A *dysplasia* is a deformity caused by abnormal growth or development, a classic example of which is achondroplasia.

Achondroplasia

The deformities of achondroplasia result from failure of cartilage proliferation in the physis. Since this disorder affects the most rapidly growing bones to the greatest extent, the humerus and femur are profoundly affected. Disproportionate shortening of the proximal segments of the limbs produces a *rhizomelic* pattern (as opposed to *mesomelic* shortening, wherein the middle segment is shortened) of dwarfism. Although achondroplasia is an heritable condition with autosomal dominant transmission, 85 to 90 percent of all achondroplasia results from spontaneous mutations.

The diagnosis of achondroplasia is made in infancy from the distinctive clinical and radiographic appearances (Fig. 8.1). The limbs are disproportionally short, and, as they age, patients develop a depressed nasal bridge and frontal bossing, with a relative increase in head size. A distinctive feature of this syndrome is the "trident hand," which precludes apposition of the fingers when they are extended, most noticeably between the middle and ring fingers. Kyphosis at the thoracolumbar junction and increased lumbar lordosis are also common.

The radiographic manifestations of achondroplasia reflect the physical appearance of the patient. The humerus and femur are shortened relative to the bones of the forearm and leg, and the pelvic outlet assumes a classic "champagne glass" appearance. Perhaps the most singular finding is gradual narrowing of the interpedicular distance from L1 to the sacrum. In the normal spine, this distance either remains the same or increases between the upper and lower lumbar segments.

Achondroplasia affects limb alignment as well as length. Tibia vara (bowed legs) may require osteotomies for correction. The most serious complications, however, involve the spine. In childhood, thoracolumbar kyphosis may progress to marked angular deformity (*gibbus*) with compression of the spinal cord, while older patients often develop nerve root impingement requiring decompression. Impingement on the spinal cord may also occur

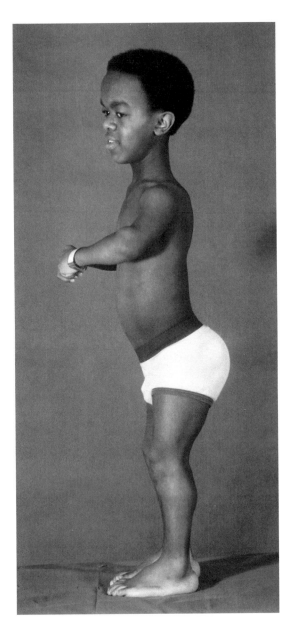

Figure 8.1   Achondroplasia. Note the distinctive cranial features and the *rhizomelic* shortening of the limbs.

at the foramen magnum or from *spinal stenosis* (narrowing of the spinal canal). These patients should be monitored closely by periodic neurologic examinations.

Multiple Epiphyseal Dysplasia

This is another generalized bone dysplasia that results in short stature, primarily from *epiphyseal* involvement. Multiple epiphyseal dysplasia (MED) has an autosomal dominant mode of inheritance and is rarely manifest clinically until the child reaches 5 to 14 years of age. Multiple epiphyseal dysplasia, like achondroplasia, causes disproportionate shortening of the limbs but is differentiated from other dwarfing syndromes by a lack of skull and facial changes.

Radiographic findings include abnormal ossification in the tarsal and carpal bones, with shortening of the metacarpals and the metatarsals. The larger epiphyses of the tibia and femur may be fragmented and abnormally shaped (Fig. 8.2). It is these changes that lead to the primary clinical concerns. Involvement of the capital femoral epiphyses can be confused with bilateral Legg-Calvé-Perthes disease if other manifestations of MED are not sought, such as limb length discrepancy and varus or valgus malalignment. Although minimal changes may be present in the spine, including scoliosis, they are not the dramatic changes associated with spondyloepiphyseal dysplasia.

Spondyloepiphyseal Dysplasia

Spondyloepiphyseal dysplasia (SED) involves the epiphyses of long bones but also, as the name implies, the growing vertebrae. The resultant shortening of the axial skeleton may take three forms. The most common type is *spondyloepiphyseal dysplasia tarda,* a sex-linked recessive trait that appears only in males. In this form, the spine and hips are the areas of primary involvement, and shortening

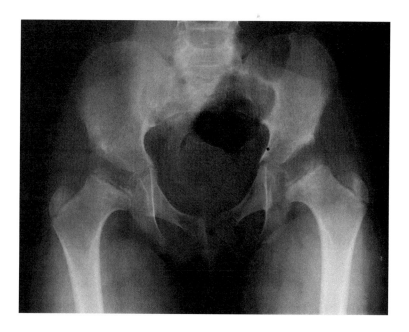

Figure 8.2 Multiple epiphyseal dysplasia. Bilateral hip involvement causes fragmentation of the capital femoral epiphyses, which can be mistaken for bilateral Legg-Calvé-Perthes disease.

is usually not apparent until 8 to 10 years of age. Radiographically, the adult spine has narrowed intervertebral disk spaces, with convexity of the vertebral end plates in the lumbar area. Changes in the hips may lead to symptomatic arthritis requiring surgery in later life.

The second form, *spondyloepiphyseal dysplasia congenita,* is usually diagnosed at birth and displays more marked involvement of the spine and long bones, although shortening may not be pronounced at birth. It is inherited in an autosomal dominant mode, is extremely rare, and the femoral heads typically do not ossify until childhood or adolescence. Ossification centers in the knees and feet, usually present at birth, are not seen until later in this syndrome. Radiographic changes in the spine are pronounced, with vertebral flattening (platyspondyly) and a hypoplastic or unossified odontoid process. Hypoplasia of the odontoid process may allow marked instability between C1 and C2, requiring fusion for stabilization. Malalignment of the femur and tibia may oc-

cur, and visual disturbances, including retinal detachment, are common.

A third variety, *pseudoachondroplastic spondyloepiphyseal dysplasia,* shows many of the radiographic changes seen in achondroplasia; however, there are no facial abnormalities, and the condition is therefore usually not diagnosed until 3 to 4 years of age. Nor is there a clearly delineated pattern of inheritance associated with pseudoachondroplasia. It may be differentiated from achondroplasia by a lack of interpedicular narrowing, the presence of radiographic wedging or platyspondyly, and epiphyseal rather than metaphyseal deformity.

Cleidocranial Dysplasia

Cleidocranial dysplasia (or *dysostosis*) is transmitted as an autosomal dominant disorder; it is named for involvement of the clavicles (cleido) and skull (cranium). Part or all of the clavicle(s) may be absent (Fig. 8.3). The lateral portion of the clavicle is most commonly absent, and the involvement is usually

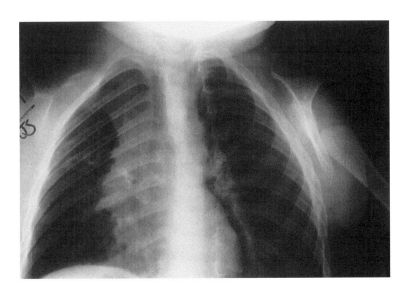

Figure 8.3 Cleidocranial dysostosis. Note the almost complete absence of clavicles.

unilateral, which leads to scapular "winging" and, in some cases, recurrent dislocation of the shoulder. The skull exhibits delayed ossification, with persistent open suture lines and large fontanels. The pelvis and hips may also be involved, with widened sacroiliac joints, delayed or absent ossification of the pubic bones, failure of closure of the symphysis pubis, and abnormal alignment of the femoral neck.

Although patients with cleidocranial dysplasia may have slightly shortened stature, scoliosis, and shoulder abnormalities, they usually do not require treatment.

Down Syndrome (Trisomy 21, or Mongolism)

Down syndrome usually results from a nondisjunction of the 21st chromosome, leaving the zygote with 47 instead of 46 chromosomes. The prevalence of this disorder increases with maternal age. Should the condition occur in one child, the mother's risk of having a subsequent child with Down syndrome is 1 in 50. Less commonly, the extra 21st chromosome translocates to a different position, leaving the normal complement of 46 chromosomes, one of which is larger. Clarifying the chromosomal abnormality is important, since the chances of a later child having Down syndrome increases to 1 in 3 when the defect is a translocation rather than a nondisjunction.

Patients with Down syndrome manifest varying degrees of mental retardation. They typically have short, stubby hands with a single palmar crease, clinodactyly, and slanted eyes with prominent epicanthal folds. Cardiac anomalies, particularly septal defects, and gastrointestinal abnormalities, such as duodenal atresia, are common. Ligamentous laxity and general hypotonia can result in dislocation of the hip and patella, atlantoaxial instability, genu valgum, and marked pes planus. With the longer life span resulting from surgical correction of the cardiac defects, there is greater need to address the orthopaedic problems in these patients.

Spontaneous dislocation of the hip occurs between 2 and 4 years of age in almost 5 percent of children with Down syndrome. The hips are usually hypermobile, and dislocations often reduce spontaneously. The dislocations are not painful. However, if this condition is persistent and remains untreated, affected patients become less active and displacement may become fixed. Nonoperative methods are generally not effective in managing spontaneous recurrent dislocations of the hip.

Patellofemoral instability occurs in about 5 percent of Down patients; it may cause frequent falling and limited ambulation, requiring surgical stabilization (Fig. 8.4).

Over 20 percent of patients with Down syndrome have atlantoaxial instability from hypoplasia of the odontoid process or laxity of the transverse ligament, which may result in neurologic compromise. Since many patients with this disorder cannot vocalize their complaints, there is frequently a delay in diagnosis. Findings include a change in gait, spasticity, weakness, bowel and bladder dysfunction, and torticollis. Lateral radiographs of the cervical spine in flexion and extension should be obtained before a patient with Down syndrome is allowed to participate in a sport that could result in injuries of the head or neck. A distance of over 4.5 mm between the odontoid process and the anterior arch of the atlas on a lateral cervical radiograph is considered ab-

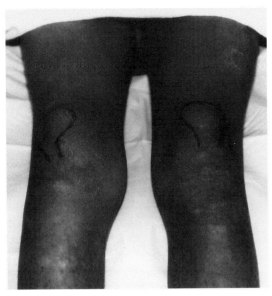

A

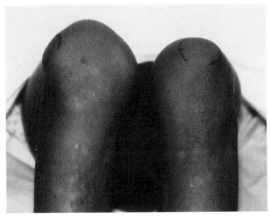

B

Figure 8.4 Down syndrome. The diffuse ligamentous laxity is manifest in this patient by *(A)* dislocation of the right patella. *B.* Patellar displacement is increased by flexion of the knee.

normal (Fig. 8.5). If radiographic abnormalities or neurologic findings are present, surgical consultation should be obtained. If cervical radiographs are normal and the patient is asymptomatic, there is no need to limit activity.

Mucopolysaccharidoses

The mucopolysaccharidoses (MPS) are a group of clinical syndromes resulting from a deficiency of one of the enzymes responsible for the degradation of three classes of mucopolysaccharides: keratan sulfate, heparan sulfate, and dermatan sulfate. These disorders occur in approximately 0.1 percent of newborns and are, with the exception of the sex-linked recessive *Hunter syndrome,* inherited as autosomal recessive traits. Tissue culture techniques have delineated 14 different enzyme deficiencies, with their clinical manifestations falling into seven categories. Although definitive diagnosis is contingent upon tissue culture, the syndromes themselves are defined by their clinical manifestations and increased mucopolysaccharide excretion in the urine (Table 8.1).

Hurler Syndrome

Hurler syndrome (MPS I-H) usually becomes manifest at 2 to 3 years of age, at which time mental retardation, dwarfing, thickened lips, wide nostrils, coarse hair, and large ears become apparent, leading to the descriptive term *gargoylism.* These patients develop joint contractures, diminished auditory and visual acuity, and hepatosplenomegaly. There are numerous radiographic findings, including a "slipper-shaped" sella turcica and premature closure of the skull sutures. Thoracolumbar kyphosis occurs frequently, with anteroinferior beaking of the vertebrae. Additional find-

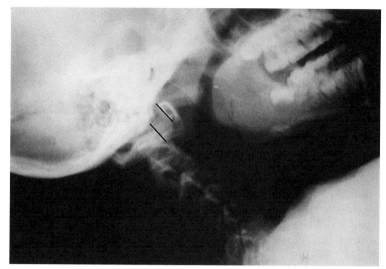

A

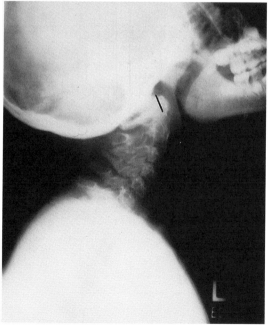

Figure 8.5 Down syndrome. Lateral flexion *(A)* and extension *(B)* radiographs of the cervical spine demonstrate C1-C2 instability, with an increased atlanto-dens interval in flexion.

B

Table 8.1 Mucopolysaccharidoses

Type	Inheritance	Enzymatic Deficiency	Urinary Excretion of MPS	Clinical Features	X-ray Findings
MPS I (Hurler)	Autosomal recessive	α-L-iduronidase	Dermatan sulfate^{2+} Heparan sulfate$^+$	"Gargoyle" facies, corneal clouding, deafness, moderate dwarfing, hepatosplenomegaly, profound retardation	Dorsolumbar kyphosis, lumbar vertebral beaking (L1 or L2), metacarpal widening, pelvic flaring
MPS I-S (Scheie)	Autosomal recessive	Sulfoiduronate sulfatase	Dermatan sulfate^{2+} Heparan sulfate$^+$	Coarse features, corneal clouding, deafness, cardiovascular (aortic valve) disease; normal mentation and height	Small hand epiphyses
MPS II (Hunter)	Sex-linked recessive	α-L-iduronidase	Heparan sulfate^{2+} Dermatan sulfate$^+$	Similar to Hurler, though milder, with less retardation and shortening and no corneal clouding	Moderate, without lumbar kyphosis
MPS III (San Filippo)	Autosomal recessive	N-heparan sulfatase or α-acetyl-glucosaminidase	Heparan sulfate^{2+}	Deafness, minimal hepatosplenomegaly, profound retardation; normal height and facies	Widening of medial clavicles, no kyphosis
MPS IV (Morquio)	Autosomal recessive	N-Ac-Gal-6 sulfate sulfatase	Keratan sulfate^{2+}	Wide mouth with prominent maxilla, progressive corneal clouding, deafness, mild aortic regurgitation, profound short stature with normal mentation	Marked changes: vertebral flattening (platyspondyly) with central tongue and irregular capital femoral epiphyses
MPS VI (Maroteaux-Lamy)	Autosomal recessive	N-Ac-Gal-4-sulfatase	Dermatan sulfate^{2+}	Coarse facies, corneal clouding, deafness, hepatomegaly, profound short stature; normal mentation	Similar to Hurler (severe)

ings are valgus deformities of the hips, inadequate acetabulae, diaphyseal widening of the long bones and metacarpals (Fig. 8.6), and distinctive flaring of the iliac wings. Treatment of the musculoskeletal manifestations of Hurler syndrome is symptomatic, since life expectancy is limited to the second decade. Atlantoaxial instability, which may follow odontoid hypoplasia, requires support with a cervical collar.

Hunter Syndrome

Hunter syndrome (MPS-II) is similar to Hurler syndrome, although symptoms are milder and later in onset. Since it is inherited as a sex-linked recessive trait, all patients with Hunter syndrome are male. These patients have cardiac defects and deafness, but they lack the

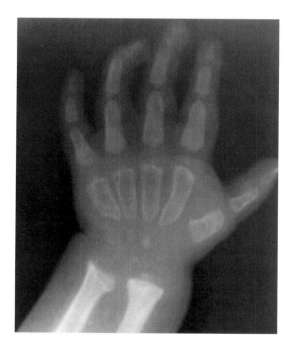

Figure 8.6 Hurler syndrome. Note the diaphyseal thickening of the metacarpals.

corneal clouding and lumbar kyphosis seen in Hurler syndrome. They usually live into adulthood and die from pulmonary hypertension and heart disease. Genetic counseling is imperative, since all daughters of involved individuals will be carriers of the trait.

San Filippo Syndrome

San Filippo syndrome (MPS-III) usually becomes evident as a result of profound mental retardation rather than serious musculoskeletal problems. There may be mild joint stiffness and shortness of stature, but the child appears normal for a few years before the onset of progressive mental retardation.

Morquio Syndrome

Morquio syndrome (MPS-IV) is the MPS most frequently seen for musculoskeletal problems. These patients have normal intelligence, but develop, around the age of 2 years, progressive genu valgum, thoracic kyphosis, a waddling gait, short stature, and deformity of the hips. Unlike other types of MPS, Morquio syndrome causes marked ligamentous laxity with planovalgus feet. There is a thoracolumbar kyphosis, with ovoid vertebral bodies in infancy that gradually become flattened and develop an anterior "tongue" projecting from the middle of the vertebral body. Atlantoaxial instability and spinal cord compression often require fusion of the upper cervical spine to the occiput. In the limbs, realignment osteotomy, wrist fusion, and triple arthrodesis may be needed for marked deformity or instability.

Scheie Syndrome

Scheie syndrome (formerly MPS-V, now MPS-I-S) is marked by poor vision and progressive corneal opacities. These patients have normal intelligence, excessive body hair, and a broad face. Despite joint stiffness and contractures of the fingers, they rarely require surgical intervention.

Maroteaux-Lamy Syndrome

Maroteaux-Lamy syndrome (MPS-VI, polydystrophic dwarfism) is usually recognized near age 3 because of marked shortening of the trunk and limbs. Bony changes include pectus carinatum, genu valgum and lumbar kyphosis. These patients have normal intelligence, with clinical and radiographic findings suggesting a mild Hurler syndrome.

Arthrogryposis Multiplex Congenita

Arthrogryposis multiplex congenita (amyoplasia) is characterized by congenitally rigid joints with decreased muscle mass, tense, glossy skin and the absence of normal skin creases. Dimpling of the skin is frequent over the knees, wrist, and elbows.

The etiology of this condition remains unclear. Since these patients have normal intelligence, a negative family history and no visceral abnormalities, the diagnosis hinges on the presence of typical facial features and characteristic, symmetrical posture of the limbs (Fig. 8.7). The child's face is typically small and oval, with a slightly upturned nose and, occasionally, a capillary hemangioma over the bridge of the nose, forehead, and eyelids. In the upper limbs, the shoulders are typically adducted and internally rotated, with the elbows fixed in flexion or extension and the wrists in flexion and/or ulnar deviation. In the lower limbs, the hips are characteristically flexed, externally rotated, and abducted.

The orthopaedic problems in arthrogryposis are related to rigid, fibrotic joints and diminished muscle mass. The most consistent path-

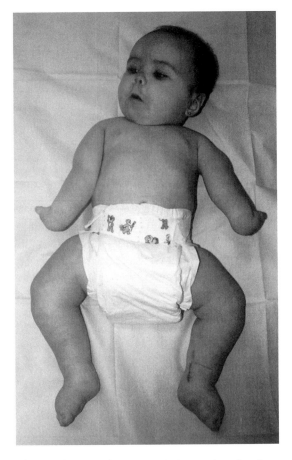

Figure 8.7　Arthrogryposis. Note the classic equinus of the feet and positioning of the upper limb, with flexion of the wrist, extension of the elbow, and adduction–internal rotation of the shoulders.

ologic findings are fibrous replacement of muscles and a reduction in the number of anterior horn cells in the spinal cord.

The goal of management is maximal function in the upper and lower limbs. The total motion in arthrogrypotic joints cannot be changed, but physical therapy, casting, orthotics, and judicious surgery enable what motion is present to be utilized in the most functional arc. Abnormalities of the lower limb that might prevent ambulation should be corrected by age 2 to avoid interference with normal development. Intervention in the upper limb focuses on placing the hands in the position of maximal function but should be deferred until the functional capacity of the upper limb is known.

Neurofibromatosis

Neurofibromatosis (von Recklinghausen disease) is an autosomal dominant disorder that occurs in 1 of every 3000 newborns. Since it is a disorder of the neural crest involving neuroectoderm, endoderm, and mesoderm, almost any organ system can be affected. Histologically, neurofibromas consist of fibrous tissue and Schwann cells that occur on the skin in protean forms or along nerves. Forty percent of these patients have a major orthopaedic problem. The diagnosis may not be apparent at birth, since café-au-lait spots are often absent during the first year of life, and the major manifestations frequently do not occur until after puberty. The diagnosis is based upon the presence of two of the four most common findings: (1) café-au-lait spots (at least five measuring more than 0.5 cm in diameter), (2) a positive family history, (3) a characteristic histologic picture, and (4) typical skeletal lesions.

Skeletal manifestations include focal gigantism (hypertrophy of a bone, digit, or limb), defects in bone cortices, bowing and lengthening or shortening of bones, and tibial or fibular pseudarthrosis. Scoliosis and kyphosis are frequent. A short scoliotic curve results from a single wedged vertebra; longer curves may be indistinguishable from idiopathic scoliosis. The skin changes in neurofibromatosis range from café-au-lait spots, nodules, and nevi to elephantiasis and verrucous hyperplasia that can be extremely disfiguring. Overall, 5 percent of patients with neurofibromatosis have associated neoplasms, and 10 percent of nevi undergo malignant degeneration. Tumors of the central nervous system include gliomas, neurosarcomas, and acoustic neuromas, while fibrosarcomas, neurofibrosarcomas, and neurogenic sarcomas develop in peripheral tissues. Older and more severely involved patients are at greater risk for malignancies.

Acrocephalosyndactylism (Apert Syndrome)

First described by Apert in 1906, acrocephalosyndactylism represents failure of mesenchymal tissue to separate into isolated ossification centers, which results in synostosis of the cranial sutures and syndactyly of the hands and feet. Increased intracranial pressure follows early cranial synostoses, but osteotomy of the cranial bones allows normalization of pressure. Many children with *Apert syndrome* are mentally retarded, although some (particularly those undergoing early neurosurgical intervention) have normal mentation.

The hands of patients with Apert syndrome exhibit varying degrees of complete, complex syndactyly—particularly of the index, long and ring fingers—which gives the hand a "mitten" or "spoon-shaped" appearance (Fig. 8.8). Surgical correction is staged, as with any complex syndactyly. It is often advisable to accept a three-fingered hand to ensure better function and adequate soft tissue coverage of the digits. Other abnormalities in the upper limbs include stiff elbows, shortening of the forearms and limited abduction of the shoulders. The feet are also involved, with varying

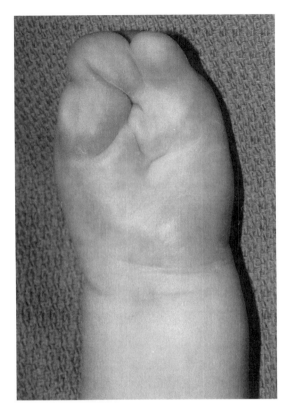

Figure 8.8   Apert syndrome. Note the complete, complex syndactyly, which creates a "mitten"- or "spoon-hand" deformity. Staged operative correction will be required to obtain a functional hand.

degrees of syndactylism and fusion of the tarsal bones.

Fetal Alcohol Syndrome

A clear association has been established between maternal alcohol abuse and fetal damage. The level of alcohol ingestion required and the biochemical mechanism of damage are unclear; however, the constellation of abnormalities is well defined and includes retarded neurologic function, disturbances in growth and facial appearance, and abnormal skeletal development.

Children with fetal alcohol syndrome start small and stay small, remaining below normal height and weight throughout life. Many are misdiagnosed as having cerebral palsy because of mental retardation, hypotonia or hypertonia, and delayed motor milestones. Approximately half of all these children have orthopaedic problems. Ten percent have dislocations of the hip; other joints exhibit restricted motion, most marked in the elbows and fingers. Congenital spinal deformities, including scoliosis and spinal dysraphism, occur in the cervical, thoracic, or lumbar spine. A unique feature of fetal alcohol syndrome is the prevalence of bony fusions in the upper limbs, especially of the proximal radioulnar and intercarpal joints.

CONNECTIVE TISSUE DISORDERS

Disorders of collagen formation and organization often cause structural abnormalities in the body. Increasingly sophisticated biochemical testing has led to specific subtyping for many of these disorders, which has produced a better understanding of the underlying structural defects. Isolated skeletal dysplasias (e.g., achondrogenesis, spondyloepiphyseal dysplasia, Stickler syndrome) have also been associated with mutations in collagen, indicating an etiologic overlap with the connective tissue disorders.

Ehlers-Danlos Syndrome

Ehlers-Danlos syndrome (EDS) is a group of clinical disorders marked by extreme ligamentous laxity, bone and soft tissue fragility, hyperelasticity and easy bruising of the skin, and varying degrees of osteopenia. Abnormalities of types I and III collagen have been identified in several types of EDS, but biochemical markers have not been elucidated in the most common forms (types I, II, and III) of the syndrome. There has been a proliferation of subtypes in EDS. The 11 most common types, their features, and their modes of inheritance are listed in Table 8.2. When joint hyperextensibility is present, recurrent dislocations of the shoulders, hips, and patellas are common, as well as pes planus and genu recurvatum. All joints are lax, which predisposes them to traumatic effusions and hemarthroses. Scoliosis and spondylolisthesis also occur in these patients.

The skin in EDS exhibits differing degrees of hyperelasticity, fragility, and bruisability, with the formation of "pseudotumors" at pressure points. The skin may become hyperpigmented and resemble parchment or cigarette paper. Tissue fragility can lead to intestinal and pulmonary ruptures and wound dehiscence following surgery. Ocular, cardiac, and gynecologic disorders are also common.

Ehlers-Danlos syndrome type I (gravis) is a severe form of this disorder characterized by joint laxity and hyperelasticity of the skin. Patients with EDS II (mitis) are similar, with less marked clinical manifestations. EDS III (benign hypermobile) forms have minimal dermal abnormalities and joint hypermobility, whereas type IV (ecchymotic) patients show hypermobility only in the interphalangeal and metacarpophalangeal joints—along with easy bruisability, pigmented scars, and occasional vascular or lower intestinal rupture.

Since the tissue itself is abnormal in EDS, recurrence is common following soft tissue surgery for joint instability. This fact, combined with problems of wound dehiscence and intraoperative hemostasis, makes surgical intervention extremely difficult and often unrewarding.

Marfan Syndrome

Both the Marfan and Ehlers-Danlos syndromes have subtypes with hypermobile joints, which creates diagnostic confusion. Although there is a defect in the organization of collagen that leads to its musculoskeletal manifestations, there is no clear biochemical marker for Marfan syndrome, so the diagnosis is made on clinical grounds. Marked variability is seen in the skeletal, ocular and cardiovascular manifestations of this syndrome.

The classic description of Marfan syndrome is as appropriate today as when Marfan, a French pediatrician, presented it in 1896. He recognized a disorder consisting of disproportionately long, thin limbs, generalized joint laxity, dissecting aneurysm or collapsed cardiac valves, dislocation of ocular lenses, and frequent hernias. Affected individuals are usually over 6 ft tall at maturity, and the length of the lower segment of the body, as measured from the top of the symphysis pubis to the sole of the foot, is greater than the length of the upper segment of the body (total height minus lower segment length.) The arm span is usually greater than the patient's height, which also illustrates the disproportionate length of the limbs. Pyeritz and McKusick have divided the physical findings into major signs (ectopia lentis, aortic dilatation, severe kyphoscoliosis, and thoracic deformity) and minor signs (myopia, tall stature, mitral valve prolapse, ligamentous laxity, arachnodactyly and the thumb,

Table 8.2 Findings in the Different Forms of Ehlers-Danlos Syndrome

Type	Biochemistry	Inheritance	Clinical Manifestations		
			Skin	Musculoskeletal	Other
I Gravis	Unknown	Autosomal dominant	Easy bruisability, hyperextensible, fragile	Laxity, dislocations, scoliosis	Prematurity, varicose veins, hernia
II Mitis	Unknown	Autosomal dominant	Mild bruising, hyperextensibility	Laxity in hands and feet	None
III Benign	Unknown	Autosomal dominant	Normal	Severe laxity, dislocations	None
IV Ecchymotic	Decreased type III collagen synthesis or secretion	Autosomal dominant or recessive	Severe bruising, thin and friable	Laxity in hands and feet, few disolcations	Aneurysms; arterial, uterine, and colonic rupture
V X-linked	Possible deficiency of peptidyl lysine oxidase	X-linked recessive	Mild bruising, fragility, profound hyperextensibility	Minimal laxity	None
VI Ocular-Scoliotic	Deficiency of peptidyl lysine hydroxylase	Autosomal recessive	Moderate bruising, fragility, hyperextensibility	Moderate laxity, dislocations, scoliosis (severe), clubfeet	Ocular fragility, floppy babies

Type	Biochemical defect	Inheritance	Skin	Joints	Associated features
VII Arthrochalasis multiplex congenita	Deficiency of procollagen *N*-protease	Autosomal dominant or recessive	Moderate fragility, hyperextensibility	Severe laxity, CDH, scoliosis, short stature	Abnormal facies
VIII Periodontosis	Possible protease-sensitive collagen	Autosomal dominant	Severe fragility, mild hyperextensibility	Moderate laxity (esp. fingers)	Periodontal disease, tooth loss
IX Occipital horns	Deficient peptidyl lysine oxidase and copper metabolism	X-linked recessive	Laxity and hyperextensibility	Elbows stiff w/ laxity of hands and feet; skeletal dysplasia w/ dislocated radial heads and occipital bony exostoses	Urinary tract dysplasia
X Platelet dysfunction	Fibronectin abnormality	Autosomal recessive	Easy bruisability, moderate hyperextensibility	Laxity of hands and feet	Defective platelet aggregation
XI Familial laxity	Unknown	Autosomal dominant	Normal	Profound laxity with frequent dislocations, patellar subluxation, CDH	None

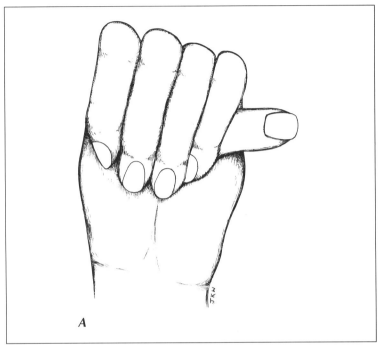

Figure 8.9 Marfan syndrome. The thumb *(A)* and wrist *(B)* signs
reflect the arachnodactyly in this entity and are two of the
major diagnostic findings.

wrist and knee sign) (Fig. 8.9). Two major
signs and multiple minor signs are necessary
for a definitive diagnosis of Marfan syndrome.

The joint laxity in Marfan syndrome results
in marked pes planus, genu recurvatum, and
recurrent dislocations of the patellas and hips.
The connective tissue abnormality also leads
to scoliosis in up to 70 percent of these patients, which is commonly apparent at an earlier age than idiopathic scoliosis and can aggravate the problems associated with cardiac
and sternal abnormalities.

Although other manifestations are debilitating, cardiovascular anomalies can cause death
in early adult life. Insufficiency of the aortic
or mitral valve, septal defects, aneurysms of
the sinus of Valsalva, and dilatation of the ascending aorta occur in patients with Marfan
syndrome. Dissecting aortic aneurysm is the
most common fatal complication.

Osteogenesis Imperfecta

Osteogenesis imperfecta (OI) is a connective
tissue disorder marked by varying degrees of
osteoporosis, bone fragility, dental abnormality, deafness, ligamentous laxity, easy bruisability and ocular abnormalities. The disorder
has been divided into four clinical types based
upon physical findings and modes of inheritance (Table 8.3). The underlying cause of all
forms of OI is a relative deficiency or abnormality of type I collagen.

Osteogenesis imperfecta type I is marked by

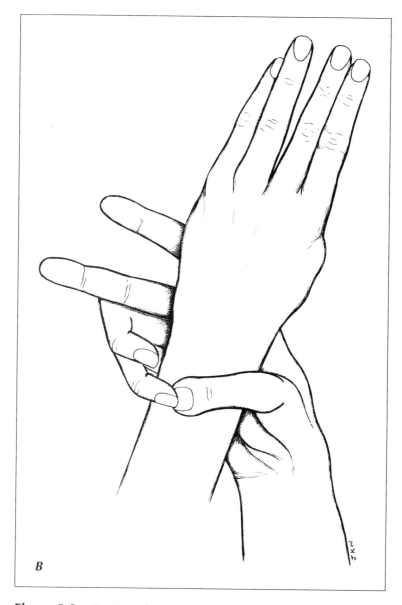

B

Figure 8.9   Continued

persistent blue sclerae, progressive hearing loss, abnormal bony fragility, and generalized osteoporosis. The presence of *dentinogenesis imperfecta* (soft, brownish, translucent teeth) is the only differentiating factor between OI subtypes IA and IB.

Osteogenesis imperfecta type II leads to death in the perinatal period or early infancy. It is marked by extreme bony fragility and delayed ossification of the skull.

Osteogenesis imperfecta type III is rare and is characterized by bluish sclerae at birth that

Table 8.3 Inheritance Patterns and Clinical Findings in Osteogenesis Imperfecta

Type	I		II	III	IV	
	A	B			A	B
Teeth	Normal	Dentinogenesis imperfecta	Unknown	Normal	Normal	Dentinogenesis imperfecta
Inheritance	Autosomal dominant		Autosomal recessive	Autosomal recessive	Autosomal dominant	
Bone fragility	Variable, less than other types		Extreme	Severe	Moderate	
Bony deformity	Moderate		Profound	Severe and progressive	Moderate	
Sclerae	Blue		Blue	Light blue at birth, white as adult	Normal	
Skull	Wormian bones		Deficient ossification	Hypoplastic		Hypoplastic wormian bones
Spine	20% scoliosis and kyphosis			Kyphoscoliosis		Kyphoscoliosis
Hearing	40% loss					Low-frequency loss
Prognosis	Fair		Perinatal death	Nonambulatory; shortened life expectancy	Fair	

become normal by adolescence, multiple fractures and progressive deformities of long bones.

Osteogenesis imperfecta type IV also has varying degrees of bluish sclerae initially; again, they become normal by adolescence. The degree of bone fragility and deformity is variable in this autosomal dominant disorder. The presence of dentinogenesis imperfecta defines the subtype IV-B classification of OI.

Radiographic findings in OI are often dramatic (Fig. 8.10). In severe cases, the long bones tend to be short and wide, with multiple fractures in varying stages of healing. It is important to differentiate these children from victims of abuse, who may have similar radiographic findings. Angular deformity results from malunion of the healing fractures. In another variation, bones are thin, with narrow medullary cavities, osteopenia, and "eggshell" cortices. Delayed and deficient ossification of the calvarium results in "wormian bones," which are detached portions of the ossification centers of the membranous bones. The clinical course and treatment of OI depend upon the degree of bone fragility in a given patient. In infancy, severely involved children require careful support and positioning to avoid fractures.

Should a patient with OI become ambulatory, progressive angular deformity of the weight-bearing long bones often develops. Fracture *healing* is not impaired in OI, but multiple fractures lead to prolonged failure of ambulation, with further weakening of the bone. Bony fragility also involves the spine, often leading to kyphosis, scoliosis, and consequent cardiopulmonary compromise. The goal in these patients is to minimize deformity and hospitalization while maximizing movement and ambulation to prevent osteoporosis.

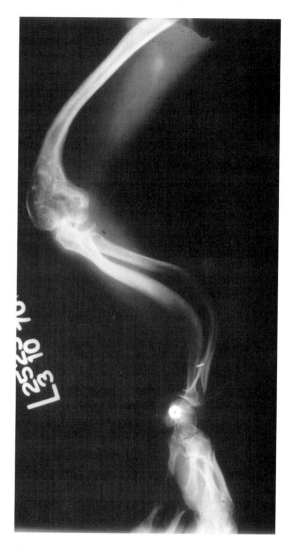

Figure 8.10 Osteogenesis imperfecta. The bony fragility has resulted in multiple fractures and deformities.

Operative intervention for spinal and long bone deformities is extremely difficult. Surgery may be complicated by failure of fixation, excessive bleeding, and hyperthermia. Realignment of long bones is possible with multiple osteotomies and intramedullary fixation, but the cornerstone of fracture care is prevention by modification of activity and the use of orthoses.

DISORDERS OF THE HEMATOPOIETIC SYSTEM

Although primarily diseases of the blood-forming elements, hemophilia, sickle cell disease, and Gaucher disease have distinctive musculoskeletal manifestations.

Hemophilia

Hemophilia is a sex-linked recessive disorder characterized by a deficiency in the activity of antihemophilic globulin factor VIII. If the blood level of factor VIII is 50 to 100 percent of the expected normal value, as with female carriers, there is usually no bleeding diathesis. In severely affected patients (factor levels < 1 percent), spontaneous bleeding occurs without antecedent trauma. Musculoskeletal compromise is a consequence of bleeding into joints and muscles.

In *hemophilic arthropathy,* joint destruction results from progressive fibrous replacement of the synovial lining and enzymatic degradation of the cartilage matrix. The most commonly affected joints are the ankles, knees, and elbows. Particularly in the severe hemophiliac, chronic arthritis may be followed by fibrous or bony ankylosis, with weakness and contracture of the surrounding musculature.

Bleeding into muscles and closed compartments can produce a compartment syndrome, with secondary myelopathy and contracture.

When a compartment syndrome is suspected, immediate replacement therapy should be undertaken, compartment pressures monitored, and fasciotomies performed as indicated (see Chap. 13). Repeated bleeding into muscles can lead to *pseudotumor* formation. These expanding masses and their surgical excision can be life-threatening events.

Maintaining a career, social life, and physical fitness requires knowledge of the treatment and prevention of bleeding episodes. Intramuscular injections and drugs that interfere with platelet function, such as aspirin, should be avoided, and dental prophylaxis should be emphasized in order to avert extractions. All patients should carry a card containing their diagnosis and blood group.

For significant bleeding episodes, transfusion of factor VIII concentrate is required. In patients undergoing surgery, factor VIII levels should be above 50 percent initially and maintained above 30 percent until the wound has healed.

Hemophiliacs treated prior to the introduction of heat-treated and recombinant concentrates have a markedly increased risk of infection by the *human immunodeficiency virus (HIV).* Approximately 70 percent of patients with severe factor VIII deficiency and 10 percent of those with mild to moderate deficiency are HIV-positive.

Synovectomy often reduces the frequency of bleeding episodes in patients with mild to moderate hemophiliac arthropathy, while joint replacement or fusion may be required for more advanced stages. The foundations of treatment, however, are education, prevention, rapid hemostasis with local measures and factor replacement, and the prevention of deformity by splinting and guided physical therapy.

Sickle Cell Disease

Sickle cell disease occurs when valine is substituted for a glutamine residue normally found at the sixth amino acid position from the *N*-terminal end of the hemoglobin molecule. The gene responsible for this mutation is found in approximately 10 percent of the African American population and is inherited as an autosomal dominant trait. Sickle cell disease occurs when an individual is homozygous for this gene, which occurs in approximately 2.5 percent of African Americans. Under reduced oxygen tension, the S hemoglobin distorts red cells into characteristic sickle-cell conformations. These "sickled" cells produce vascular stasis and progressive localized deoxygenation, resulting in more sickling and a vicious cycle of pain and organ damage. Such *sickle cell* crises may be triggered by alterations in local tissue perfusion, such as trauma or infection, but they also occur spontaneously and can be extremely painful. Management consists of the elimination of causative factors, administration of fluids, and analgesia. Bone infarcts in sickle cell disease are often responsible for avascular necrosis of the femoral and humeral heads (Fig. 8.11). If these areas of infarction progress to collapse and joint destruction, joint replacement may become necessary.

Children with sickle cell disease are typically short, with delayed bone age and sexual maturation. Children under age 2 are prone to *dactylitis,* with pain and swelling of the hands and feet. They are also vulnerable to *salmonella* osteomyelitis, manifest by fever, pain, and swelling of the limb. This condition is differentiated from a sickle cell crisis, which may have identical symptoms, by needle aspiration.

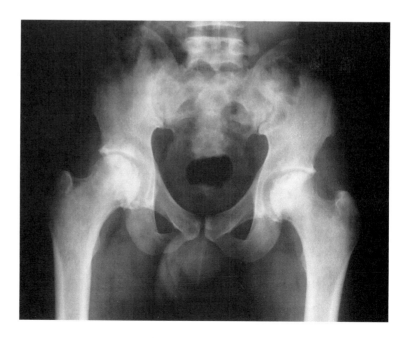

Figure 8.11 Sickle cell disease. Note the multiple infarcts within the sclerotic femoral heads, which may lead to collapse and secondary arthritis.

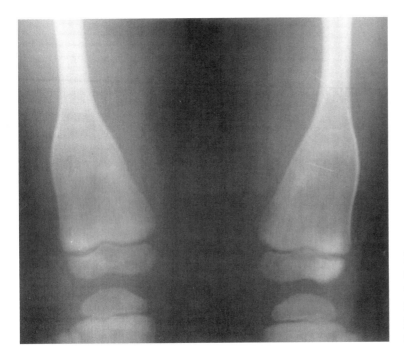

Figure 8.12   Gaucher disease. Note the typical widening of the distal femoral metaphyses producing an "Erlenmeyer flask" appearance.

Management may require surgical drainage, along with administration of appropriate systemic antibiotics.

Gaucher Disease

Gaucher disease, a disorder occurring most commonly in Ashkenazi Jews, stems from a deficiency of the glucocerebroside-cleaving enzyme beta-glucosidase. This defect leads to an accumulation of glucocerebroside-kerasin in reticuloendothelial cells.

Most patients with this disease are diagnosed before 10 years of age as a result of symptoms from splenomegaly (fatigue, bleeding diathesis, abdominal distention) or skeletal involvement (bone pain). The femur is the bone most commonly involved, with enlargement of the distal metaphysis producing an "Erlenmeyer flask" appearance (Fig. 8.12). Infiltration and replacement of bony trabeculae by the kerasin-containing reticulum cells often causes avascular necrosis of the hip, shoulder, knee, or spine.

Patients with Gaucher disease occasionally develop crises similar to those of patients with sickle cell disease. The onset of pain in these crises is acute, with fever, swelling, and tenderness of the involved limb. Management of these crises, as with sickle cell disease, consists mainly of rest, fluids, analgesics, and ruling out infection.

REGIONAL DISORDERS

Spine

Os Odontoideum

Os odontoideum is an ossicle of varying size located at or near the normal location of the odontoid process of C2 (Fig. 8.13). Compared

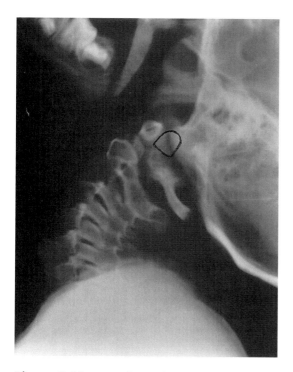

Figure 8.13 Os odentoideum (outlined). Note the associated C1-2 instability.

to the general population, anomalies of the odontoid occur more often in patients with Down syndrome, Klippel-Feil syndrome, Morquio syndrome, and other congenital disorders. Although the topic is included here, it has not been established whether the condition is congenital or acquired. Embryologically, the odontoid process originates as part of the first cervical vertebra, from which it separates, moves caudally, and ultimately fuses with the second cervical vertebra. These points suggest a congenital origin. Other investigators, however, feel that the condition is traumatically acquired. In one series, 17 of 35 patients had a history of cervical trauma sufficient to warrant immobilization, and 9 of these patients had prior radiographs showing a normal odontoid.

The clinical significance of os odontoideum rests with the associated subluxation and instability between C1 and C2. The coupling of instability with limited space for the spinal cord may cause neurologic problems. The diagnosis of an os odontoideum is made radiographically; the instability and space for the cord are assessed with plain radiographs, tomograms, or magnetic resonance imaging (MRI) with the neck in flexion and extension.

Individuals with an os odontoideum may be asymptomatic or complain of headache, neck pain, shoulder pain, transient paresthesias, and/or unsteadiness. The primary treatment options are observation or surgical fusion of C1 to C2. The decision to operate is based primarily on the space available for the spinal cord and the presence of neurologic symptoms or findings. Progression of either instability or neurologic involvement adds urgency to the need for surgery.

Klippel-Feil Syndrome

The term *Klippel-Feil syndrome* is applied to patients with congenital fusion of at least one level in the cervical spine (Fig. 8.14). The significance of the condition depends on the extent of cervical involvement and on the presence or absence of anomalies in addition to those in the cervical spine. The classic manifestations of the syndrome are a short neck with limited motion and a low posterior hairline; however, many affected individuals will not have all three signs. If the number of fused levels is few or if significant compensatory motion develops at unfused levels, cervical motion may be nearly normal. Loss of motion is also less apparent in lower cervical segments, which contribute less to motion than those in the upper cervical spine.

Evaluation of cervical involvement is primarily radiographic. Adequate plain radiographs may be difficult to obtain owing to lim-

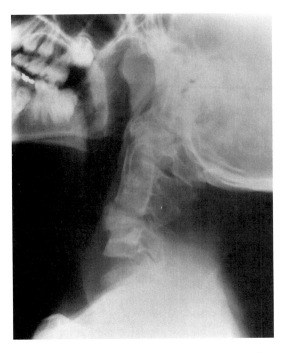

Figure 8.14 Klippel-Feil syndrome. Note the congenital failure of separation (fusion) of multiple cervical vertebrae. This patient also has Sprengel deformity (see Fig. 8.22).

ited motion and deformity, in which cases tomograms and computed tomography (CT) scans may be helpful. Films in flexion and extension are important to assess instability from excessive motion at unfused levels. In very young patients, flexion-extension views may indicate a fusion that is not otherwise apparent because of incomplete ossification of the vertebral bodies.

The clinical problems that develop in the cervical spine usually occur at levels that are initially normal. Fusions within the cervical spine place greater mechanical demands on unfused levels. This accelerates the development of degenerative changes and/or creates hypermobility at unfused levels, with the as-

sociated risks and symptoms of instability. The cervical anomaly most likely to cause clinical problems is a single open level with fused vertebrae above and below, such as fusion of C2-C3 coupled with occipitalization of C1, which leads to excessive wear and/or instability at C1-C2.

The Klippel-Feil anomaly is characterized as a syndrome because of its frequent association with other abnormalities. The most commonly associated condition, found in over half of the patients, is congenital scoliosis. As discussed elsewhere in this chapter, congenital deformities of the spine warrant careful monitoring during skeletal growth. Renal anomalies are found in up to one-third of patients with Klippel-Feil syndrome. Awareness of this association is particularly important, since the renal abnormality is usually asymptomatic in the young. The most common renal anomalies are absence of a kidney, a double collecting system, renal ectopia, and ureteropelvic obstruction. Congenital cardiac anomalies typically involve an interventricular septal defect or patent ductus arteriosus. Hearing impairment has also been reported, with both conductive and sensorineural hearing losses described. Another occasional finding is *synkinesis,* or mirror motions, consisting of involuntary paired movements of the hands. Involvement may be subtle and manifest only as difficulty with two-handed activities such as typing. Sprengel deformity, which is discussed later in this chapter, is frequently associated with Klippel-Feil syndrome.

Congenital Muscular Torticollis

Congenital muscular torticollis or "wry neck" is a condition characterized by unilateral contracture of the sternocleidomastoid muscle, which results in the head being tilted toward the involved side, with the chin rotated to the opposite side and slightly raised (Fig. 8.15). In the first few weeks of life, a localized enlargement or mass is often palpable within the sternocleidomastoid muscle, but it disappears quickly. The differential diagnosis includes torticollis caused by congenital vertebral anomalies, a neurogenic problem (such as a central nervous system tumor or syringomyelia), and fracture or subluxation. Upper respiratory infections may also lead to rotary subluxation at C1-2. Stability of the hips must be carefully assessed, since instability occurs in roughly 20 percent of patients with this condition.

The etiology of congenital muscular torticollis is uncertain. The most compelling theory is that positioning of the head in utero impairs venous outflow from the sternocleidomastoid muscle, resulting in a compartment syndrome within the muscle that ultimately leads to fibrosis and contracture.

The most significant clinical problem with congenital muscular torticollis is *plagiocephaly* (asymmetry of the face and skull). Affected infants who sleep prone apply pressure primarily to one side of the head, which contributes to the deformity. When instituted during the first year of life, stretching of the affected muscle is effective treatment for most patients. Surgical release of the muscle is generally recommended for children over 1 year of age with persistent, significant restriction of motion. Delaying surgery beyond infancy is likely to result in less complete restoration of facial symmetry.

Syringomyelia

Syringomyelia is a condition in which a fluid-filled, longitudinal cavity *(syrinx)* develops in the spinal cord (Fig. 8.16). Treatment of the lesion itself comes under the purview of the neurosurgeon, but orthopaedic manifestations are common and varied. Symptoms are pain in the head, neck, back, or limbs. Physical findings include wasting of intrinsic muscles in the hands, cavus deformities of the feet, and altered deep tendon reflexes. Neurologic findings are often subtle and asymmetrical, involving the upper or lower limbs. The most commonly associated orthopaedic finding is scoliosis, present in up to half of the patients with syringomyelia. Left thoracic curves associated with pain and neurologic abnormalities are atypical in idiopathic scoliosis and

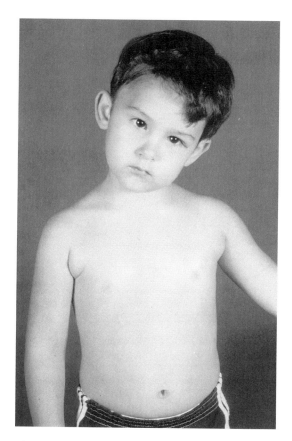

Figure 8.15   Congenital muscular torticollis. Contracture of the left sternocleidomastoid muscle has tilted the head to the left and rotated the chin to the right.

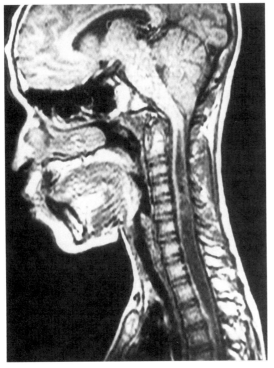

A

Figure 8.16   Syringomyelia. *A.* An MRI scan showing an extensive syrinx in the spinal cord. *B.* A radiograph showing atypical left-sided scoliosis, which is often associated with syringomyelia.

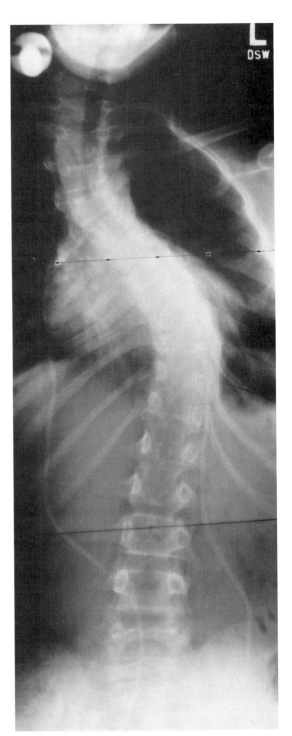

B

should make intraspinal pathology suspect. Plain radiographs may be normal, may show scoliosis, or may display only subtle abnormalities, such as widening of the distance between pedicles. An MRI scan is the best means of identifying the syrinx. Neurosurgical drainage of the cavity often improves neurologic function and makes surgical treatment of the scoliosis safer if such treatment is required. The effect of drainage on the scoliosis is unpredictable.

Congenital Spinal Deformities

Congenital spinal deformities result from uneven growth of congenitally malformed vertebrae. Deformity in the sagittal plane (excessive kyphosis or lordosis) or frontal plane (scoliosis) often is not apparent at birth. Subsequent growth, if asymmetric, produces the deformity. For this reason, affected individuals must be carefully monitored until skeletal maturity is reached. Idiopathic scoliosis, whether infantile, juvenile, or adolescent, is distinguishable from congenital scoliosis by the absence of intrinsic vertebral anomalies.

Abnormalities of the vertebrae typically consist of failure of a vertebra to form fully or to separate normally from adjacent vertebrae (Fig. 8.17). Failure of formation of the lateral portion of a vertebra may be partial (wedged vertebra) or complete (hemivertebra). The consequences of the malformation depend on growth. For example, if both sides of a wedged vertebra grow at the same rate, there will be no increase in the deformity. If only the formed side of a hemivertebra grows, there will be progressive scoliosis.

Failure of formation may also differentially affect the anterior or posterior portion of a vertebra. With anterior deficiencies, posterior exceeds anterior growth, leading to progressive kyphosis. Minor failures of posterior forma-

tion, such as spina bifida occulta, are common and generally have no clinical significance. Major failures of posterior formation are rare without associated anomalies of adjacent neural elements (myelodysplasia) and overlying soft tissues. The spinal problems of individuals with myelomeningocele are more complex because they include both osseous and neuromuscular elements.

Failure of vertebrae to separate may also lead to angular deformities. Incomplete separation on one side of adjacent vertebrae is called a bar. The bar may tether growth asymmetrically, leading to progressive deformity. Complete failure of separation, block vertebra, causes little deformity unless associated with other anomalies. Failures of formation and separation may coexist, with the complexity and extent of vertebral anomalies varying widely (Fig. 8.18).

Individuals with congenital anomalies of the spine frequently have other abnormalities as well. Additional ribs, missing ribs, and fused or misshapen ribs are common although rarely of clinical consequence. Of greater potential concern are anomalies of the genitourinary tract, which are present in up to 20 percent of patients with congenital anomalies of the spine. The association is sufficiently frequent that all children with congenital spinal disorders should undergo renal ultrasound or an intravenous pyelogram (IVP). Anomalies of the collecting system may cause an obstructive uropathy that requires treatment. Other anomalies, such as a single kidney or renal ectopia, do not necessarily require treatment, but the patient should be made aware of the disorder. Cardiac anomalies are also associated with congenital spinal anomalies in up to 15 percent of patients. Occult spinal dysrhaphism, such as diastematomyelia (fibrous or bony cord in the spinal canal) and tethering of the

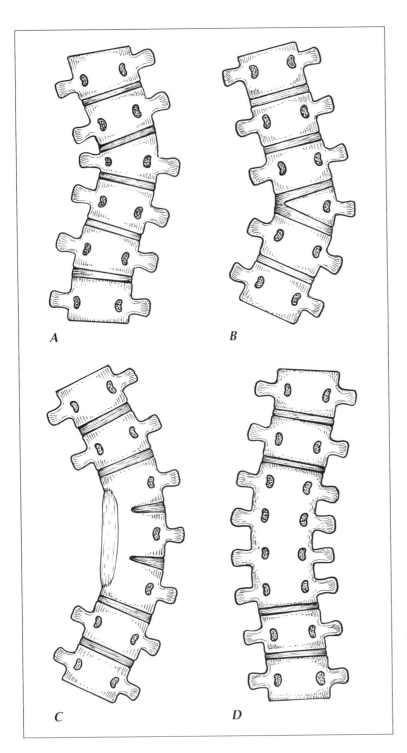

A

B

C

D

Figure 8.17 Congenital vertebral anomalies. Failures of formation include (A) wedge vertebra and (B) hemivertebra. Failures of separation include (C) a bar and (D) block vertebrae.

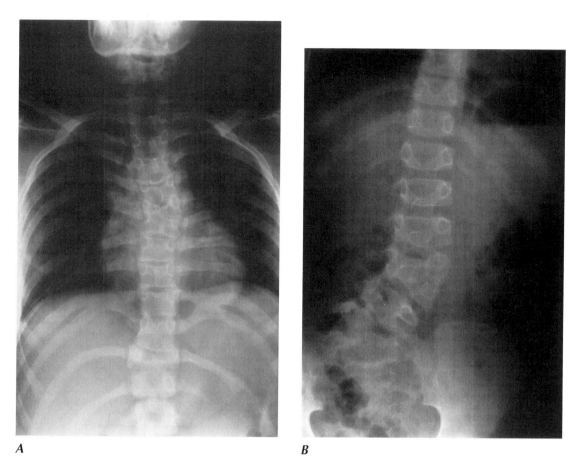

A   *B*

Figure 8.18   Congenital scoliosis. *A.* Congenital spinal abnormalities and
   fused ribs, causing insignificant scoliosis. *B.* Lumbar vertebral anomalies
   causing scoliosis, with imbalance of the trunk.

cord, are suggested by the presence of a hairy patch, a hemangioma, or a dermal sinus overlying the spine. Neurologic deficits associated with spinal dysrhaphism may be subtle and progressive.

It is important to obtain high-quality anteroposterior (AP) and lateral radiographs of the spine to identify specific abnormalities and to quantify the magnitude of the deformity in both sagittal and frontal planes. In very young children, incomplete ossification of the vertebrae often makes it difficult to delineate the pathoanatomy. Failure of separation in the form of a cartilaginous bar may lead to rapidly progressive deformity, yet no bar is visible on routine radiographs. Progression of the deformity is best assessed by serial radiographs at 6- to 12-month intervals.

Curves that are small and nonprogressive do not require treatment. The risk of progression of the deformity is highly dependent on the specific vertebral anomalies. For most patients, the most appropriate initial management is serial radiographs, watching closely for progression. Treatment is usually necessary for progressive deformities, particularly if skeletal growth remains. A unilateral, unsegmented bar opposite hemivertebrae is virtually certain to result in progressive deformity. It is appropriate to proceed directly with surgical treatment if this constellation of anomalies is present in a skeletally immature patient. Surgery should also not be delayed for a physically immature patient who, when initially evaluated, already has a curve of 40° or more and a clinical history of developing deformity.

Surgical treatment usually entails fusion of the affected area, without correction of existing deformity, to prevent worsening of the curve. Surgical risks and technical difficulties are greatly increased by attempts to correct existing deformities. Even in a very young child, early fusion is preferable to waiting until the child is older and has more marked deformity. Bracing, often used in treating idiopathic or neuromuscular scoliosis, has little role in the management of congenital deformities of the spine.

Idiopathic Scoliosis

Idiopathic scoliosis is the most common cause of spinal curvature, yet the diagnosis is largely one of exclusion. Extensive investigations for abnormalities of proprioception, motor control, biomechanics, connective tissue, and genetics have shown a familial predisposition but revealed no definitive causative factors. The diagnosis of idiopathic scoliosis depends upon recognizing the distinctive clinical appearance and ruling out other causes of spinal curvature.

The deformity of idiopathic scoliosis is three-dimensional. Lateral curvature is accompanied by changes in the normal kyphosis and lordosis of the spine. These changes reflect the spinal rotation that occurs with this entity and are responsible for the findings of shoulder asymmetry and rib prominence sought on scoliosis screening examinations (Fig. 8.19). Idiopathic scoliosis is classically divided into three groups that are determined by age at the onset of deformity.

Infantile idiopathic scoliosis occurs prior to 3 years of age and has an 85 percent likelihood of spontaneous resolution. Patients who do not get better on their own require prolonged orthotic treatment and, in the "progressive" type, may need surgical intervention. In many cases, bracing will not eliminate the need for surgery but may delay it sufficiently to allow spinal fusion to be performed closer to skeletal maturity, thereby increasing the patient's height and decreasing the risk of postoperative recurrence.

Juvenile idiopathic scoliosis becomes manifest after 3 years of age but prior to puberty. Its treatment is similar to that of the infantile form, with bracing for curves greater than 20° to avoid or delay the need for spinal fusion. Recent investigations have disclosed a higher percentage of intraspinal pathology (e.g., syringomyelia and diastematomyelia) in this patient population, necessitating a careful physical examination for any signs of neurologic impairment or structural abnormalities.

Adolescent idiopathic scoliosis is by far the most common form of spinal deformity. It begins at the onset of puberty and usually has a right thoracic component to the curve. There may be variable left or right, lumbar or thoracic curves in addition (Fig. 8.20), but isolated left thoracic curves are extremely un-

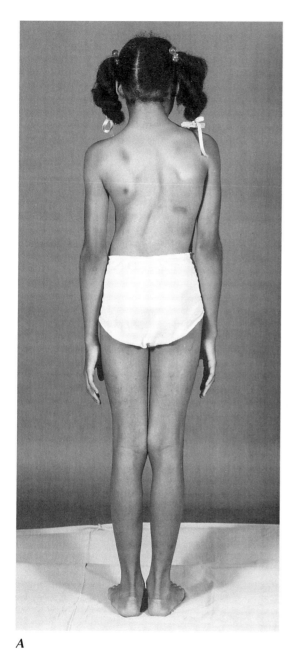

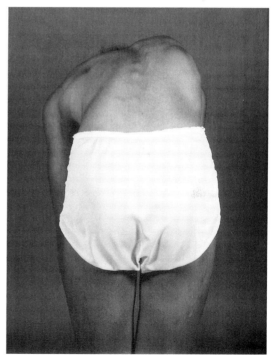

A   *B*

Figure 8.19   Idiopathic scoliosis. Note *(A)* the typical right thoracic curve
   and *(B)* the posterior prominence of the right rib cage (produced by
   vertebral rotation) with forward bending.

usual and should arouse suspicion of an underlying cause, such as syringomyelia.

School screening programs have increased our understanding of the incidence and natural history of idiopathic scoliosis. Although the incidence is nearly equal for each gender, with a female-to-male ratio of 1.5 to 1, girls are eight times more likely to have a progressive curve that requires treatment. The reasons for this discrepancy are unclear. What is clear is that many treatment modalities in the past have shown no impact on the natural history of idiopathic scoliosis. Exercises, electrical stimulation and stretching have no documented efficacy in the prevention of curve progression.

Bracing and surgery are the only effective treatment modalities for idiopathic scoliosis. A curve of greater than 20° or less than 40° may be considered for bracing, although studies indicate that bracing influences curve progression in only 20 percent of these patients. Most progression occurs prior to skeletal maturity, but curves of greater than 50° tend to increase at a rate of 1° per year, even after maturity. To prevent increasing deformity and morbidity, spinal fusion is usually indicated in these patients.

Spondylolisthesis

The slippage of one vertebral body relative to the subjacent body is known as *spondylolisthesis.* Many conditions lead to this disorder, including congenital, isthmic, traumatic, degenerative, and pathologic causes. The degenerative form is common in the elderly (see Chap. 14). In children, the most common type is *isthmic spondylolisthesis,* which stems from a defect *(spondylolysis)* in the *pars interarticularis,* the segment of bone connecting the pedicle and superior facet to the lamina and inferior facet (Fig. 8.21). Isthmic spondylolisthesis tends to develop insidiously; in contrast, *traumatic spondylolisthesis* results from a discrete, violent incident, and the injury often involves multiple bony elements. Isthmic spondylolisthesis is sometimes diagnosed acutely after an injury, but it is difficult to prove that the patient did not already have an asymptomatic spondylolysis, which is relatively common in the general population and present in approximately 5 percent of all children. Isthmic spondylolisthesis should also be distinguished from the rare *congenital* (or *dysplastic*) *spondylolisthesis,* which is associated with congenital inadequacy of the disk and

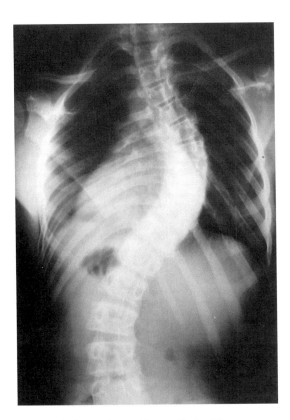

Figure 8.20 Idiopathic scoliosis. The curve is decompensated, which occurs when the compensatory upper and lower curves fail to balance the primary thoracic curve.

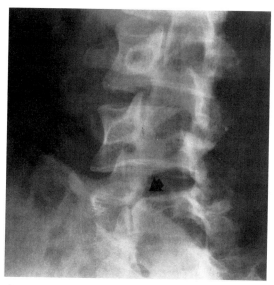

A

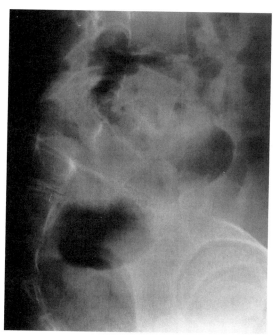

B

Figure 8.21   Spondylolisthesis. *A.* Defect in the pars interarticularis, seen on the oblique view *(arrow). B.* Marked spondylolisthesis of L5 on S1.

facet joints without a defect in the pars interarticularis.

The cause of isthmic spondylolisthesis is not known. Autopsies of infants who expire in the perinatal period have failed to show defects in the pars interarticularis, which therefore must develop sometime during childhood. Many believe that it is a stress fracture of the pars interarticularis that fails to unite, perhaps resulting from a congenital defect in the cartilage anlage. The stress on the pars is maximal in the lordotic lower lumbar segments; as a result, isthmic spondylolisthesis is most common in the L5 vertebra. Athletes who hyperextend the spine, such as gymnasts, offensive linemen in football, and butterfly swimmers seem especially prone to develop spondylolisthesis.

The degree of displacement of the vertebral body can vary from none to complete displacement. Most children are asymptomatic and never come to medical attention. Symptomatic patients usually complain of mild low backache, but in advanced cases patients may develop severe pain, deformity, and limitation of motion. Pain may radiate into the buttocks and thighs, and sciatica occasionally occurs. On examination, the lumbar lordosis is exaggerated and flexion of the spine is limited. Hamstring spasm is another hallmark of the disorder and can be demonstrated by the straight leg–raising test (Fig. 14.5). In severe cases, the torso is shortened, with skin creases between the rib cage and the pelvis. Oblique radiographs of the lumbar spine show the defect in the pars interarticularis most clearly. The lateral view shows the amount of displacement (Fig. 8.21).

Most patients respond to nonoperative treatment, consisting of limitation of activities, stretching exercises for the back and hamstrings, and analgesics. Orthotic support for the lumbosacral spine provides symptomatic relief for some patients. Patients with significant slippage should be closely monitored by an orthopaedist for further displacement during growth, especially if they are engaged in strenuous activities. Occasionally, surgical intervention is required for intractable pain.

Upper Limb

Sprengel Deformity

Sprengel deformity, or congenital elevation (or, more correctly, failure of descent) of the scapula, is caused by incomplete caudal migration of the scapula early in embryonic development (Fig. 8.22). The faulty development usually includes a small scapula and absent, hypoplastic, or fibrotic periscapular muscles.

Sprengel deformity is usually unilateral, sporadic, and nonfamilial. Over half of affected individuals have one or more associated anomalies, most commonly in the cervical spine, thoracic spine, or rib cage, producing deformities such as Klippel-Feil syndrome, congenital scoliosis, cervical ribs, and fused or absent ribs. Other associated anomalies include cleft palate, renal anomalies, diastematomyelia, and congenital heart disease.

Clinical concerns are primarily cosmetic (prominence of the scapula and shoulder asymmetry) and functional (restriction of shoulder motion, particularly abduction). Normal shoulder abduction involves smoothly coordinated glenohumeral and scapulothoracic movement in a ratio of roughly 1° of scapular rotation for every 2° of glenohumeral abduction. In Sprengel deformity, an abnormal cartilaginous or bony connection, the *omovertebral bone,* tethers the superomedial corner of the scapula to the posterior elements of the lower cervical spine. The omovertebral bone, present in 30 to 40 percent of patients, restricts

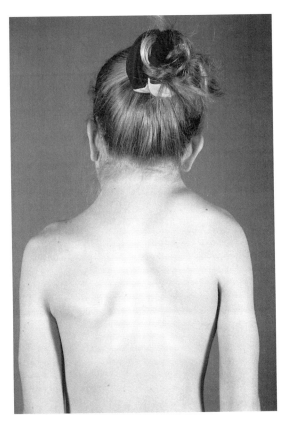

Figure 8.22   Sprengel deformity. Note the failure of descent of the right scapula.

the scapulothoracic component of shoulder motion. In addition, the affected scapula is typically smaller and malrotated as well as elevated. Rotation of the inferomedial corner of the scapula toward the midline orients the glenoid inferiorly and thereby decreases the glenohumeral component of shoulder abduction.

Surgery is the only effective treatment. With minimal degrees of deformity, cosmetic and functional concerns generally are not sufficient to warrant surgical treatment. In more marked cases, surgical correction consists of repositioning the scapula more caudally with simultaneous correction of the malrotation. Typically such surgery is done between 3 and 8 years of age.

Congenital Pseudarthrosis of the Clavicle

Congenital pseudarthrosis of the clavicle is an anomaly consisting of atrophy or absence of the central third of the clavicle (Fig. 8.23). The defect is usually present at birth, and the associated deformity tends to be progressive. The disorder usually involves the right side, but up to 10 percent are bilateral, and there are sporadic reports of involvement only on the left side. Typically the condition occurs without associated anomalies.

The etiology of congenital pseudarthrosis of the clavicle is uncertain. Reports of familial involvement suggest that the condition is inherited through a Mendelian recessive pattern. Alternatively, the condition may develop because separate ossification centers fail to coalesce. The most popular theory is that pulsations of the subclavian artery inhibit development of the central third of the clavicle. The right subclavian artery is more superiorly located and in closer proximity to the central third of the clavicle than the left.

The primary clinical problem with congenital pseudarthrosis of the clavicle is cosmesis. Bulbous ends of the clavicle at the pseudarthrosis produce a visible prominence. The shoulder on the affected side is lower, positioned more anteriorly, and closer to the midline than that of the contralateral side. Mild to moderate discomfort may result in functional limitations. The defect in the central third of the clavicle is apparent on plain radiographs and most easily distinguished from a fracture by the absence of callus.

Although the consequences of the condition are not serious, the recommended treatment is usually surgical repair with a bone graft and internal fixation between 3 and 6 years of age. If done later, restoration of symmetry is less complete.

Congenital Dislocation of the Radial Head

Congenital dislocation of the radial head occurs both in isolation and in association with other anomalies. The associated anomalies may be limited to the same limb, such as a radioulnar synostosis or radial ray defect, or may be part of a broader condition, such as the nail-patella syndrome or arthrogryposis. The radial head can be dislocated anteriorly, laterally, or, most often, posteriorly (Fig. 8.24). One or both sides may be involved.

Despite the dislocation, motion is surprisingly good, with loss of supination being the most significant deficit. The condition is often

Figure 8.23 Congenital pseudarthrosis of the clavicle. Note the defect in the midportion of the right clavicle with smooth, bulbous ends, which distinguishes congenital pseudarthrosis from a fracture.

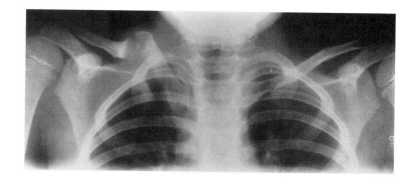

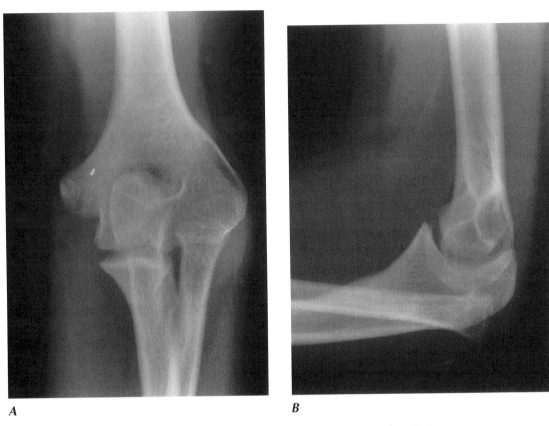

A   *B*

Figure 8.24 Congenital posterior dislocation of the radial head. The radial head, which normally points toward the capitellum on all projections, is posterior to the capitellum on the lateral view (see also Fig. 8.25).

not recognized for several years, owing to minimal functional limitations. When it is diagnosed late, the question often arises as to whether the dislocation is congenital or acquired. Associated anomalies, bilateral dislocations, a family history of congenital anomalies of the upper limb, and the absence of significant trauma suggest congenital dislocation. Radiographic findings that distinguish congenital dislocation include hypoplasia of the capitellum, an ulna that is short proximally and long distally relative to the radius,

and a dome-shaped deformity of the radial head.

Patients generally do not benefit from surgery aimed at reducing the dislocation. Treatment is excision of the radial head for adults who find the prominence cosmetically objectionable or who have significant discomfort. Motion is usually not improved by surgery. Removal of the radial head should be delayed until after skeletal maturity; otherwise, continued growth of the radius may cause recurrent symptoms.

Congenital Radioulnar Synostosis

Normally, by 6 weeks of gestation, the cartilaginous anlage of the radius and ulna have separated. Failure to separate completely results in the uncommon anomaly of radioulnar synostosis (Fig. 8.25). Typically the synostosis is located proximally and is bilateral. Occasionally the condition is familial, with an autosomal dominant inheritance pattern. The most commonly associated anomaly is ipsilateral dislocation of the radial head.

The shoulder can compensate to a remarkable degree for the loss of forearm rotation, especially pronation. For this reason, the restriction of motion is often unrecognized until school age. In most cases the forearm is fixed

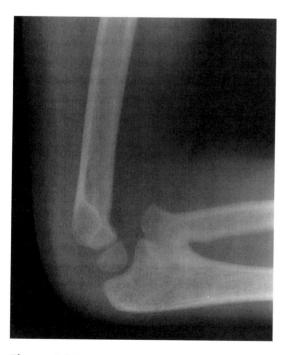

Figure 8.25   Congenital radioulnar synostosis. Note the association with congenital anterior dislocation of the radial head.

in pronation. There is relatively little functional limitation unless the condition is bilateral and both sides are in marked pronation. Therefore, for most affected individuals, treatment is unnecessary. Poor results commonly follow attempts to separate the radius and ulna, owing to reformation of the bony connection. If treatment is needed for marked malposition of the forearm, a rotational osteotomy that leaves the bones united but more functionally positioned is the procedure of choice.

Madelung Deformity

Madelung deformity is a congenital disorder characterized by diminished growth of the ulnar and volar portion of the distal radial physis (Fig. 8.26). This growth abnormality leads slowly to shortening and dorsoradial bowing of the radius. The ulna is relatively long, resulting in dorsal subluxation and prominence of the head of the ulna. Although the disorder is congenital, Madelung deformity generally does not become clinically apparent until the child is 8 or 9 years old. The cause of the abnormal growth pattern is unknown. The condition is typically transmitted as an autosomal dominant trait and both forearms are usually affected. It is sometimes found in association with other orthopaedic anomalies, such as scoliosis, or as part of generalized conditions, such as Hurler mucopolysaccharidosis or Turner syndrome. Slight restriction of motion and discomfort are common, but in most cases surgical treatment is unnecessary. The surgical approach depends upon the degree of deformity and the amount of growth remaining.

Trigger Digits

Trigger digits in infants are similar to those in adults. One difference, however, is that in infants the thumb is much more commonly af-

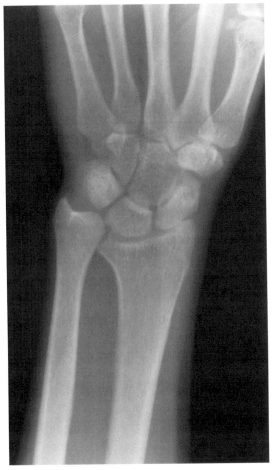

A

Figure 8.26 Madelung's deformity. Note *(A)* the deformity of the distal radius and *(B)* the dorsal subluxation of the distal ulna.

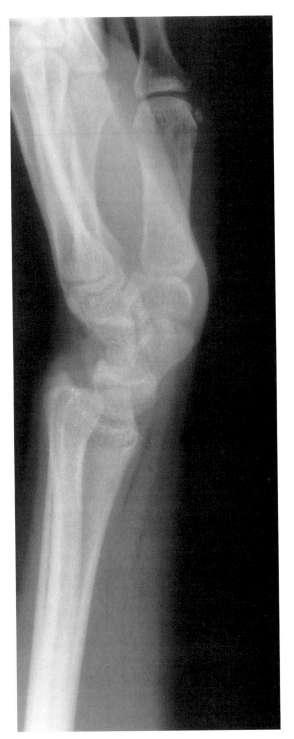

B

fected than the fingers. Approximately one-fourth of the cases are diagnosed at birth. In the remainder, the condition is either absent or not noted until as late as 6 or 7 years. Typically the condition occurs spontaneously, with a negative family history and no associated anomalies. Roughly one in four cases is bilateral.

The most common presentation is that of a fixed flexion deformity of the interphalangeal (IP) joint of the thumb. Less commonly, clicking or snapping is noted with movement, or there is fixed extension of the IP joint. The condition results from restricted movement of the flexor tendon through the pulleys or "tunnels" in which it lies. Most commonly the A-1 pulley near the metacarpophalangeal (MCP) joint is affected. The pulley may be constricted, the tendon may be enlarged by a nodule (often palpable), or both structures may be involved.

Congenital trigger digits noted at birth have a 30 percent chance of spontaneous resolution. Those that develop or are not recognized until after 6 months of age resolve without surgery in roughly 10 percent of patients. Trigger digits that disappear spontaneously or undergo surgical release before 3 to 4 years of age typically have no residual stiffness or other sequelae. Surgical release of the pulley is a relatively simple procedure with excellent results and should be recommended when the disorder persists beyond the age of 3. Splinting is probably not effective.

Hypoplastic Thumb

Hypoplasia of the thumb is variable in extent, ranging from complete absence to mild, insignificant shortening (Fig. 8.27). The bones, joints, and intrinsic and extrinsic muscles of the thumb may be involved. The presence of

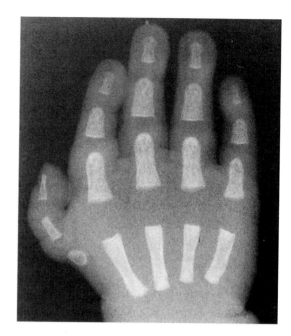

Figure 8.27 Hypoplastic thumb. Note the marked involvement of the first metacarpal.

a hypoplastic thumb mandates a careful search for associated ipsilateral limb as well as cardiovascular, gastrointestinal, vertebral, or other anomalies. The condition is also found in association with many syndromes for which evaluation by a geneticist may be warranted.

Treatment must be tailored to the specific clinical situation and focused on improving function. Simple shortening of the digit is rarely of sufficient functional significance to warrant treatment. Tendon transfer, joint stabilization, widening of the web space, and pollicization of the index finger are operative procedures used to address these deficiencies.

Congenital Clasped Thumb

Clasped thumb describes a position of fixed thumb adduction, usually with flexion of the metacarpophalangeal and interphalangeal joints (Fig. 8.28). A normal neonate typically postures the hand with the thumb in the palm, but spontaneous active extension of the thumb is present, and by 3 to 4 months of age, the thumb is no longer clasped. Congenital clasped thumb is usually bilateral and twice as common in males, suggesting a sex-linked recessive inheritance pattern. Associated anomalies are rare, the most common being clubfoot. Congenital clasped thumb is quite

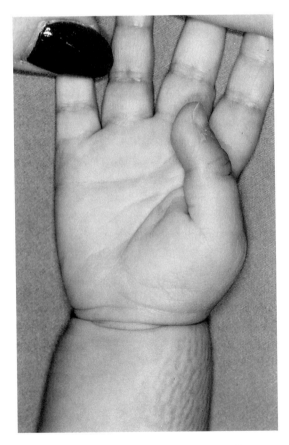

Figure 8.28 Congenital clasped thumb. Note the limited extension.

different from the thumb-in-palm posture of children with severe cerebral palsy. The two conditions are easily distinguished, since other manifestations of cerebral palsy are usually obvious.

The underlying pathoanatomy of congenital clasped thumb is variable. In most patients, there is hypoplasia or absence of the extensor pollicis brevis; occasionally, the extensor pollicis longus may also be deficient. The anomalous extensor tendons are sometimes associated with joint contractures and abnormalities of the flexor tendons. Rarely, the clasped thumb is hypoplastic and better grouped with congenital hypoplasia of the thumb. During the first 6 months of life, splinting the thumb in extension usually yields good results. Protecting the deficient thumb extensors from more powerful thumb flexors allows the extensors to develop and function adequately; however, splinting may be necessary for up to 6 months. If casting or splinting during the first year of life is inadequate, one should assume that the thumb extensors are absent or severely hypoplastic and proceed with surgical reconstruction.

Camptodactyly

Camptodactyly means "bent finger" and refers to a flexion deformity, typically of the proximal interphalangeal (PIP) joint of the little finger (Fig. 8.29). Camptodactyly usually develops during infancy, but there is a rare type in which the deformity develops during adolescence. It sometimes occurs spontaneously; at other times, there is an autosomal dominant inheritance pattern. Males and females are equally affected, and roughly 70 percent of cases are bilateral. Unilateral cases usually involve the right side. Isolated camptodactyly

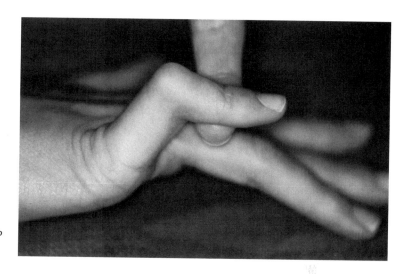

Figure 8.29
Camptodactyly. Note the flexion contracture of the PIP joint in the little finger.

must be distinguished from curved digits caused by trauma, arthrogryposis, congenital absence of extensor tendons, and Dupuytren contracture. Camptodactyly also occurs in association with many syndromes, including trisomy 13. The degree of deformity usually worsens with growth, particularly during infancy and adolescence, when growth is most rapid. Typically, progression ceases with completion of skeletal growth. Flexion deformity of the PIP joint rarely impairs function, owing in great part to compensatory hyperextension of the metacarpophalangeal (MCP) joint. Splinting can improve mild deformities and prevent progression. Surgical treatment should be considered if and when functional impairment warrants. Since multiple structures may be involved in the deformity, surgical treatment must be individualized according to underlying pathoanatomy.

Clinodactyly

Clinodactyly is angular deformity of the finger, but, in contrast to camptodactyly, clino-

dactyly involves angulation in the mediolateral plane. Most commonly the deformity involves ulnar angulation of both little fingers at the distal interphalangeal (DIP) joint (Fig. 8.30). The condition is part of numerous syndromes, including Down syndrome, in which an association of 40 percent has been reported. The condition occurs sporadically, but more commonly it is inherited as an autosomal dominant trait with variable penetrance. Seldom is there significant functional impairment, even with considerable angulation. Treatment is therefore warranted primarily for cosmetic improvement. It is difficult to splint this deformity in small children, nor is it of proven benefit. Surgical correction, particularly if done for cosmetic reasons, is best undertaken at or near skeletal maturity.

Polydactyly

Polydactyly, duplication of all or part of a digit, is one of the most common congenital musculoskeletal anomalies. The extent of duplication is wide ranging, from a small, soft

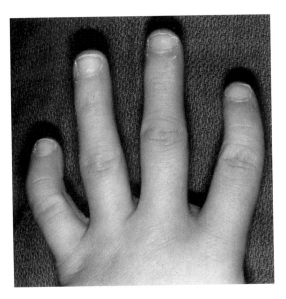

Figure 8.30   Clinodactyly. Note the angular deformity of both the little and index fingers.

tissue mass to complete duplication of a digit, including the metacarpal (Fig. 8.31). Postaxial polydactyly (duplication on the ulnar side of the hand) is the most common form. In blacks, who are affected 10 times more frequently than whites, the condition is inherited as an autosomal dominant trait with variable penetrance and usually occurs without associated anomalies. Preaxial polydactyly (duplication of the thumb) is most often an isolated, unilateral anomaly that occurs spontaneously. Central polydactyly is less common, usually bilateral, inherited as an autosomal dominant trait, and frequently associated with complex syndactyly.

Function and cosmesis are likely to be significantly improved by surgery in most patients with polydactyly. If the duplication involves only hypoplastic soft tissues with no skeletal connection, amputation can easily be accomplished in the neonatal period. With more extensive and complicated duplications, reconstruction is technically more demanding and better delayed until the child is between 6 months and 3 years of age.

Syndactyly

The term *syndactyly* refers to failure of separation of adjacent fingers or toes. It is described as complete or incomplete and as simple or complex. In complete syndactyly, the connection between digits extends to the tips.

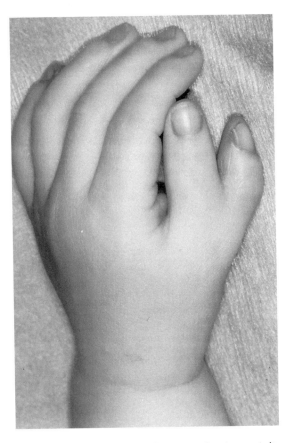

Figure 8.31   Polydactyly. Note the (preaxial) duplication of the thumb.

With incomplete syndactyly, the digits are separate for at least part of their length. Simple syndactyly involves only the soft tissues, whereas in complex syndactyly, bony elements are included in the fusion. The clinical significance of syndactyly ranges from mild webbing of the fingers that does not come to medical attention to the severe "mitten-hand" associated with Apert syndrome (Fig. 8.8).

Syndactyly is bilateral in roughly half of the patients and, when so, is usually symmetrical. It most often occurs sporadically, although familial involvement is seen. Males are predilected in a ratio of approximately 2 to 1. Most affected individuals do not have other anomalies, although associated defects, such as cranial synostoses, congenital constriction bands, and other mesodermal, ectodermal, and endodermal anomalies have been reported.

Surgical treatment is indicated for all but those patients with minimal functional or cosmetic concerns, and each surgical procedure must be carefully individualized. Anatomically conjoined neural or vascular structures may limit the extent of separation that can be accomplished. The timing of surgery depends upon the specific anomaly and the presence of associated problems, but it is usually performed between the ages of 3 months and 3 years. Treatment is begun earlier in patients who will require staged surgical procedures or when the syndactyly involves the borders of the hand (thumb and index or ring and little fingers). In these cases functional impairment may be significant, and the relatively large difference in the normal length of the fused digits causes additional problems with growth.

Congenital Constriction Bands

The anomalies associated with congenital constriction bands are varied and usually multiple, making it appropriate to consider this condition as a syndrome. Annular constricting rings typically involve two or more limbs and are more common distally than proximally, with the digits most frequently affected. The index and long fingers are involved most often, with the thumb least likely to be involved (Fig. 8.32). The condition is not familial.

The three primary manifestations of the syndrome are acrosyndactyly, annular constricting rings, and amputations. *Acrosyndactyly* is a peculiar form of syndactyly in which the digits are fused distally but separated proximally. These digits should be separated surgically in the first 6 months of life. Roughly 80 to 90 percent of patients with a congenital band have hand anomalies, and clubfoot is found in 20 to 30 percent of affected individuals, with or without an ipsilateral proximal constricting ring. The clinical consequences depend upon the depth of the ring. Shallow grooves usually cause no distal disturbances; deeper rings result in peripheral lymphedema and neurologic, vascular, or motor deficits. Surgical release of the constricting band is generally recommended for digits with distal abnormalities and may be required emergently for an infant with distal vascular insufficiency. In less severe cases, the surgery is done on an elective basis during the first year of life. *Amputations* are thought to be the result of a deep constricting ring in utero, as is acrosyndactyly, in which healing at the site of the band results in fusion of the digits distally. Amputations without associated abnormalities are less likely to benefit from surgical treatment.

Lower Limb

Many disorders of the lower limb that are present at birth are not apparent at that time.

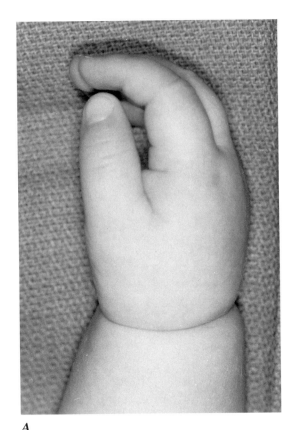

A

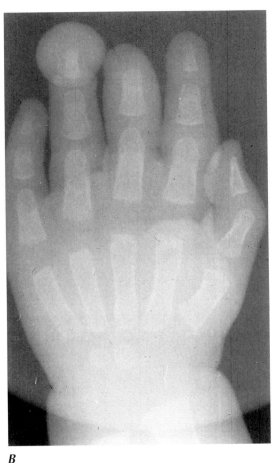

B

Figure 8.32   Congenital constriction bands. *A.* Note the annular
constriction band at the wrist. *B.* Radiograph of another patient with
bulbous soft tissue swelling at the distal end of the ring finger and partial
amputation of the long finger caused by congenital constriction bands.

Certain deformities, such as polydactyly and
syndactyly, are obvious; others, however, especially those involving the hip, require considerable diagnostic skill and management to
avoid devastating consequences.

Developmental Dysplasia of the Hip

Developmental dysplasia of the hip (DDH) is
the currently accepted term for abnormalities
of the hip joint that, untreated, lead to faulty
development and disability. Included in this
heading are hips that are frankly dislocated at
birth, those that are unstable or dislocatable,
and those that appear normal but become dysplastic with growth.

Approximately 12 of every 1000 children
are born with instability of the hip. Of those
12, about 10 percent will have dislocated hips

at birth, and 10 percent more will have a hip that is dislocatable. Factors that greatly increase the likelihood of DDH include breech positioning, a family history of DDH, female gender, and being a firstborn child. Almost 3 percent of girls with a breech presentation have a dislocation of the hip at birth. Children with congenital foot deformities or torticollis also are at greater risk for DDH.

For the hip joint to develop normally, the femoral head must be centered in the acetabulum. The acetabular growth centers respond to the pressure of the femoral head by forming a spherical, congruent surface. Incongruent positioning during the first 4 years of growth leads to dysplasia and degenerative arthritis of the hip; therefore, early detection and remediation are imperative.

In 1936, Ortolani described the test for instability of the hip that bears his name. With gentle hip abduction and anterior translation, the dislocated hip may be felt to enter the acetabulum with a palpable "clunk" (positive *Ortolani sign*). This test is usually combined with the *Barlow maneuver* to confirm neonatal hip instability (Fig. 8.33). A child with a dislocated hip may also appear to have a leg-length discrepancy *(Galeazzi sign),* which is most obvious when both hips and knees are flexed, with the feet on the examining table. Practice is necessary to appreciate the clinical subtleties of hip instability. Not infrequently, children noted later to have unstable or dislocated hips were recorded as having "normal" neonatal examinations. Equivocal clinical findings require a combination of radiographs and ultrasound for resolution (Fig. 8.34).

Developmental dysplasia of the hip detected through newborn screening programs is followed by treatment with abduction and flexion of the hips; usually with a Pavlik harness (Fig. 8.35). Properly applied, this method is 85 per-

cent successful in achieving and maintaining reductions. If it fails, traction, closed reduction, or operative intervention may be necessary. Patients in whom the diagnosis is made late often require osteotomies of the femur and/or pelvis to position the hip properly for normal development.

Congenital Displacement of the Knee

Congenital displacement of the knee presents a spectrum of extension deformities from genu recurvatum, wherein the tibia can be passively hyperextended, to frank dislocation. More severe cases are regularly associated with other congenital abnormalities (e.g., DDH, clubfoot, or arthrogryposis) and require manipulation, traction, serial casting and, usually, operative intervention. The milder form (knee hyperextension) is far more common and usually responds to stretching. Rarely, serial splinting or casting in increasing flexion is needed.

Deficiencies of the Limbs

Deficiencies of the limbs occur between the fourth gestational week, when the origins of the limb buds are detectable, and the seventh week, by which time the embryonic skeleton is well formed. It is less clear whether these abnormalities result from arrested development of the embryonic limb or a destructive process. Congenital deficiencies of the limbs are broadly classified as *terminal,* wherein all parts of the limb distal to a certain point are affected, or *intercalary,* in which there is normal distal anatomy but a deficient intervening segment. These two larger headings are subdivided into *transverse* and *longitudinal* deficiencies. With a transverse deficiency, the defect involves the entire width of the limb, whereas a longitudinal defect involves only the preaxial (tibial or radial) or postaxial (fibular

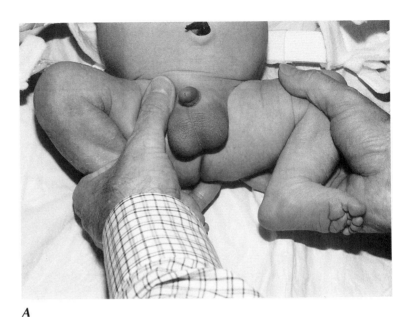

A

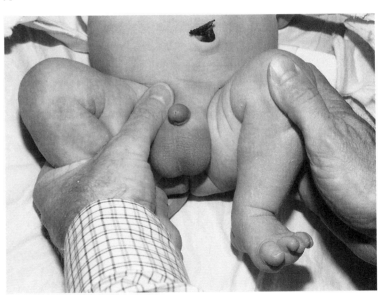

Figure 8.33   The Ortolani *(A)* and Barlow *(B)* tests for hip instability in DDH. Note that the pelvis is stabilized while these evocative tests for relocation (Ortolani) and hip dislocation (Barlow) of the hip are performed.

B

or ulnar) segments of the limb (Fig. 8.36). Terminal, transverse deficiencies (congenital amputations) are the most common deficiencies of the lower limb. They are treated in much the same way as traumatic amputations,

with appropriate stump care and prosthetic fitting.

FIBULAR HEMIMELIA   Fibular hemimelia is the most common longitudinal deficiency of

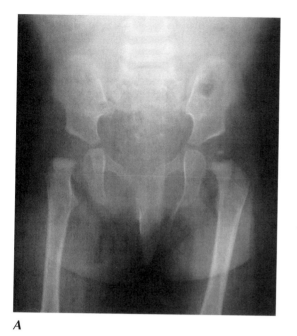

A

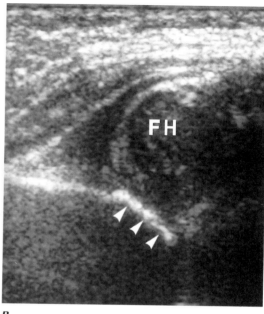

B

Figure 8.34   Imaging changes in DDH. Radiograph of the pelvis demonstrates *(A)* delayed ossification of the right femoral head in a child with DDH. Ultrasound of an unstable hip shows *(B)* subluxation of the femoral head (FH) from the acetabulum *(arrows)* with adduction of the hip and *(C)* improved position with abduction and flexion.

C

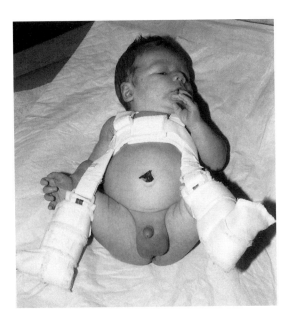

Figure 8.35 Developmental dysplasia of the hip. The Pavlik harness reduces the hip and maintains the femoral head within the acetabulum by the anterior straps holding the hip in flexion and the posterior straps preventing adduction.

the long bones. Although fibular deficiency is the most obvious abnormality, the entire limb is involved. The involvement is commonly unilateral (Fig. 8.37).

The foot may be normal in fibular hemimelia, but more typically there are deficiencies of the lateral rays of the foot and characteristic tibial defects, including shortening, antero-medial bowing and a deformed distal tibial physis. The femur may also be affected, with involvement ranging from minimal shortening to marked proximal femoral deficiency.

Numerous bony and soft tissue reconstructive procedures have been utilized to address the leg-length inequality, malalignment, insta-bility, and foot deformities associated with this

entity. The most satisfactory results, however, are frequently achieved by a Syme amputation of the foot and early prosthetic fitting.

TIBIAL HEMIMELIA   As with fibular hemimelia, tibial hemimelia involves more than the named bone. The knee is unstable, the foot an-gulated and deficient medially, and, in 20 per-cent of cases, the hip is dislocated. Both limbs are involved in nearly 30 percent of patients. The deformity is usually greater than that found with fibular hemimelia, and, although attempts have been made to salvage the limb by using the fibula as the primary weight-bear-ing bone of the limb, the failure rate is such that amputation and early prosthetic fitting is the preferred treatment.

CONGENITAL DEFICIENCIES OF THE FEMUR
Congenital deficiencies of the femur range from complete intercalary deficiency (congen-ital absence of the femur) to minimal hypopla-sia (congenitally short femur). For prognostic and therapeutic purposes, this disorder can be divided into three categories: *proximal femo-ral focal deficiency (PFFD), congenital coxa vara,* and *congenital short (bowed) femur.*

PFFD has four subclasses: Patients with class A deficiency have an adequate acetabu-lum and femoral head but no connection be-tween the shaft and head before maturity, by which time a pseudarthrosis has developed. In class B, no connection develops between the shaft and the head of the femur. Patients with class C deficiencies have no femoral head, and the acetabulum is markedly dysplastic, while in Class D there is no acetabulum or femoral head.

All classes of PFFD have severe shortening of the thigh, which is flexed, abducted, and externally rotated. The soft tissues about the

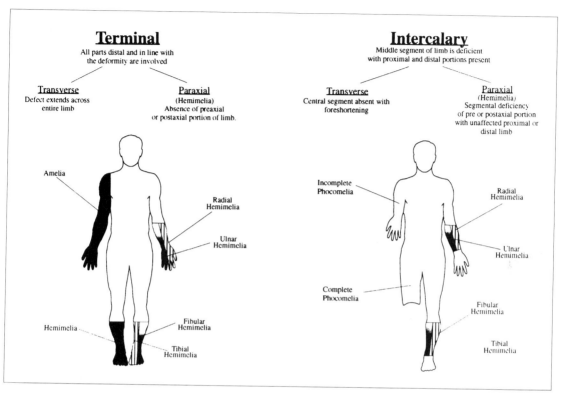

Figure 8.36 Nomenclature for congenital limb deficiencies.

upper thigh are bulky and taper, funnellike, toward the knee. One in eight patients has bilateral involvement, and 75 percent of patients have associated fibular hemimelia.

Treatment of PFFD usually involves fitting with an unconventional prosthesis. In patients with class A or B deformity, surgical stabilization of the proximal deficiency permits the ankle, which, because of profound shortening, is near the level of the contralateral knee, to substitute for the knee joint. Allowing the patient to ambulate as a below-knee amputee affords increased mobility and decreased expenditure of energy.

Congenital coxa vara is a decrease in the neck-shaft angle of the femur (Fig. 8.38). This rare deformity (1 in 25,000 live births) results from abnormal growth of the proximal femur. The proximal femur grows initially from a continuous physis that separates into trochanteric and cervical growth plates during the first postnatal year. Defective growth of the medial cervical physis allows relative overgrowth of its lateral counterpart, with tilting of the physis into a more vertical orientation. Although this abnormal angulation may be present at birth, it usually develops with growth, becoming apparent between the ages of 3 and 5 years. In many instances, this disorder is more a developmental than a congenital abnormality. Coxa

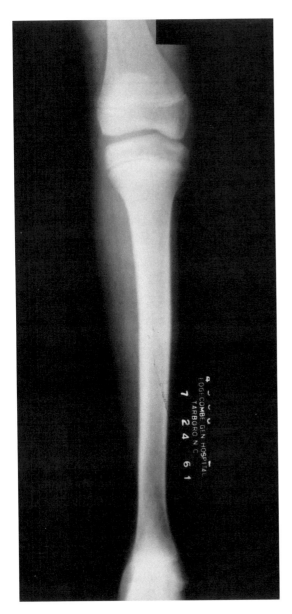

Figure 8.37 Fibular hemimelia. Note the complete absence of the fibula.

Radiographs reveal a neck-shaft angle of less than 120°, with increased vertical orientation of the cervical physis and proximal migration of the greater trochanter. There is usually a small triangular fragment of bone on the inferomedial aspect of the femoral neck. The most important radiographic measurement is *Hilgenreiner's epiphyseal angle,* which is formed by the intersection of a line parallel to the epiphyseal plate and Hilgenreiner's line, which is drawn horizontally through the triradiate cartilage of both hips (Fig. 8.39). This angle is less than 25° in normal hips, and an angle of less than 45° usually corrects spontaneously with growth. An angle over 60° predicts continued progression into varus, which warrants surgical intervention. The "gray zone" between 45 and 60° requires individualized treatment based on consideration of such mitigating factors as age, weight, severity of limp, neck-shaft angle, and progression of deformity. Congenital coxa vara can also be associated with a congenitally short or bowed femur, in which case the overall deformity is greater than that expected solely from the coxa vara.

The most common longitudinal deficiency of the femur is simple shortening, *congenitally short (bowed) femur,* which may be associated with inconsequential bowing of the femoral shaft that diminishes with growth. As with proximal femoral focal deficiency, the percentage of shortening of the femur relative to the unaffected side remains constant throughout growth and development, allowing prediction of eventual absolute discrepancy. This inequality is treated in the same manner as leg length discrepancies of other etiologies.

Congenital Pseudarthrosis of the Tibia

Congenital pseudarthrosis of the tibia with anterolateral bowing must be differentiated from

vara is usually diagnosed as a result of a limp or leg-length discrepancy. Additional clinical findings are decreased abduction and internal rotation of the hip.

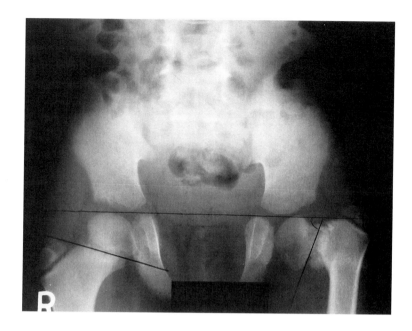

Figure 8.38   Congenital coxa vara. Note the decreased neck-shaft angle in the left femur. Lines indicate an increase in Hilgenreiner's epiphyseal angle (see Fig. 8.39).

the less ominous *posteromedial bowing* of the tibia and fibula. In the latter condition, approximately 50 percent of the initial angulation corrects spontaneously during the first 2 years of life, and surgical correction is rarely necessary. Associated with the bowing are a calcaneovalgus posture of the foot, minimal calf atrophy, tightness of the anterior musculature, and a leg-length discrepancy. The soft tissue components of the deformity are of no clinical

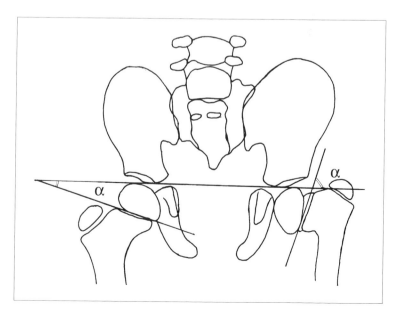

Figure 8.39   Hilgenreiner's epiphyseal angle (α). This angle is subtended by a line through the triradiate cartilages (the line of Hilgenreiner) and a line paralleling the physeal plate. In congenital coxa vara, a measurement of greater than 60° predicts continued progression into varus and necessitates surgical intervention.

concern and resolve with gentle stretching. The leg-length discrepancy, however, is progressive and may require surgical equalization. The final discrepancy is fairly predictable, since the percentage of shortening in the tibia remains constant. Thus, if the involved tibia is 85 percent as long as the uninvolved tibia when the child is first seen, it will also be 85 percent as long at skeletal maturity. Since the overall length of the tibia is greater at that time, the absolute value of the discrepancy will also be greater.

Bowing of the tibia in an anterolateral direction is potentially a more serious deformity, since it is often associated with pseudarthrosis of the tibia, which requires operative intervention and occasionally amputation (Fig. 8.40). Patients with this deformity are usually classified into one of four types, depending upon their clinical and radiographic appearance. Type I patients have anterolateral bowing with increased bone density but a normal medullary canal. They usually do not fracture or develop a pseudarthrosis and require surgery only if a leg length discrepancy develops. Type II patients have a sclerotic medullary canal initially but eventually fracture, requiring surgical intervention. Type III patients have associated cystic lesions that resemble fibrous dysplasia. They are more susceptible to early fracture and therefore require prophylactic operative treatment. Patients with type IV lesions have fractures, cysts, and pseudarthroses. Repair of the defect is extremely difficult, with high failure and reoperation rates. Multiple interventions—including electrical stimulation, bone grafting, vascularized bone transplantation, external fixation, and intramedullary fixation—have been used; but high complication and failure rates have led some to recommend early below-knee amputation. Most pseudar-

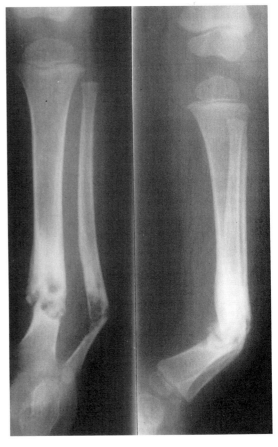

Figure 8.40   Congenital pseudarthrosis of the tibia. Note the anterior angulation, with both cystic and sclerotic changes at the pseudarthrosis site.

throses of the tibia are associated with neurofibromatosis, although neurofibromatotic tissue has rarely been found at the site of the pseudarthrosis. The cause of neither the bowing nor the pseudarthrosis is clear.

Clubfoot (Congenital Talipes Equinovarus)

Congenital clubfoot is one of the most common (1 per 1000 live births), widely discussed, and least well understood of all congenital musculoskeletal deformities. The deformities in clubfoot consist of plantar flexion of the foot and ankle (equinus); inversion (varus) of the heel, forefoot, and midfoot; and adduction of midfoot and forefoot. Most feet fall into one of two categories, those that are supple and manually correctable to normal alignment and those that are stiff and resistant to manipulative correction. The latter group is characterized by a transverse plantar crease in the midfoot, a smaller foot, and atrophy of the calf. These feet represent approximately 25 percent of patients seen with the deformity and are extremely resistant to stretching, taping, or casting. The more supple feet usually correct with early serial casting, while the resistant variety commonly require surgical intervention.

Flexible clubfeet are thought to be "postural," the result of intrauterine malposition. The etiology of resistant clubfeet is multifaceted, with ultrastructural abnormalities noted in muscles, ligaments, and tendons of the involved limb. A neurogenic causation, with sec-ondary muscle imbalance, has been posited, as has a primary germplasm defect that causes bony deformity and soft tissue contracture. The genetics of clubfeet appear to be multifactorial, with the incidence of clubfeet in children of affected parents being as high as 25 percent. Siblings of patients with clubfeet have a 3 percent chance of being similarly affected.

The pathologic anatomy of clubfoot involves medial and plantar dislocation of the navicula, cuboid, and calcaneus relative to the talus. This displacement can cause the navicula to abut the medial malleolus, while the calcaneus rotates medially and tilts into equinus under the talus (Fig. 8.41). These changes are reflected in radiographs of the foot, with parallelism of the talus and calcaneus on both AP and lateral radiographs (Fig. 8.42). The normal AP talocalcaneal angle is between 20 and 35°; on the lateral view, the angle should measure at least 25°. The structure of the bones themselves is also abnormal in congenital clubfoot, with shortening of the

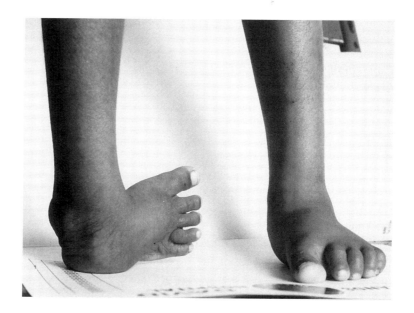

Figure 8.41 Untreated clubfoot. The midfoot and forefoot are displaced medially, with weight-bearing on the head of the talus.

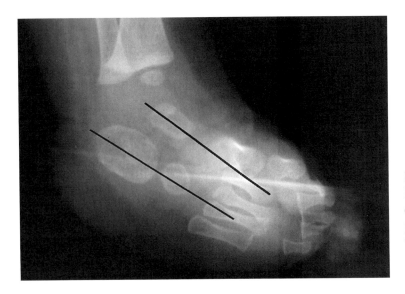

Figure 8.42 Clubfoot. The lateral radiograph demonstrates near parallelism of the talus and the calcaneus. The normal lateral talocalcaneal angle is 25 to 50°.

calcaneus, medial angulation of the talar neck, and a wedge- shaped navicula. Most of the abnormal bony architecture develops from the presence of persistent deforming forces in a patient with uncorrected deformity.

Surgical correction in the resistant clubfoot requires extensive release of contracted ligaments and joint capsules to reposition the involved bones.

Congenital Vertical Talus (Congenital Convex Pes Valgus)

Convex pes valgus deformity presents almost the opposite deformity of congenital clubfoot. In this entity, the talus is markedly plantar-flexed, with dorsal dislocation of the navicula on the talus. Tightness of the Achilles tendon and an equinus posture of the calcaneus give the foot a "rocker-bottom" appearance. The long axis of the talus is nearly collinear with the tibia, and the prominent talar head is palpable on the plantar aspect of the foot medially, producing an extremely rigid flatfoot that cannot be passively corrected. Congenital vertical talus is extremely rare as an isolated entity; more commonly it occurs in association with myelodysplasia, arthrogryposis, or other syndromes.

The radiographic appearance of congenital vertical talus is equally distinctive, with vertical orientation of the talus and an increase in the lateral talocalcaneal angle that does not correct with forced plantar flexion (Fig. 8.43).

Manipulation of the foot stretches contracted soft tissues but is inadequate definitive treatment for congenital vertical talus. Surgical release of soft tissue contractures and bony repositioning are mandatory. Lengthening of the Achilles tendon is required to position the foot properly; in selected cases, lengthening or transfer of other tendons may be indicated.

Congenital Metatarsus Varus (Metatarsus Adductus)

Metatarsus adductus is one of the most common referrals to pediatric orthopaedists. It consists of medial (varus) angulation and supination of the forefoot. The lateral border of the foot is convex, with normal alignment of the hindfoot. The vast majority of these feet cor-

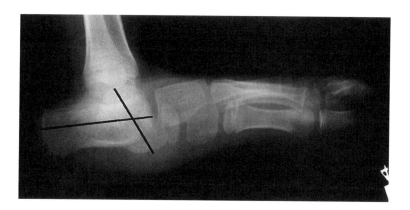

Figure 8.43 Congenital vertical talus. The lateral radiograph demonstrates near colinearity of the talus with the tibia and a marked increase in the lateral talocalcaneal angle (normal: 25 to 50°).

rect spontaneously if the deformity is passively correctable to neutral alignment or beyond. Unlike clubfeet, even resistant metatarsus adductus deformities can usually be corrected by manipulation, casting, or orthotic treatment. Surgical intervention is rarely considered prior to 4 years of age.

Calcaneovalgus Foot

One of the most dramatic clinical findings in the newborn is the calcaneovalgus foot. Intrauterine malpositioning causes profound ankle dorsiflexion, often such that the entire foot lies along the anterior aspect of the tibia. Fortunately, this is a flexible deformity that responds to gentle stretching. It is important to document active plantar flexion, since neurologic abnormalities, such as myelodysplasia, can cause similar posturing. The incidence of residual flatfootedness is increased in patients with marked calcaneovalgus deformities.

Polydactyly

Duplication of the toes is most common on the postaxial (fibular) side of the foot. It predilects blacks and females and is transmitted as an autosomal dominant trait. Supernumerary digits may be associated with other syndromes, making complete examination of the child mandatory. If osseous structures are duplicated, surgical excision is performed between 9 and 12 months of age for cosmesis and ease of shoe wear. A supernumerary digit consisting entirely of soft tissue can be removed by ligation in the nursery.

Syndactyly

Isolated confluence of the toes is of little functional or cosmetic significance. Surgical intervention is unnecessary unless the condition includes osseous or soft tissue deformity that compromises function.

Macrodactyly

Isolated hypertrophy of one or more toes is of such rarity that any involved child should be evaluated for neurofibromatosis or a soft tissue tumor. Surgical excision or reduction is indicated when the hypertrophied digit interferes with shoe fitting or weight-bearing or when the appearance is cosmetically unacceptable.

Congenital Curly Toe

This most common congenital deformity of the lesser toes consists of medial deviation, plantar flexion, and supination deformities (Fig. 8.44). The involvement is usually bilateral and symmetrical and has a familial pre-

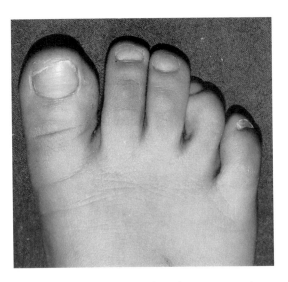

Figure 8.44 Congenital curly toe. Note the rotation and deviation of the phalanx. This anomaly occurs typically in the fourth toe.

disposition. Twenty-five percent improve spontaneously, and intervention is necessary only if abnormal pressure and callus formation interfere with function. Stretching and splinting do not help; surgical correction, if needed, is deferred until long after weight-bearing has begun.

Congenital Overriding of the Fifth Toe (Digitus Minimus Varus)

Congenital overriding of the fifth toe, like curly toe, is a common deformity with a familial predisposition that does not respond well to nonoperative treatment. The metatarsophalangeal joint is contracted dorsally with shortening of the extensor tendon. Shoe wear frequently causes painful callus formation on the dorsum of the fifth toe.

SUGGESTED READINGS

GREEN DP (ED): *Operative Hand Surgery,* 3d ed. New York, Churchill Livingstone, 1993.

McKUSICK VA: *Heritable Disorders of Connective Tissue,* 4th ed. St. Louis, Mosby, 1972.

MORRISSEY RT (ED): *Lovell and Winter's Pediatric Orthopaedics,* 3d ed. Philadelphia, Lippincott, 1990.

TACHDJIAN MO: *Pediatric Orthopedics,* 2d ed. Philadelphia, Saunders, 1990.

WENGER DR, RANG M: *The Art and Practice of Children's Orthopaedics.* New York, Raven Press, 1993.

Chapter *9*

Vascular and Epiphyseal Disorders

Edmund R. Campion and H. Robert Brashear

Bone is not the inert substance encountered in the laboratory skeleton; it is a dynamic, living tissue that constantly remodels and reorganizes in response to the physical and metabolic demands of the body. Bones are provided with an elaborate vascular system for access to their abundant mineral supplies, particularly calcium and phosphorus. The circulation nourishes the blood-forming elements of the marrow and maintains the cells that form bone (osteoblasts) and the cells that destroy it (osteoclasts).

VASCULARITY

The Blood Supply of Bone

There are four sources of blood vessels to a typical long bone: the nutrient artery, vessels that enter through the many small openings in the metaphysis, vessels that penetrate the epiphysis, and the periosteal vessels.

The *nutrient artery* enters a long bone through an oblique channel. The direction of the channel is determined by the relative amount of growth that has occurred at the proximal and distal ends of the bone. Nutrient channels are directed away from the faster-growing end of the bone and therefore slope away from the knee in the femur, tibia, and fibula and toward the elbow in the radius, ulna, and humerus. After reaching the medullary cavity, the nutrient artery divides, sending branches in proximal and distal directions. Some of these branches supply the marrow substance; others, coursing close to the endosteal surface, enter the cortex to supply the haversian systems of the inner two-thirds or more. Several major ascending and descending

branches continue in somewhat parallel alignment to the metaphysis. In the growing child, these vessels terminate at the metaphyseal side of the growth plate, where they participate in endochondral ossification. (Fig. 9.1).

The presence of the epiphyseal plate and the requirements of growth necessitate different patterns of circulation in the child and in the adult. As the terminal branches of the nutrient artery (augmented peripherally by the metaphyseal vessels) approach the growth plate, they branch repeatedly, maintaining a parallel relationship. When the vessels reach the growth plate, branches are so numerous that there is one vessel for nearly every column of cartilage cells. In the final few millimeters before the terminal arteriole reaches the cartilage, it is encased in a tube of enchondral bone. As the vessel extends to the last cartilage cell of the column, it makes an abrupt 180° turn to enter a larger venule. (It is here that slowing of the circulation may permit the lodgment and proliferation of bacteria, producing an early focus of hematogenous osteomyelitis.) The function of this extensive vascular supply on the metaphyseal side of the growth plate is to supply nutrition for the active cells involved in endochondral ossification.

Disruption of the nutrient artery in growing bone results in necrosis of part of the marrow and the inner portion of the cortex. (The anastomosing epiphyseal-metaphyseal collateral circulation present at maturity limits this necrosis in adults.) Loss of circulation in the terminal vessels of the nutrient artery of growing bone results in changes in the epiphyseal plate that interfere not with growth of the cartilage plate but with endochondral ossification. New cartilage continues to form, but it is not resorbed and replaced by bone. Thus, the growth plate becomes thicker until the metaphyseal

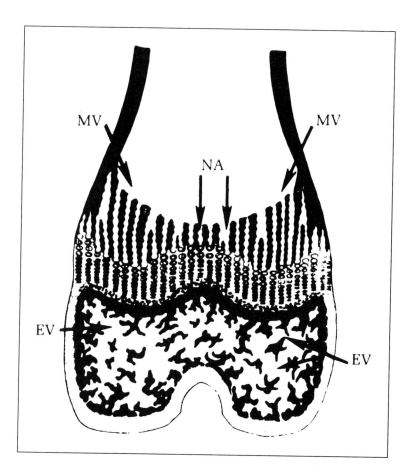

Figure 9.1   Blood supply to the epiphyseal plate. Vessels are derived from the nutrient artery (NA), metaphyseal vessels (MV), and epiphyseal vessels (EV).

circulation is restored, which usually occurs rapidly.

Examination of the metaphyseal portions of long bones reveals numerous small foramina through which pass vessels that enter the marrow cavity to anastomose with vessels derived from the nutrient artery. Most of these metaphyseal channels, however, contain veins that permit egress of blood from the marrow cavity.

Similar openings in the epiphysis permit the passage of vessels into and out of the ossification centers. In the growing child, these epiphyseal vessels are isolated from those of the rest of the bone, but with closure and obliteration of the cartilaginous growth plate, extensive anastomoses develop between the epiphyseal-metaphyseal vessels and the terminal branches of the nutrient artery.

Vessels that enter the epiphyseal ossification center send branches to bone underlying the articular cartilage, where, in the child, they participate in the slower-paced endochondral ossification by which the epiphysis enlarges. Other branches of these vessels reach the epiphyseal side of the growth plate and come to lie in small cavities among the resting cartilage cells of the plate. These vessels are extremely important, since they supply the dividing cells of the growth plate that provide longitudinal bone growth.

Obliteration of the epiphyseal blood supply results in necrosis of the epiphysis and deprives the deeper cartilage cells in the growth plate of their nutrition. Longitudinal growth ceases, and if collateral circulation is not restored, permanent closure of the epiphyseal plate occurs.

The fourth source of blood to the long bones is the vasculature of the periosteum. This extensive network of vessels covers the entire length of the shaft. During youth, while the periosteum is actively engaged in circumferential bone growth, the circulation in this area is much more abundant than it is during adulthood. Periosteal vessels send small branches through minute channels in the cortex to supply, at most, the outer third of the cortex. Loss of the periosteal circulation by stripping the periosteum from the shaft results in the death of osteocytes in the outer third of the cortex. This situation occurs in *scurvy,* when subperiosteal hemorrhage lifts the periosteum from the shaft, and in acute pyogenic infection, when pus elevates the periosteum.

There are certain areas of bone in which the vascular supply is precarious. The head of the femur, the scaphoid, and the body of the talus have a large portion of their surface covered with articular cartilage, which is impervious to blood vessels. Their blood supply enters through restricted spaces, with limited collateral circulation. These areas are subject to infarction when their principal route of circulation is interrupted by trauma or disease.

The venous drainage of bone is complex and less well understood than the arterial supply. The arterioles on the metaphyseal side of the growth plate, after making their hairpin turn, enter venules, which in turn open into larger venous sinusoids. These sinusoids empty into a large central vein that has a much greater capacity than the nutrient artery. Much of the outflow from bone is through the many venous channels in the metaphyseal-epiphyseal system.

The Physiology of Blood Flow to Bone

Study of the physiology of bone blood flow has been difficult because of the numerous vascular channels in bone and the several sources of its blood supply. Attempts to isolate the arterial and venous circulation of a single bone have required such extensive and precise dissection that a true physiologic condition for testing has not been obtainable. Indirect information from radioisotopic studies suggests that the rate of blood flow through bone is approximately 10 mL/min per 100 g of wet bone, including its marrow.

Pressure within the marrow cavity of the long bones varies with the systemic blood pressure and is in synchrony with respiration. The pressure in the diaphysis is much higher than in the epiphysis and is one-fourth to one-half the systemic blood pressure. Metaphyseal pressure is less than that in the diaphysis but greater than epiphyseal pressure. Muscular activity, by compressing the veins of the periosteum, causes a rise in marrow pressure and exerts a pumping effect on bone circulation.

Blood Supply in Healing and Repair

The details of fracture healing and bone repair are outlined in Chap. 13. Vascularity is a vital part of that process during each phase.

At the time of injury, vessels of the periosteum, marrow, cortex and surrounding soft tissues are disrupted, with consequent hemorrhage. It is largely the extent of vascular injury, rather than the fracture itself, that determines the ease with which a bone will heal. Extensive disruption makes the cleanup and repair phases of the healing process more difficult.

Vessels near the fracture site dilate, with an outpouring of exudate, polymorphonuclear cells, and macrophages that participate in the cleanup process. Fibrin strands within the clot act as a scaffold for vessel ingrowth. The adjacent bone, which has undergone varying amounts of necrosis, is resorbed by osteoclasts and cleared from the area along with soft-tissue debris. New vascular tissue begins to invade the fracture area within 48 h following injury. These vessels come mostly from surrounding soft tissues, with contributions from the marrow cavity. A consequent increase in blood flow is seen in the entire bone.

The repair phase is made possible by the influx of pluripotential cells into the fracture callus. These cells are capable of producing collagen, fibrous tissue, cartilage, and bone. The microcirculation of the callus and the resultant oxygen tension, pH, and accumulation of metabolites determine how well the fracture progresses toward union. Bones with abundant blood supply, such as the femur and clavicle, heal in a predictable manner, while those with more problematic circulation (tibial shaft, scaphoid, etc.) are more susceptible to nonunion.

Disorders of the Circulation to Bone

Appreciation of bone as a dynamic organ system rather than a static, structural scaffold explains how alterations in vascularity can lead to marked changes in growing bones as well as in the mature skeleton. In the femoral head, an interruption of blood supply results in *osteonecrosis (avascular necrosis)*.

Legg-Calvé-Perthes Disease

This idiopathic form of necrosis of the femoral head results from avascularity of the femoral head in a skeletally immature individual. It occurs in approximately 1 per 1500 children, with a male-to-female ratio of 4:1. Eighty percent of these patients are between the ages of 4 and 9, and 10 percent have bilateral involvement.

While the cause of the interruption of blood supply to the femoral head is unclear, it has become apparent that repeated insults are necessary to produce this distinctive picture in children. The progressive deformity of the femoral head and its associated clinical manifestations are caused not by interruption of the blood supply per se but rather by the resorption of necrotic bone that accompanies revascularization.

The pain and limp of Legg-Calvé-Perthes disease (LCPD) may be present for several months prior to medical consultation. The pain is frequently referred to the medial knee or thigh and is frequently associated with limited hip motion, particularly abduction and internal rotation.

Radiographic changes depend upon the stage of the disease. Initially, a smaller ossific nucleus and slight widening of the articular cartilage space may be the only findings. The patient is usually asymptomatic at this stage. Subsequently, a subchondral lucency is observed, which indicates a fracture through the subchondral bone weakened by the resorptive process. This finding, the *crescent sign* or *Caf-*

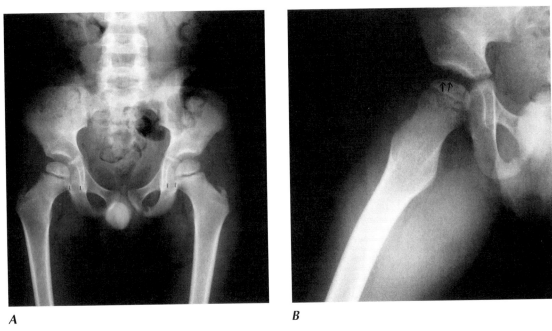

A   *B*

Figure 9.2 Legg-Calvé-Perthes disease (early). The AP view *(A)* has subtle changes with widening of the joint space on the right, while the lateral view *(B)* clearly demonstrates a "crescent sign" *(arrows),* indicative of subchondral fracture.

fey's sign, varies in extent with the degree of involvement of the femoral head (Fig. 9.2). Later radiographic changes include fragmentation of the epiphysis, loss of sphericity, partial extrusion of the femoral head from the acetabulum, and degenerative changes (Fig. 9.3).

Fifty percent of all femoral heads with LCPD heal spontaneously with no sequelae. The likelihood of a successful outcome is determined primarily by a younger age at onset, less extensive involvement of the femoral head, and the absence of lateral extrusion from the acetabulum. Children under 6 years of age have a good prognosis, while those over 9 at the start of their disease are more likely to have residual deformity and early arthrosis. In-volvement of less than 50 percent of the femoral head is a good prognostic sign and may be estimated either by the size of the crescent sign, or later by the amount of epiphyseal fragmentation.

Osteonecrosis in the Adult Hip

Osteonecrosis of the femoral head in adults can occur as an isolated finding, in conjunction with systemic disorders, or following fractures and dislocations of the hip joint (Fig. 9.4). Clinical conditions associated with osteonecrosis of the femoral head include Gaucher disease, alcoholism, hemoglobinopathies, corticosteroid use, dysbaric ischemia (the "bends"), and diabetes mellitus. The same

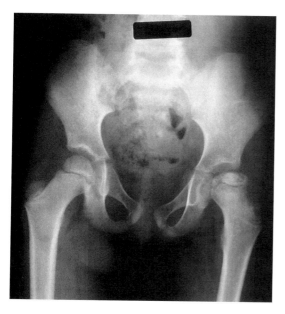

Figure 9.3   Legg-Calvé-Perthes disease (late). Note sclerosis, fragmentation, and collapse of the left capital femoral epiphysis.

clinical and radiographic picture, without known predisposing factors, is termed *adult idiopathic osteonecrosis.* There is experimental evidence that coalescence of endogenous lipoproteins and subsequent fat embolism play a causative role in the interruption of blood flow to the femoral head and may be the final common pathway for all nontraumatic osteonecroses. A tendency toward increased intraosseous pressure has also been documented in these patients.

Patients with osteonecrosis may be quite symptomatic, with pain and limp preceding changes on plain radiographs. In these stage I patients, a technetium bone scan or magnetic resonance imaging (MRI) may facilitate diagnosis (Fig. 9.5). Stage 0 has a negative MRI but a positive bone biopsy. Stage II osteonecrosis shows increased bone density on plain radiographs but no collapse or fracture, whereas stage III is marked by the crescent sign of subchondral fracture, and stage IV exhibits flattening of the femoral head. In stage

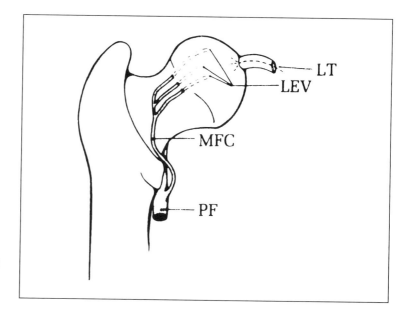

Figure 9.4   Vascular supply to the adult femoral head. There is a minor contribution through the ligamentum teres (LT); the major blood supply comes from the lateral epiphyseal vessels (LEV), which are terminal branches of the medial femoral circumflex artery (MFC) that arises from the profunda femoris artery (PF).

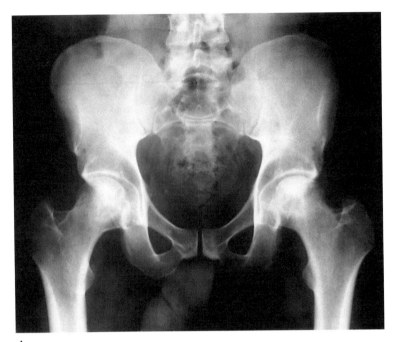

A

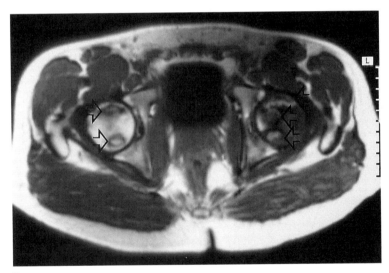

B

Figure 9.5 Avascular necrosis of the hips. *A.* Plain radiographs show changes in the femoral head on the left, with questionable involvement of the right (asymptomatic) hip. *B.* Magnetic resonance imaging reveals osteonecrosis also in the right hip (the "silent hip" of AVN).

V disease, there are degenerative changes in the acetabulum; advanced arthrosis is seen in stage VI disease.

The percentage of patients progressing from early (stages I and II) osteonecrosis to the more advanced stages has never been elucidated. It has therefore been difficult to evaluate the efficacy of treatment regimens. Drilling of the femoral head (to relieve intraosseous pressure and facilitate neovascularization), bone grafting, and vascularized bone transfer have been tried with inconsistent results.

Bone Infarct

Infarction of bone can also occur in the shafts of long bones, often in association with steroid use, sickle cell disease, Gaucher disease, or dysbaric phenomena *(Caisson disease),* which occurs when nitrogen bubbles formed in the bloodstream by rapid depressurization become entrapped in the marrow vessels. Bone infarcts can cause intense pain and, rarely, secondary malignancies in old marrow infarcts. Typically, however, bone infarcts have no long-term clinical consequences.

Kienböck Disease

Kienböck described osteonecrosis of the lunate in 1910, attributing its changes to avascularity of the bone. Despite the intervening decades, the cause of the vascular compromise is still unclear, although it has been associated with *ulnar minus variance,* in which the distal ulna is shorter than the adjacent radius. This disparity leads to increased loading of the lunate, with secondary vascular changes (Fig. 9.6). Equalizing the length of the two bones, either by shortening the radius or lengthening the ulna, often ameliorates the disease and prevents the development of degenerative arthritis.

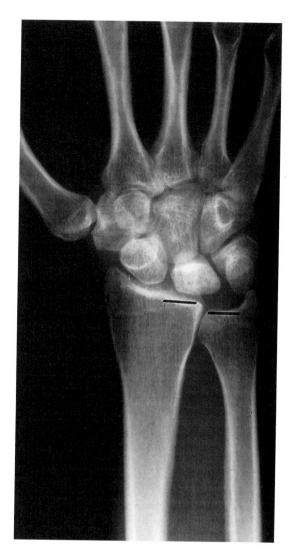

Figure 9.6 Kienböck disease. Note sclerosis of the lunate caused by osteonecrosis, with associated negative ulnar variance (shortening of the ulna relative to the radius).

Hypervascularity

Increased blood flow to bones is less often of clinical concern than diminished circulation. The most common manifestation of hypervascularity occurs in children following fracture of a long bone. The increased blood flow to the physes resulting from the healing process can induce permanent overgrowth of the entire limb, which is of greater clinical import in the lower than in the upper limbs. Stimulation of growth can also result from infection and arteriovenous fistulas, both of which increase blood flow to the affected bone. In the adult, Paget disease may increase the blood flow to involved bones to such an extent that cardiac output is significantly increased, occasionally to the point of cardiac failure.

DISORDERS ABOUT THE PHYSIS

A more detailed description of growth and development of the human skeleton is provided in Chap. 2. Here we will examine instances in which the normal process is somehow confounded. These disorders occur in the growth plate itself, in articular and epiphyseal cartilage, and at sites of nonarticular bone growth. When the normal process of growth is disturbed by an idiopathic alteration of enchondral ossification, it is termed an *osteochondrosis*.

Abnormalities of the Physis

Tibia Vara (Blount Disease)

Medial (varus) angulation of the tibia was first described by Erlacher in 1922 and further elu-

cidated by Blount in 1937. It is divided into infantile (early-onset) and late-onset forms of the disease, with late onset defined as from 4 years of age until skeletal maturity. In both forms the etiology is probably repetitive loading of a malaligned physis. The resultant shear, compressive, and distractive stresses lead to retarded growth of the medial physis, with subsequent angular deformity.

Infantile tibia vara is associated with internal tibial torsion; it occurs most frequently in

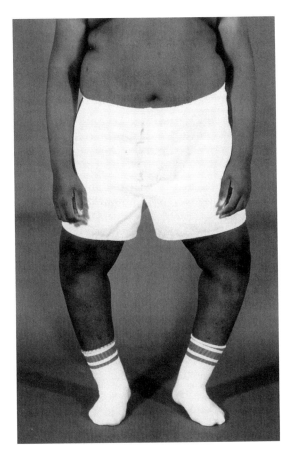

Figure 9.7 Late-onset tibia vara. This entity is seen most often in obese African American males.

African American girls who are early walkers (prior to 11 months of age). Late-onset tibia vara, however, does not commonly include tibial torsion and is seen most commonly in obese African American males (Fig. 9.7). The difficulty lies in differentiating Blount disease, which will progress to marked deformity, from physiologically bowed legs, which will straighten spontaneously. Clinical evaluation can be misleading, and radiographs are necessary for differentiation.

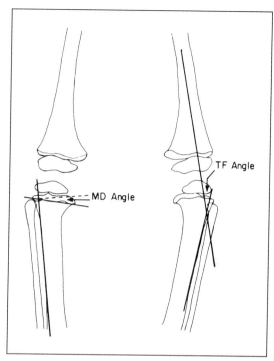

Figure 9.9   The metaphyseal-diaphyseal angle of Drennan (MD angle) is formed by a line across the proximal "beak" of the tibial metaphysis and a line perpendicular to the diaphysis. The tibiofemoral (TF) angle reflects the relative position of the tibial and femoral diaphyses.

In true Blount disease the deformity can progress from simple medial angulation of the physis to profound articular angulation and medial physeal growth arrest (Fig. 9.8). The most reliable early marker for Blount disease is the *metaphyseal-diaphyseal angle* of Drennan (Fig. 9.9). Angulation of more than 11° makes progression of the deformity very likely.

The efficacy of nonoperative treatment for tibia vara is controversial. Bracing may prevent progression in mild, infantile cases; how-

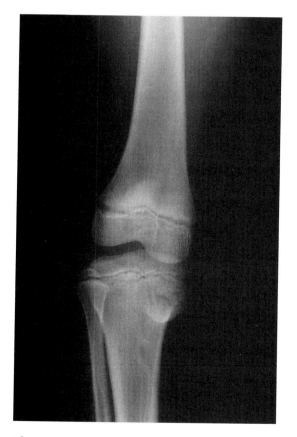

Figure 9.8   Idiopathic tibia vara. Note the changes in the medial tibial physis, with secondary valgus alignment of the distal femur.

ever, operative intervention is necessary to avoid progressive deformity in more severe or late onset patients.

Slipped Capital Femoral Epiphysis

Another disturbance of the physis caused by repetitive loading and shear stress is slipped capital femoral epiphysis (SCFE). In this entity, there is failure through the hypertrophic zone of the proximal femoral physis, with displacement of the femoral neck relative to the femoral head, which remains in the acetabulum.

Slipped capital femoral epiphysis occurs most commonly during the adolescent growth spurt. At that time the physis is widened, and the *perichondrial ring,* which accounts for 50 to 75 percent of physeal resistance to shear stress during childhood, becomes markedly thinner and less resilient. Obese adolescents are much more likely to develop SCFE, lending credence to the theory that slippage results from mechanical stress on a weakened physis.

This entity occurs most commonly in males and African Americans and, if radiographs are carefully examined, is bilateral in almost 50 percent of patients. When SCFE occurs outside of the normal adolescent growth spurt, an underlying endocrine abnormality should be suspected, since systemic processes—such as hyper- and hypothyroidism, hypoparathyroidism, excessive growth hormone or testosterone, and hypogonadism—also predispose to SCFE.

This most common of adolescent hip disorders is usually manifest by a painful limp that may have been present for days to months. The pain is typically localized to the hip but is referred to the knee in about 20 percent of cases, which may lead to diagnostic error. Dis-

placement of the neck relative to the head causes the affected limb to rotate externally when the hip is flexed. Anteroposterior and lateral radiographs of the hip are necessary both to make the diagnosis and to grade the slip (Fig. 9.10). The severity of the slip is determined by measuring the percentage of the head of the femur that has displaced from the physis. A grade I (mild) slip has displaced less than one-third of the width of the neck, while a grade II (moderate) slip measures between 33 and 50 percent displacement. More than 50 percent displacement is considered a grade III (severe) slip (Fig. 9.11).

Slipped capital femoral epiphysis is divided broadly into acute and chronic types. Between 80 and 95 percent of all slips are chronic, i.e., have had symptoms longer than 3 weeks. This delineation is important, because attempts to improve the position of chronic slips by manipulative reduction often lead to avascular necrosis of the femoral head, whereas this complication is extremely uncommon in chronic SCFE without manipulation. Almost 50 percent of acute slipped capital femoral epiphyses develop avascular necrosis following manipulation.

Chondrolysis is another potential complication of SCFE. This acute necrosis of articular cartilage occurs in 1 to 28 percent of all patients, depending upon the series cited. Factors implicated in chondrolysis include prolonged cast immobilization, intraarticular pin penetration, severe slippage, and African American heritage.

Late reconstruction of profound deformity may be necessary in patients with severe slips, but because of the increased and devastating complications of manipulative reduction, the treatment of choice for chronic SCFE is usually in situ pin fixation of the epiphysis.

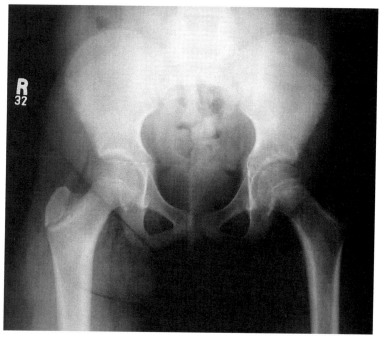

A

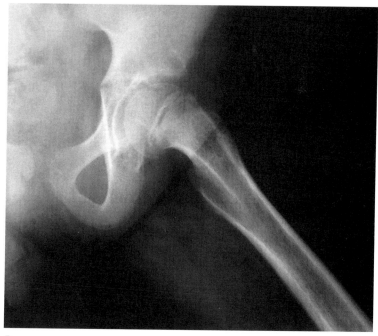

Figure 9.10 Slipped capital femoral epiphysis. *A.* The AP radiograph shows only a widened and less distinct physis on the left. *B.* Obvious displacement is present on the lateral view.

B

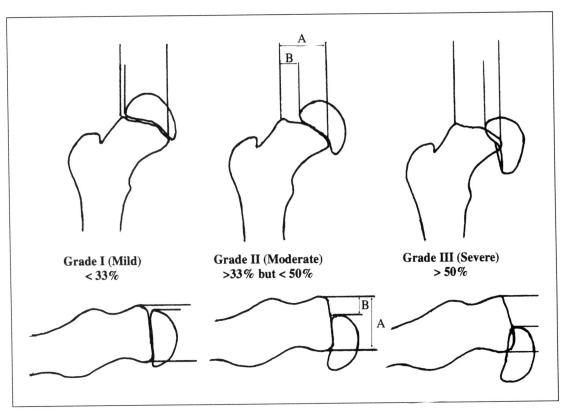

Figure 9.11   Slipped capital femoral epiphysis. The slip can be mild (<33 percent), moderate (33 to 50 percent), or severe (>50 percent) relative to the neck on either the AP or lateral radiograph. (Redrawn with permission from Tachdjian MD: *Pediatric Orthopaedics,* 2d ed. Philadelphia, Saunders, 1990, p 2868.)

Limb-Length Discrepancy

Many clinical entities result in *anisomelia* (limb-length inequality), but all result from growth stimulation, growth retardation, or mechanical shortening (as in excessive loss of length due to fracture) (Table 9.1). In addition to these pathologic situations, unexplained discrepancies of up to 2 cm have been observed in 75 percent of U.S. Army recruits. Although these differences can lead to disorders of gait, the degree of clinical difficulty cannot be predicted accurately from the degree of discrepancy.

Despite extensive study, no clear correlation has been drawn between inequality of limb length and either the incidence of adult back pain or the development of structural scoliosis. The management of disparate lower limb lengths must therefore be based upon the projected discrepancy at maturity, its possible functional significance, and the consequences of treating or not treating the asymmetry.

Table 9.1   Causes of Lower Limb-Length Discrepancy

Categories	Limb Shortening	Limb Lengthening

Congenital	Congenital hemiatrophy
	Congenital hip dislocation
	Congenital longitudinal deficiencies:
	    Amputations
	    Tibial and fibular hemimelia
	Congenital short femur
	Proximal femoral focal deficiency
	Profound malformations (e.g., severe
	    clubfoot)
		Congenital hemihypertrophy
		Localized gigantism

Developmental and tumorous	Neurofibromatosis Dysplasia epiphysealis hemimelica Enchondromatosis (Ollier disease) Fibrous dysplasia (Albright syndrome) Multiple hereditary exostoses Punctate epiphyseal dysplasia	Neurofibromatosis Arteriovenous fistula Soft tissue hemangiomatosis
Infectious and inflammatory	Osteomyelitis Pyarthrosis Tuberculous arthritis	Osteomyelitis (metaphyseal or diaphyseal) Rheumatoid arthritis Hemophilic hemarthrosis

Traumatic	Physeal injury
	Fracture malposition (overlap or
	    angulation)
	Severe burns
		Fracture (overgrowth after
		    metaphyseal or diaphyseal
		    fracture, especially of the femur)
		Traumatic arteriovenous fistula or
		    aneurysm

Neuromuscular	Brain or spinal cord lesions (trauma, tumor, or abscess) Cerebral palsy Myelomeningocele Nerve injury (femoral, sciatic, or peroneal) Poliomyelitis	

Other	Legg-Calvé-Perthes disease
	Lack of weight-bearing
	Slipped capital femoral epiphysis
	Radiation with physeal injury
		Iatrogenic trauma
		    Bone graft harvest
		    Periosteal stripping
		    Osteosynthesis

In the adult, marked discrepancies in length between the lower limbs are addressed by (1) shortening the long limb, (2) lengthening the short limb, (3) amputation and prosthetic fitting, (4) shoe or heel lifts, or (5) "benign neglect." The decision as to which option to pursue is predicated upon the clinical impairment of the limb, the general health of the patient, and the needs and expectations of the patient and family.

In the growing child, one must also take into account the etiology of the inequality, the patient's skeletal age and projected adult height, and the anticipated progression of the discrepancy. In most congenital syndromes, the percentage of limb shortening will remain constant throughout growth, e.g., if the left lower limb is 85 percent as long as the right lower limb at 5 years of age, it will remain so at skeletal maturity, although the absolute discrepancy will be much greater. If several measurements are made during growth, the pattern of inhibition can be charted and reasonable predictions made of the final limb-length inequality. Clinical examination is unreliable; therefore, radiographic measurement—by computed tomography (CT) or plain radiograph—is necessary to chart progression (Fig. 9.12). Other causes of asymmetry, such as trauma, infection, inflammation, and tumors, may not result in a fixed percentage of shortening throughout growth, in which cases close monitoring of discrepancies is even more important.

The rate of growth in the lower limbs is not constant throughout childhood. The periods of most rapid growth occur during infancy and the adolescent growth spurt, which is from age 10 to 12 in girls and 12 to 14 in boys. In addition, different growth centers in the lower limb contribute variable amounts to the overall length of the limb. The proximal femur ac-counts for approximately 15 percent of growth in the limb, while the distal femur and proximal tibia contribute 35 and 30 percent respectively. Knowledge of these facts makes plotting of expected growth in normal limbs possible and allows predictive comparisons for affected limbs. Despite pooled data from large groups, predicted normal values have wide standard deviations and therefore function as general guidelines for treatment rather than absolute indicators.

Once the final discrepancy has been projected and clinical evaluation of the patient completed, equalization should be considered. Discrepancies of less than 2 cm are usually left alone or treated by a shoe lift. If the expected discrepancy is more than 2 cm, operative equalization may be warranted. Surgically induced cessation of growth in the distal femoral and/or proximal tibial physis by *epiphyseodesis* at the appropriate time lessens the discrepancy, but, given the inherent inaccuracies in assessment of the eventual discrepancy, exact equalization is infrequent. Overcorrection with excessive shortening is a consequence of premature epiphyseodesis.

If the anticipated discrepancy is over 5 cm, shortening of the longer limb may lead to excessive loss of height, in which case operative lengthening of the shorter limb should be considered. Numerous techniques have been utilized, all of which are lengthy, technically demanding, and associated with high rates of complication (Fig. 9.13). A cooperative patient and family and relatively normal surrounding soft tissues are prerequisites for operative limb lengthening.

Scheuermann Juvenile Kyphosis

It is unclear what causes the disruption of enchondral ossification and longitudinal growth of vertebrae seen in Scheuermann kyphosis.

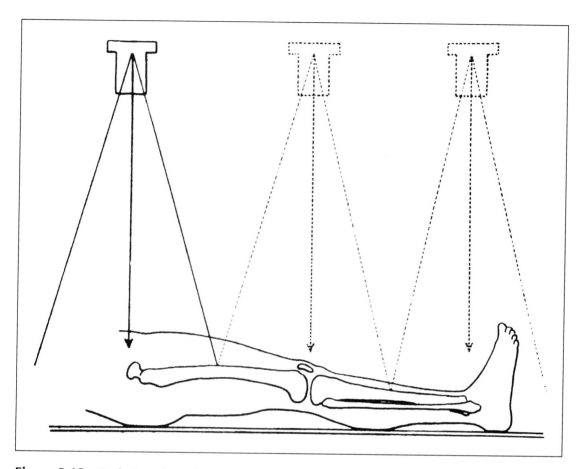

Figure 9.12   Technique for orthoroentgenographic measurement of leg-length discrepancies. Separate radiographs of the hip, knee, and ankle minimize magnification, limit radiation to the patient, and allow different exposures at each level. A radiographic ruler remains over all cassettes for consistent measurement.

Repeated studies have refuted Scheuermann's theory, proposed in 1920, that aseptic necrosis led to the distinctive wedge-shaped vertebrae and characteristic vertebral end-plate abnormalities associated with the entity that bears his name.

The diagnosis of Scheuermann disease is confirmed by a lateral radiograph that shows a kyphotic deformity of three or more adjacent vertebrae, with at least 5° of wedging in each vertebra (Fig. 9.14). These changes occur in from 1 to 8 percent of the population and are usually detected between the ages of 10 and 17. Occasionally, the patient is seen because of pain or fatigue; more commonly poor posture is the reason for consultation. In contrast to "postural round back deformity," patients with Scheuermann disease have a more acute,

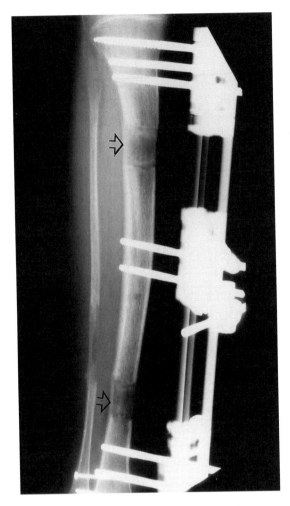

Figure 9.13 Limb lengthening by *callotasis.* New bone is formed *(arrows)* as the bone is lengthened by an external fixator after cutting of the bony cortex *(corticotomy).*

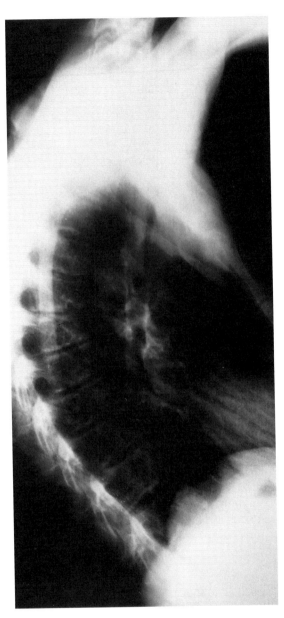

Figure 9.14 Scheuermann disease. Note the increased thoracic kyphosis.

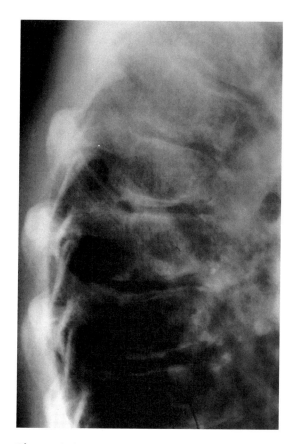

Figure 9.15 Scheuermann disease. Note the vertebral wedging and end-plate abnormalities.

fixed curvature. Marked tightness of the hamstring and iliopsoas muscles are frequently associated findings.

In addition to kyphosis and anterior vertebral wedging, radiographs reveal irregularity of the vertebral end plates, narrowing of the intervertebral disk spaces, and often concavities of the end plates resulting from localized protrusions of intervertebral disks into adjacent vertebrae *(Schmorl nodes)* (Fig. 9.15).

Orthotic treatment, which entails bracing in extension, has proven successful in the treatment of Scheuermann disease; surgical correction is rarely necessary.

Abnormalities of the Apophysis

Osgood-Schlatter Disease

One of the commonest causes of knee pain in the adolescent, this condition was described independently by Osgood and Schlatter in 1903. Although originally thought to be caused by avascular necrosis of the tibial tubercle, it is rather the result of repeated stress on a physis undergoing rapid growth (Fig. 9.16). It occurs during the adolescent growth spurt and is three times more common in boys than girls.

Pain, tenderness, and enlargement of the tibial tubercle are the clinical hallmarks of Osgood-Schlatter disease. Symptoms are exacerbated by repetitive stressful activities, such as running and jumping. The disorder is self-limited, and cessation of symptoms coincides with closure of the apophyseal physis. Symptomatic relief follows stretching of the quadriceps muscle and reduction of activity levels. In severe or resistant cases, immobilization in a cylinder cast may be necessary.

Sinding-Larsen-Johannson Syndrome

Although frequently grouped with Osgood-Schlatter disease, Sinding-Larsen-Johannson syndrome represents infrapatellar tendinitis with ossification. The clinical presentation and treatment are similar to those of Osgood-Schlatter disease except that the tenderness is at the proximal rather than the distal end of the infrapatellar tendon.

Sever Disease

Also termed *calcaneal apophysitis,* it is unclear whether the posterior calcaneal pain and

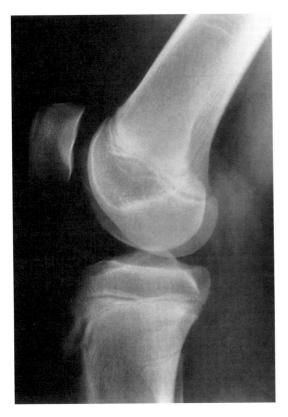

Figure 9.16 Osgood-Schlatter disease. Note the elevation and irregularity of the tibial tubercle.

tenderness in this condition have anything to do with the apophysis. Variable density and fragmentation of the calcaneal apophysis are normal findings that may or may not be associated with heel pain. This form of heel pain occurs most commonly in 6- to 10-year-old males and responds to activity restriction, heel cord stretching, and a heel lift. Occasionally a short period of immobilization in a below-knee walking cast may be necessary.

Little League Elbow

The medial epicondyle of the distal humerus is frequently the site of acute and chronic injuries, especially in throwing athletes and tennis players. The mechanism of injury is valgus stress at the elbow. The term *Little League elbow* usually refers to these injuries and should be distinguished from other elbow disorders, such as *osteochondritis dissecans of the capitellum,* which is also common in young throwers. Occasionally, an acutely avulsed medial epicondyle is entrapped in the joint, which requires surgical removal. Widely displaced fragments may necessitate operative repair to restore stability. Most injuries, however, can be treated with splinting, protected motion, and modification of activities.

Abnormalities of Articular and Epiphyseal Cartilage

Osteochondritis Dissecans

Separation of a fragment of articular cartilage and associated subchondral bone from the surrounding tissue defines osteochondritis dissecans (OD). Although interruption of blood supply to the region has been proposed as the etiology, it is unclear whether avascular necrosis is the proximate cause or the result of a traumatic event leading to OD. Whatever the cause, the effect is avascular necrosis of a segment of bone, which undergoes subsequent revascularization and repair by creeping substitution. If stresses in the area are excessive during the healing phase, the subchondral bone and overlying hyaline cartilage may separate from the parent bone. This syndrome occurs in the elbow, hip, and shoulder, but the most common sites are the knee and ankle.

In the knee, OD most commonly occurs on the lateral aspect of the medial femoral condyle (Fig. 9.17). Males are three times more likely to be affected than females. The presenting complaints may be indistinguishable

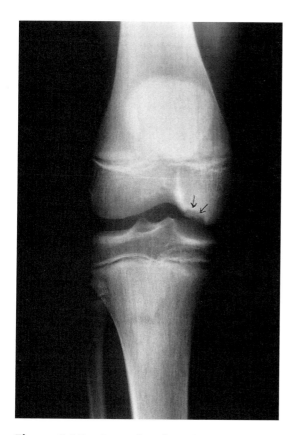

Figure 9.17 Osteochondritis dissecans. Note the involvement of the lateral aspect of the medial femoral condyle *(arrows)* and the sclerotic rim that surrounds the lucent lesion.

require surgical intervention for persistent pain or mechanical symptoms. Patients over age 20 have a poor prognosis and regularly require surgical intervention.

Osteochondritis dissecans of the talus can occur in either the medial or lateral angle of the talar dome. Lateral lesions usually have a clear history of antecedent trauma, which may be lacking with medial lesions. If the fragment is not completely detached or causes no mechanical symptoms, nonoperative treatment is indicated. Medial lesions, even if completely detached, usually heal with nonoperative treatment if they remain within the defect. Lateral fragments that are completely detached rarely consolidate without operative intervention.

Freiberg Infraction

Avascular necrosis of the second metatarsal head is usually manifest by localized pain and swelling. Prolonged weight-bearing, especially in high heels, frequently precedes this condition. Radiographically, the metatarsal head is flattened and irregular, with sclerosis followed by osteolysis. Relief of pressure under the second metatarsophalangeal joint is often helpful, but removal of loose bodies or the metatarsal head may be necessary if symptoms persist.

from those of a meniscal tear or a loose body, with stiffness, swelling, and mechanical symptoms (locking, popping, and giving way). Children under 13 years of age typically have smaller lesions that heal spontaneously. Treatment depends largely upon the age of the patient. Girls under 11 years of age and boys under 13 years usually do not require operative intervention. A short course of immobilization is often followed by healing of the lesion. Patients who are older but still under 20 years

Köhler Disease

Avascular necrosis of the tarsal navicula occurs most commonly in females about 4 years of age and in males near 6 years. Minor trauma often precedes the onset of pain and tenderness. Despite radiographic changes of increased density and fragmentation, the bone invariably heals with full reconstitution and without sequelae (Fig. 9.18). Treatment is entirely symptomatic, consisting usually of no more than an arch support.

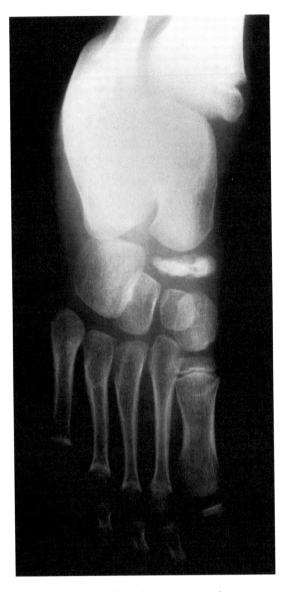

Figure 9.18   Köhler disease. Note the fragmentation and sclerosis of the navicula.

SUGGESTED READINGS

MORRISSEY RT (ED): *Lovell and Winter's Pediatric Orthopaedics,* 3d ed. Philadelphia, Lippincott, 1990.

TACHDJIAN MO: *Pediatric Orthopedics,* 2d ed. Philadelphia, Saunders, 1990.

WENGER DR, RANG M: *The Art and Practice of Children's Orthopaedics.* New York, Raven Press, 1993.

WILSON FC (ED): *The Musculoskeletal System,* 2d ed. Philadelphia, Lippincott, 1985.

Chapter **10**

Neuromuscular Disorders

Thomas G. Braun and Patrick P. Lin

ANATOMY AND PHYSIOLOGY

Neuroanatomy

The nervous system is divided into the *central nervous system*, composed of the brain and spinal cord, and the *peripheral nervous system*, which includes spinal and cranial nerves. Those aspects of the nervous system pertinent to motor and sensory innervation of the limbs are reviewed in this chapter.

Motor control depends on three components of the central nervous system: the pyramidal motor system, the extrapyramidal system, and the cerebellum. Gross voluntary movement is generated by the pyramidal system, whereas smooth, coordinated movement requires the input of the extrapyramidal system and cerebellum.

The *extrapyramidal system* includes the basal ganglia and several subthalamic and midbrain structures. Its output is directed primarily to the cerebral cortex via the thalamus. The basal ganglia are involved in the initiation of movement. The best known disorder of the basal ganglia is *Parkinson disease*, characterized by rigidity, bradykinesia (slowness of movement), and tremor. Other disorders of involuntary movement include tremor, athetosis (axial writhing), chorea (rapid movements of the limbs), and ballismus (violent flailing).

The *cerebellum,* like the extrapyramidal system, does not project directly onto the spinal cord. The deep cerebellar nuclei send their output to the thalamus, cerebral cortex, and nuclei in the brainstem. The cerebellum contains a complete sensory and motor representation

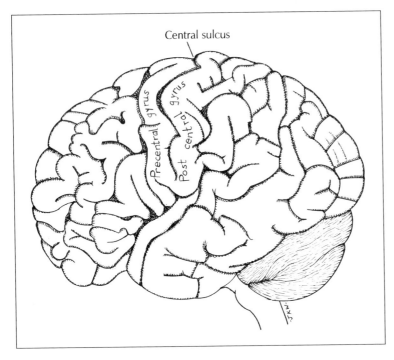

Figure 10.1   Primary motor cortex. Most of the cell bodies of the pyramidal tract reside in the precentral gyrus anterior to the central sulcus. The primary sensory cortex is in the postcentral gyrus.

of the body. Much of the input to the cerebellum is from stretch receptors, such as Golgi tendon organs, which are involved in unconscious control of muscle tone. Injury to the cerebellum does not result in weakness or sensory deficit but in tremor, dysarthria, loss of balance, and loss of coordinated action of agonist and antagonist muscles.

The *pyramidal system* begins in the primary motor cortex of the cerebrum, which generates most of the fibers of the corticospinal tract (Fig. 10.1). Significant contributions to the tract are also made from adjacent areas and the parietal lobe. The corticospinal tract is often called the *pyramidal tract* because of its appearance on the ventral portion of the medulla. Each pyramid contains approximately 1 million fibers. Near the junction of the medulla and spinal cord, the corticospinal tract splits into a large lateral tract and a much smaller anterior tract. The lateral corticospinal tract decussates before entering the spinal cord, whereas the anterior tract remains uncrossed (Fig. 10.2). Thus, for the most part, the right brain moves the left side of the body and vice versa.

Upper motor neuron lesions involve the corticospinal tract. These disorders are characterized by paresis (weakness) or paralysis of voluntary movements, followed usually by spasticity, hyperactive myotactic reflexes, muscular atrophy, and a Babinski sign. Spasticity and hyperreflexia reflect the loss of inhibitory signals from the extrapyramidal system. The *lower motor neuron,* or motor unit, includes the anterior horn cell, its axon, and skeletal muscle. Injury of the lower motor neuron results in *flaccid* paralysis, with diminished muscle tone and loss of myotactic reflexes. Muscle atrophy is more profound than in upper motor neuron lesions.

The primary sensory tracts in the spinal cord include the dorsal columns and the lateral and anterior spinothalamic tracts (Fig. 10.3). The dorsal columns are responsible for proprioception, vibration sense, and deep pressure. The lateral spinothalamic tract transmits temperature sense and sharp pain. The anterior spinothalamic tract carries fibers for light touch. The axons for the lateral and anterior spinothalamic tracts cross to the other side of the spinal cord before ascending, whereas the dorsal columns do not cross until after synapse in the medulla. Knowledge of spinal cord tracts and where they cross is important to understanding the various spinal cord syndromes (Fig. 10.4).

The *peripheral nervous system* comprises 12 cranial nerves and 31 segmental spinal nerves: 8 cervical, 12 thoracic, 5 lumbar, 5 sacral, and 1 coccygeal. The spinal nerves are mixed nerves containing sensory, motor, and sympathetic fibers. The axons of sensory nerves run from the periphery to the spinal cord, entering through the dorsal ramus. The cell bodies of sensory nerves reside in adjacent dorsal root ganglia outside the spinal cord. Cell bodies of the peripheral motor nerves are located in the anterior horn of the cord, from which axons run to muscles. The axons exit the cord through the ventral spinal ramus and join the dorsal ramus to form the spinal nerve. The sympathetic nervous system originates in the intermediolateral column of the spinal cord from T1 to L2. Axons leave the cord via the ventral roots of spinal nerves.

In the thoracic region, each spinal root provides sensory, motor, and sympathetic innervation for one intercostal level. In the cervical

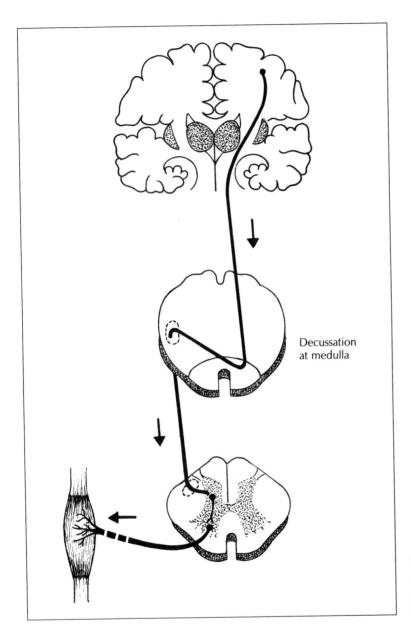

Decussation
at medulla

Figure 10.2   The lateral
corticospinal tract. Note
decussation (crossing) at the
medulla.

and lumbar areas, the dermatomal and myoto-
mal distributions are not so neatly divided.
Groups of spinal nerves join in a plexus, which
in turn forms the named peripheral nerves of
the limbs. Muscles are therefore often innervated by more than one spinal level.

Peripheral nerves frequently exhibit anatomic variations. A well-known example is the

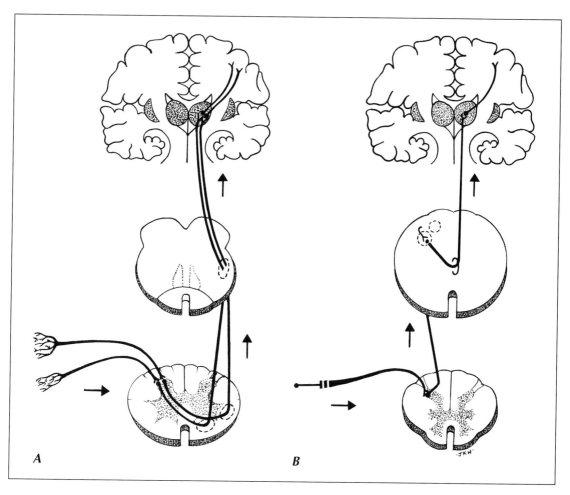

Figure 10.3 The sensory pathways. *A.* The lateral and anterior spinothalamic tracts contain fibers for light touch, sharp pain, and temperature sensation. Note fibers cross before ascending. *B.* The dorsal columns transmit vibration, pressure, and position sense. Note the synapse and decussation at the medulla.

variable course of the motor branch of the median nerve in the palm, which renders it vulnerable to injury during carpal tunnel release. Anatomic variations may also lead to erroneous diagnosis. For example, in 10 to 30 percent of people, the Martin-Gruber anastomosis connects the median or anterior interosseous nerve to the ulnar nerve in the proximal forearm, an anomalous link that can mask injury to these nerves.

Peripheral nerves are covered with *epineurium,* a layer of dense fibrous connective tissue

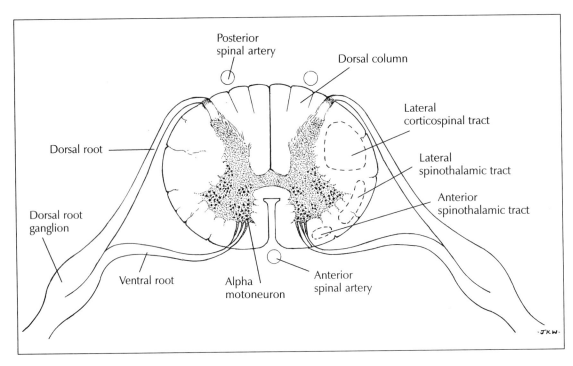

Figure 10.4   Cross section of the spinal cord at the level of the first thoracic vertebra.

(Fig. 10.5). Within the nerve, discrete fascicles of fibers are surrounded by *perineurium.* While both the epineurium and perineurium are strong enough to hold sutures, the *endoneurium,* which covers axons and Schwann cells, is too delicate for surgical repair. The Schwann cell is a specialized neuroglial cell that supports and forms a tube around the axon.

The speed of conduction is determined by the diameter of the axon and the presence or absence of a myelin sheath. As the diameter increases, speed increases, but there is a limit to the size of axons. Myelin, which is formed by Schwann cells and envelops most axons greater than 1 μm in diameter, increases con-

duction velocity by insulating the axon and allowing depolarization to spread farther. Regular interruptions, known as *nodes of Ranvier,* occur in the myelin sheath at discrete intervals. In a myelinated nerve, action potentials propagate only at the nodes of Ranvier.

Injury and Regeneration

Injuries of the nervous system are often temporary and without structural damage. For example, when the brain sustains a concussion, there is a transient loss of consciousness. Similarly, in spinal shock, function of the entire cord is temporarily lost. In peripheral nerves,

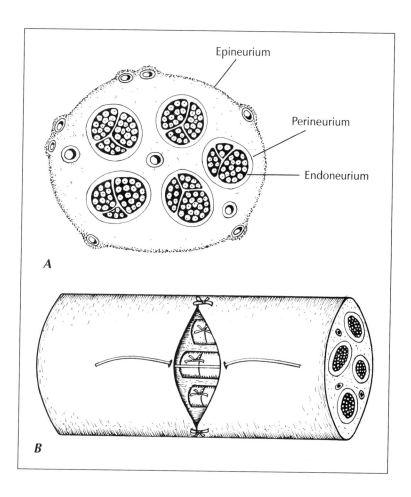

Figure 10.5 Peripheral nerve. *A.* Cross section of the nerve shows several fibrous connective tissue sheaths. *B.* Nerve repair involves suturing the tough epineurium and sometimes the perineurium of large fascicles.

contusion or pressure can cause palsies lasting from a few minutes to several days.

Physical damage to the central nervous system usually results in gliosis, or scarring. Although sprouting of nerve fibers occurs, there is no effective regeneration. In contrast, when peripheral nerves are injured, the axons and Schwann cells may respond in a number of different ways. *Wallerian degeneration* occurs after transection of an axon. The distal axon is digested by Schwann cells and macrophages over a period of weeks. Degeneration of the

proximal stump of the axon is limited to several internodal segments, after which it attempts to regenerate the distal end. *Axonal degeneration* describes progressive destruction of an axon in a distal to proximal direction ("dying back"), reflecting impaired metabolism of the cell body and its inability to maintain viability of the axon—a process that may end with death of the cell body. *Segmental demyelination* occurs when Schwann cells die in a localized region, while the denuded axon remains viable. Surrounding Schwann cells eventually proliferate and regenerate the myelin sheath, but it is thinner and has shorter internodal distances than normal. Segmental demyelination often follows prolonged pressure on nerves, as occurs in the carpal tunnel syndrome.

Damage to motor neurons results in paralysis of muscles. Muscle atrophy is rapid during the first 2 months, then gradually slows. Complete fibrosis eventually occurs but may take years. If reinnervation occurs, return of muscle function proceeds in a proximal-to-distal fashion.

Damage to sensory nerves produces loss of sensation, which may not be immediately apparent, since there is great overlap in sensory nerve distribution. Areas supplied exclusively by one nerve are called *autonomous* or isolated zones. In the hand, these areas include the tip of the index finger (median nerve), the first

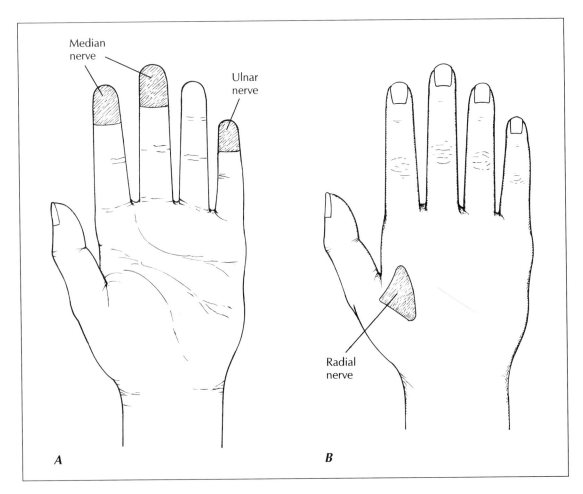

Figure 10.6   Autonomous sensory zones of the hand. *A.* Palmar. *B.* Dorsal.

dorsal web space (radial nerve), and the tip of the small finger (ulnar nerve) (Fig. 10.6). Sensory examination should focus on autonomous zones when possible so as to avoid ambiguous findings. The *intermediate zone* corresponds to the anatomic distribution of a nerve on gross dissection. The *maximal zone* can be appreciated by blocking surrounding nerves and can extend surprisingly far beyond the intermediate zone.

Injury to sympathetic nerves results in a number of changes. There is loss of pilomotor responses or "goose pimples." *Anhydrosis* can be documented by the starch-iodine or ninhydrin test, but a simpler test is the *wrinkle test.* Skin fails to wrinkle after immersion in water. Vasomotor disturbances are prominent. Initially, the affected area appears pinker and warmer than surrounding areas, since there is vasomotor paralysis and vasodilatation. In the ensuing weeks, vasoconstriction occurs, and the limb becomes cold, pale, mottled, or even cyanotic. Eventually, the skin becomes thin, atrophic, hairless, and shiny; nails appear deformed and brittle; and pressure sores or ulcers may develop (see "Reflex Sympathetic Dystrophy" in Chap. 13).

Of the several classification schemes for acute, traumatic neural injuries, Seddon's classification is probably the most widely used. *Neuropraxia* refers to physiologic, segmental block of a nerve without disruption of axons. Action potentials can propagate above and below the block but not across it. *Axonotemesis* occurs when the axon is disrupted but the connective tissue sheath remains intact. *Neurotmesis* occurs when both the axon and the connective tissue sheath are interrupted.

With any type of injury, there is immediate conduction block at the site of damage. During the first week after injury, electrophysiologic

studies (see below) cannot differentiate grades of injury. After 2 to 3 weeks, distal conduction remains normal in neuropraxia but not in neurotmesis or axonotmesis. At 6 to 8 weeks, the appearance of reinnervation potentials is characteristic of axonotmesis. Absence of neural function at this time does not preclude recovery, but chances of a normal outcome diminish.

Regeneration occurs to a variable degree in peripheral nerves, depending on the type and severity of the injury. A *regeneration unit,* which is composed of new neurites, sprouts from the cut ends of axons and nearby nodes of Ranvier. *Growth cones* are terminal swellings of the neurites that possess motile filopodia and respond to chemotactic influences. Sprouts that reach target organs survive; those that fail to reach their destination degenerate. Target organs, such as muscles, exert a trophic effect on the new axons, enabling them to increase in diameter and become remyelinated; however, the sheath is thinner and the internodal distance shorter than before injury. Under optimal conditions, regeneration progresses at about 1 mm/day.

The mechanisms controlling neural regeneration are not well understood. The ability of the regeneration unit to enter the distal end of the transected nerve is the first requisite for success. Once the growth cones find the track of the old axon, they are subjected to numerous biological influences. *Nerve growth factor,* which is secreted by muscles and Schwann cells, stimulates regeneration but does not act alone. Other growth factors are involved, as well as proteins in the matrix of the myelin sheath and endoneurial tube. Young patients tend to have better functional results, even though the density of regenerated axons is the same in young and mature patients. Reorganization of the the motor cortex and other areas in the central nervous system may account for the difference in functional outcome.

Diagnostic Studies

Electrophysiologic studies are adjunctive to a thorough history and physical examination. In many situations, however, these studies are es-

sential for diagnosis or alerting the physician to an entity that may not have been in the differential diagnosis. The two most commonly used tests are nerve conduction velocity and electromyography.

Nerve conduction velocity (NCV) measures the speed of neural conduction. Typically the test requires a stimulator and several electrodes (Fig. 10.7). For motor evaluation, the

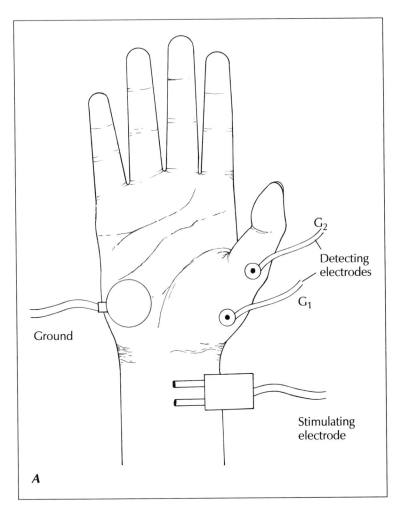

Figure 10.7 Nerve conduction tests. *A.* Distal motor latency of the median nerve is the interval between stimulation of the nerve proximal to the wrist and contraction of the thenar muscles. *B.* Distal sensory latency of the median nerve at the carpal tunnel is measured by stimulating the skin of the palm (or fingers) and measuring the time delay until the action potential is detected at the wrist.

stimulator is placed over the nerve and the recording electrodes over the target muscle. For sensory evaluation, the electrodes may be arranged either orthodromically (to stimulate distally and record proximally) or antidromically (to stimulate proximally and record distally). Measurements include *latency* [to the onset (motor) or peak (sensory)] of the action potential and *amplitude* of the negative peak. Latency, the time delay between stimulation and response, increases as the distance between electrodes increases and the speed of

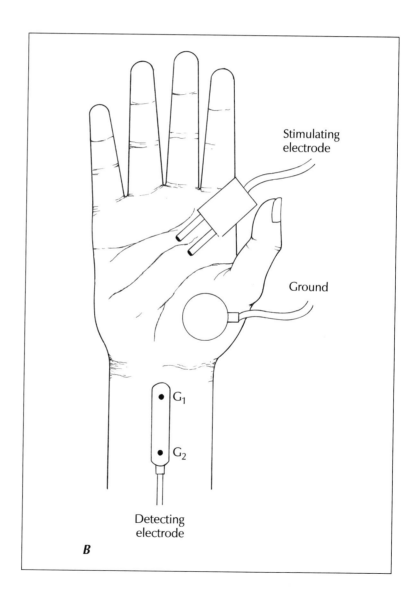

Figure 10.7   Continued

conduction decreases. The amplitude of the waveform reflects the number of axons present. Normal values of latency and amplitude are available for commonly tested sensory and motor nerves.

Electromyography (EMG) examines the characteristics of the motor unit with a concentric needle that contains both the active and reference electrodes in a single unit. Insertional activity is seen when the needle enters the muscle. Normally, there is a slight burst of activity that lasts about 20 ms. The *motor unit action potential* (MUAP) is recorded on an oscilloscope as the patient gently contracts the muscle. The amplitude of the wave varies with the number and size of fibers firing. *Recruitment* of fibers refers to the increase in active muscle fibers that occurs with increasing force of contraction.

Various pathologic processes can be detected with EMG studies. Denervation of muscle is characterized by increased insertional activity and spontaneous muscular activity, such as fibrillation potentials and positive sharp waves. In myopathy, the MUAP shows greater polyphasia, smaller amplitudes, shorter duration of action potentials, and earlier firing of motor unit action potentials. In neuropathy, there are fewer and larger motor unit action potentials firing at a rapid rate.

A biopsy of muscle is useful in distinguishing myopathy from neuropathy. *Myopathy* is characterized by central nuclei and widespread muscle degeneration; *neuropathy* is distinguished by scattered areas of fiber atrophy and more subtle changes. Specimens have to be obtained at a center where histochemistry is available, as well as the ability to store samples at $-70°$ C for subsequent enzyme analysis. The muscle must be carefully chosen and should reflect the disease at an intermediate rather than a late stage, when muscles have been replaced by scar tissue.

GENERALIZED DISORDERS OF THE NEUROMUSCULAR SYSTEM

Although many generalized neuromuscular diseases benefit from operative treatment, most entail only supportive measures, such as exercises, to maintain joint movement. Those diseases that require more specific orthopaedic management are addressed below.

Diseases of Upper Motor Neurons

Cerebral Palsy

Patients with cerebral palsy are the largest group of patients with neuromuscular disorders in the United States. Cerebral palsy is a static encephalopathy that occurs at an early age and affects motor control. Although the encephalopathy does not worsen with age, abnormal muscle balance and tone can cause progressive deformities of the spine and limbs. Patients with cerebral palsy often have associated problems, including diminished sensation, mental retardation, blindness, deafness, hydrocephalus, congenital malformations, and feeding problems. About 30 percent have epilepsy.

Cerebral palsy has been divided into several subgroups. *Spastic* cerebral palsy is the most common type, representing two-thirds of all patients, followed by the *dyskinetic* group (25 percent), and the *ataxic* type (3 percent). A *mixed* group makes up the remainder. Many other classifications exist, varying mostly in the subdivisions of dyskinetic cerebral palsy, which is characterized by athetosis, rigidity, posturing, or ballismus. Patients with ataxia have difficulty with balance and coordination and typically have diminished muscle tone.

Cerebral palsy may affect one limb or the entire body. *Hemiplegia* refers to involvement of one side of the body. Most hemiplegic patients are spastic, with the upper limb often more affected than the lower. *Diplegia* refers to primary involvement of the legs, with mild involvement of the arms. Patients have trunk control and can sit independently. Total body involvement or *quadriplegia* refers to involvement of all four limbs, with poor control of the head, neck, and trunk (Fig. 10.8). Although other patterns occur, such as *monoplegia* (involvement of one limb) and *triplegia* (involvement of three limbs), they are much less com-

mon than the patterns above. True *paraplegia,* which involves only the lower limbs, is rare.

The incidence of cerebral palsy varies among geographic areas and populations, with a range from 0.6 to 5.9 per 1000 live births. There has been a slight increase in recent decades because of greater survival in neonatal intensive care units. The great majority of cases arise prenatally or near the time of birth.

Potential causes of cerebral palsy are many, but it has been difficult to prove that any given factor is responsible for the disorder. Prenatal risk factors include *abruptio placentae,* pla-

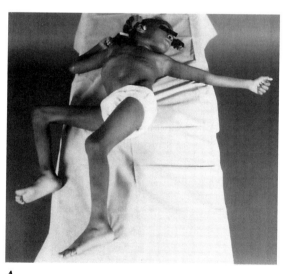
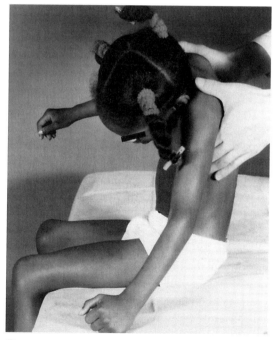

A   *B*

Figure 10.8   Spastic quadriplegia. Note the scoliosis and flexion contractures of the hip and knee. The patient lacks sufficient head and trunk control to sit unsupported.

cental infarction, diabetes, metabolic derangements, and viral infections, such as rubella. Maternal use of alcohol and drugs has been associated with cerebral palsy. *Erythroblastosis fetalis,* caused by Rh incompatibility and subsequent kernicterus, is a risk factor for athetosis, but this form of dyskinetic cerebral palsy has become less frequent in recent decades as a result of better screening programs for Rh antigens. The two risk factors with the most predictive value for the development of cerebral palsy are low birth weight (less than 2000 g) and congenital malformations.

Hypoxic damage to the brain is believed to be important in the pathogenesis of cerebral palsy, especially in premature infants, whose brains are less developed and more vulnerable to lack of oxygen. Computed tomography, magnetic resonance imaging, ultrasound, and autopsy have provided evidence of brain damage in neonates with cerebral palsy. Although the critical period of hypoxia is difficult to ascertain, it can occur prior to labor and delivery. Only 20 percent of patients with cerebral palsy show signs of intrapartum asphyxia, such as a low Apgar score, acidosis, or bradycardia. Furthermore, 15 to 20 percent of patients display no gross abnormality on imaging studies or autopsy, indicating a derangement of development at the microscopic level rather than damage to a normally developed brain.

Cerebral palsy can also arise in the postnatal period, but the limits of this period are difficult to define, and there is disagreement as to which patients to include. Some authors state that the period ends between 2 and 3 years of age, when myelinization is complete; others contend that the brain continues to mature throughout childhood. Regardless of the temporal definition, it is clear that insults to the brain during infancy and childhood can cause

spasticity and problems with motor control. These insults include meningitis, encephalitis, stroke, trauma, and any condition that causes a sustained period of hypoxia.

Early diagnosis, important for optimal care, can be challenging in infants, especially those not severely affected. Parental complaints may seem innocuous, e.g., toe walking or a delay in sitting up. The history of the mother's pregnancy and delivery are critical, as are significant illnesses in the neonatal period. Prematurity, low birth weight, and fetal distress requiring emergent cesarean section suggest the possibility of hypoxia. Developmental milestones provide important diagnostic leads. Infants usually have head control at 3 months, sit independently at 6 months, pull to a stand at 9 months, and start walking at 12 months. They should not develop right- or left-handedness before 12 months.

Examination begins with observation. The child's speech and behavior should be checked for appropriateness to age. Asymmetric movements or favoring the use of one side over the other should be noted. Gait abnormalities include limping, intoeing, and toe walking. In the upper limbs, abnormal posturing is frequent; for example, the elbow and wrist are often held flexed, and the arm may not swing naturally during ambulation.

The persistence of infantile reflexes into childhood years has been correlated with a poor prognosis for ambulation. The *Moro reflex* is a response to sudden extension of the neck or a loud noise, in which the infant moves the arms away from the body and then toward the body in an embracing fashion. The *extensor thrust* is characterized by extension of the lower limbs as the child is picked up and held vertically. The *parachute reaction,* present in normal children, may be absent in cerebral palsy. As the child is pulled from a crouched position off the table and suddenly lowered, the arms and legs extend outward toward the table in a protective manner.

An important part of the examination is the assessment of muscular tone. Patients with ataxia are born hypotonic and remain that way throughout life. Those with athetosis, who are hypotonic at birth, eventually become hypertonic as they develop abnormal postures and movements. Patients with spasticity are hypertonic from birth. One must keep in mind that tests for muscle tone are qualitative, since muscle tone can vary greatly depending on the patient's mood and alertness. Excessive muscle tone can be appreciated in several ways. Clonus can be elicited in the foot by sudden dorsiflexion of the ankle. Resistance to movement, or even rigidity, can be felt with passive motion. A useful maneuver is gentle shaking of a limb. Children are often tense in the examining room, but in a normal patient, gentle shaking of a limb usually results in relaxation.

Patients with spasticity have exaggerated deep tendon reflexes as well as Babinski, Chaddock, and Hoffmann reflexes. The *Babinski reflex* is obtained by stroking the sole of the foot, which causes dorsiflexion of the great toe and spreading of the lesser toes. The *Chaddock reflex* is obtained by stroking from the heel to the toes on the outer edge of the foot, which produces a response similar to the Babinski reflex but tends to cause less withdrawal of the foot. The *Hoffmann reflex* is elicited with gentle flicking of the terminal phalanx of the middle finger, which induces a pincer movement of the index finger and thumb.

Long-standing, untreated spasticity results in muscle tightness and deformities, particularly of the spine, hips, knees, and ankles. *Equinus* is the most common deformity and is

demonstrated by inability to dorsiflex the ankle passively to neutral. Equinus prevents the foot from being placed flat on the ground during ambulation and manifests itself as toe walking (Fig. 10.9).

Toe walking occurs in normal children, especially when they begin to walk, and it may persist, as *habitual toe walking (idiopathic toe walking)*, which is distinguished from other causes of toe walking by the absence of asso-

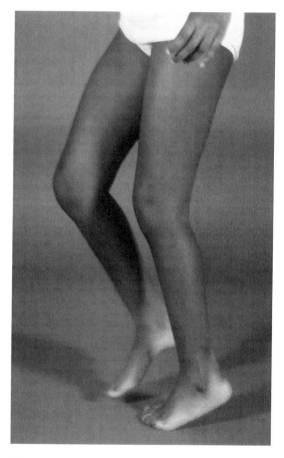

Figure 10.9 Spastic diplegia. Toe walking results from equinus contractures and spastic calf muscles

ciated findings, such as spasticity or fixed deformity.

Flexion deformity of the knee is often related to tightness of the hamstrings and contractures of the hip. The former can be measured by the *popliteal angle,* which in a normal child should be less than 10 to 20° (Fig. 10.10). With the patient supine, the hip is flexed 90° and the knee extended maximally. The residual knee flexion is the popliteal angle. Hip contractures can be appreciated by the *Thomas*

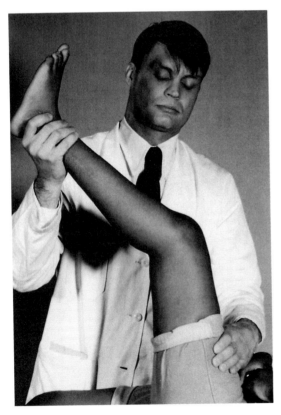

Figure 10.10   The popliteal angle. This angle, which gauges hamstring tightness, is normally less than 10 to 20° and is formed by the tibia and a line extending vertically along the femur.

test, in which both knees are first brought to the chest to reduce compensatory lumbar lordosis (Fig. 10.11). The hip in question is then extended and the persisting flexion deformity noted. Hip and knee contractures produce a crouched gait. Tightness of the adductors limits hip abduction and is associated with a scissoring gait.

Dislocation of the hips can be detected by the Ortolani and Barlow maneuvers in the neonate (Chap. 8). In older infants and children, these tests are not reliable, and other clues must be sought. Signs of dislocation include a discrepancy in leg lengths and asymmetrical ranges of movement in the hips, particularly limitation of abduction. Spastic patients with overactive adductors and weak abductors are likely to develop coxa valga and increased femoral anteversion, two deformities that promote dislocation of the hip. Increased anteversion of the femur is manifest by increased internal and decreased external rotation of the hip and intoeing during ambulation.

There is a close relationship between dislocation of the hips, pelvic obliquity, and scoliosis. *Pelvic obliquity,* which can be appreciated by palpating the iliac crests in the supine position, impairs sitting ability. It may be caused by or cause scoliosis, which is present in 7 percent of mildly affected children and in 35 percent of those severely affected. Minimal curves are difficult to appreciate, since many children are unable to bend over to demonstrate a rib hump. The need for radiographs should be guided by the physical examination. When scoliosis or subluxation of the hip is suspected, spinal, pelvic, and hip films should be obtained.

The treatment of cerebral palsy must be directed to the patient as a whole. Past efforts have concentrated on walking; however, am-

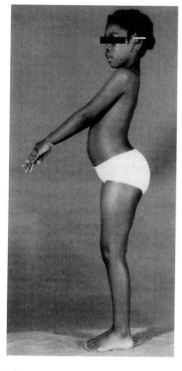
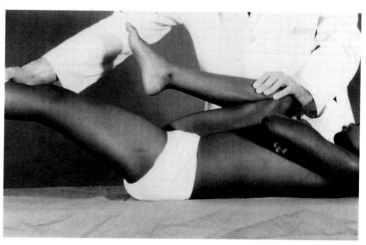

Figure 10.11   Spastic diplegia. Flexion contracture of the hip is masked by excessive lumbar lordosis and is revealed by the Thomas test.

bulation is not the sole measure of success. The goals of treatment are, in descending order, (1) communication of needs, (2) performance of activities of daily living, (3) mobility, and (4) ambulation. Severely affected patients tend to have poor expressive language abilities and often seem mentally retarded; however, many have good *receptive* language skills and are intelligent. Surgery is indicated to facilitate nursing care and provide resting comfort as well as to correct deformities and improve function. Mental retardation alone, no matter how severe, is not a contraindication to surgery.

Management of musculoskeletal problems varies with the type of cerebral palsy. Patients with ataxia benefit from intensive physical therapy, biofeedback, strengthening of muscles, and exercises to improve coordination. Bracing the lower limbs may help ambulation by compensating for the lack of motor control. Surgery is rarely indicated.

Patients with dyskinesia benefit from physical therapy and relaxation techniques. Severe rigidity is especially difficult to manage, and deformities in these patients are usually not responsive to bracing or surgery. If control over involuntary movements can be achieved, purposeful voluntary motions can be taught.

Spastic cerebral palsy is more responsive to operative intervention than other types of cerebral palsy. A combination of physical therapy, bracing, and surgery is often necessary for optimal function. Physical therapy helps preserve movement and prevent contractures. Bracing and casting can stabilize passively correctable deformities and are most commonly employed for equinus deformity. Polypropylene ankle-foot orthoses (AFOs) are worn inside the shoe to maintain a plantigrade foot and improve gait.

Certain deformities are not amenable to correction with physical therapy and braces. Subluxation or dislocation of the hip that fails closed reduction requires surgical correction; likewise, scoliosis that cannot be controlled with bracing needs operative stabilization. In many instances, surgery can improve function and prevent major deformities by correcting muscle imbalances. For example, patients with spastic diplegia typically have overpowering adductors and flexors of the hip. Judicious tenotomies of the overactive muscles not only improve posture and gait but also prevent subluxation of the hip by relieving the forces that cause coxa valga and increased femoral anteversion.

Diseases of Lower Motor Neurons

Poliomyelitis

Poliomyelitis was once the most common cause of crippling disease in childhood, but it is now rare in the United States because of successful immunization programs. Only 76 cases of paralytic poliomyelitis were reported between 1969 and 1978; however, there remains a significant residual population of patients who contracted the disease prior to the era of immunization, and poliomyelitis in the third world is still a major health problem.

Poliovirus is a member of the enterovirus family. It is transmitted through the fecal-oral route and infects primarily the alpha motor neurons of the spinal cord. The motor nuclei of the cranial nerves may also be affected, but their involvement is usually minimal. Paralysis is caused by the death of motor neurons, which is followed by gliosis, although some infected nerve cells recover and continue to function. Contractures and deformities develop in the limbs as a consequence of muscle weakness and resultant imbalance.

Most acute infections are subclinical and do not come to medical attention. In *abortive poliomyeltis*, patients have a nonspecific febrile illness for 2 or 3 days without neurologic involvement. In *nonparalytic poliomyelitis*, a brief aseptic meningitis occurs with subsequent full recovery. *Paralytic poliomyelitis*, characterized by permanent paralysis, occurs in only 10 percent of patients. In the rare cases of *fulminant poliomyelitis*, there is widespread infection of the central nervous system and a fatal outcome.

The clinical hallmark of paralytic poliomyelitis is asymmetrical flaccid paralysis with sparing of sensation (Fig. 10.12). The disease can be confused with *Guillain-Barré syndrome*, which is usually manifest by paresthesias in the distal limbs, followed by ascending paralysis that is usually symmetrical; reflexes are absent, and the spinal fluid contains an elevated protein level but no cells. Nerve conduction is slowed, with increased distal motor latencies and prolonged F waves. In some cases, the sensory parameters are normal. The prognosis is undoubtedly better than for polio. In paralytic poliomyelitis, the maximal extent of paralysis becomes evident within a few days. During the convalescent stage of the dis-

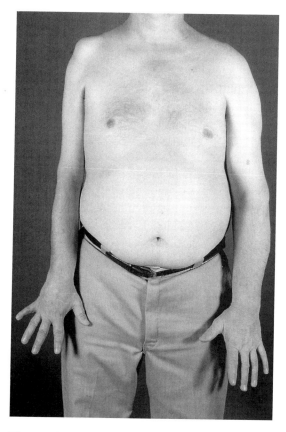

Figure 10.12 Poliomyelitis. Note asymmetrical, flaccid paralysis and profound atrophy of the proximal muscles in the right arm.

ease, which lasts 6 to 24 months, improvement in motor function occurs. After this period, paralysis is permanent.

Poliomyelitis can produce a multitude of orthopaedic problems, including impairment of growth, contractures, deformities of the foot, kyphosis, and scoliosis. In the convalescent stage, physical therapy and braces are used to slow progression of deformities. Surgery should be deferred until neuromuscular recov-

ery has reached a plateau. Tendon transfers and arthrodeses are effective means of stabilizing joints, correcting deformities, and relieving pain, often allowing braces and crutches to be dispensed with. Scoliosis should be treated aggressively.

Decades after the initial illness, a *postpolio syndrome* develops in 20 to 80 percent of patients. The disorder is characterized by renewed fatigue, weakness, and pain. Muscles previously mildly affected show progressive weakness, perhaps due to an acceleration of the normal aging process. Patients with poliomyelitis have limited numbers of muscle fibers performing the work of entire muscles. Since there is less reserve capacity, degeneration of only a few muscle fibers may result in appreciably more weakness. The postpolio syndrome should probably be distinguished from late lower motor neuron disease, also referred to as *postpoliomyelitis progressive muscular atrophy* (PPMA). Patients with this disorder experience recrudescent, progressive lower motor neuron disease, characterized by new areas of weakness, atrophy, and fasciculation.

Spinal Muscular Atrophy

In addition to poliomyelitis, there are several other diseases of the alpha motor neuron in the spinal cord. Certain viruses, such as herpes zoster and coxsackievirus, occasionally produce a syndrome similar to poliomyelitis. In the United States, alpha motor neuron dysfunction is most commonly caused by spinal muscular atrophy, a group of inherited disorders characterized by muscular weakness and wasting. Unlike amyotrophic lateral sclerosis and other motor neuron diseases, the upper motor neuron and spinal tracts are not involved in spinal muscular atrophy; however, motor nuclei in the brainstem are affected. Most cases are inherited in an autosomal recessive manner.

Several forms of spinal muscular atrophy are recognized. Type I *(Werdnig-Hoffmann disease)* is the most common, with an incidence of 1 per 25,000. It is a severe, infantile disease, usually evident at birth and fatal by 2 years. Type II disease becomes symptomatic at 3 months to 1 year and is compatible with a longer life, although with episodic deterioration. Type III *(Kugelberg-Welander disease)* begins in childhood and has a relatively benign course. Type IV disease has its onset in adulthood, can progress rapidly, and is very rare, with an incidence less than 0.5 per 100,000.

Examination reveals weakness, especially of the proximal muscles, without sensory involvement or signs of upper motor neuron involvement, such as hyperreflexia. Electromyography and muscle biopsy are necessary for diagnosis. Characteristic microscopic findings include sheets of small round atrophic muscle cells punctuated by occasional hypertrophic cells.

Orthopaedic treatment is usually for scoliosis, which affects a high proportion of patients, especially those who are nonambulatory. Braces are employed in childhood but, because of their weight, may have a deleterious effect on the patient's ability to walk. Patients with progressive curves uncontrolled by braces should have spinal fusion and instrumentation. Early mobilization after surgery is important, since many patients have a poor cough and diminished respiratory effort. For the same reason, anterior spinal fusion is more hazardous than posterior fusion in these patients.

Spinocerebellar Degeneration

Friedreich Ataxia

Friedreich ataxia is a disorder characterized by progressive degeneration of the spinocerebellar tracts, with involvement of other long spinal tracts, including the dorsal columns and pyramidal tracts. The clinical picture is striking. Patients exhibit ataxia, loss of proprioception in the legs, absent deep tendon reflexes, and cardiac abnormalities. The disease is usually inherited as an autosomal recessive disorder, although an autosomal dominant form also exists. The aberrant gene has been localized to chromosome 9. The prevalence is estimated to be 1 in 50,000.

Friedreich ataxia typically begins in early adolescence. Ataxia, one of the first symptoms, is followed by clumsiness in the hands, which develops as position sense is lost. Other manifestations include spasticity, weakness, dysphagia, deafness, blindness, epilepsy and dementia. Nerve conduction studies show absent or low-amplitude action potentials in sensory nerves. The prognosis is poor, and death usually occurs in the third or fourth decade from myocarditis and cardiomyopathy.

Orthopaedic problems involve the foot and spine. Cavus, equinovarus, and claw-toe deformities are common. Early, severe deformities impair ambulation and may be amenable to surgical correction. Scoliosis, occurring in nearly all patients, may also require surgical stabilization, since the deformity is difficult to control with bracing. Current techniques, such as sublaminar wiring, have made early mobilization after surgery possible.

Peripheral Neuropathy

Charcot-Marie-Tooth Disease

Charcot-Marie-Tooth disease, also known as *peroneal muscular atrophy,* is a slowly progressive peripheral neuropathy that affects both sensory and motor nerves. At least two forms of the disorder exist. The *hypertrophic* form is more severe and more common. It is usually inherited as an autosomal dominant trait, which has been linked to a duplication of a small region on chromosome 17, but it can also be inherited as a recessive trait or occur sporadically. Pathologically, it is distinguished by peripheral nerve enlargement and "onion bulb" formation, which reflect repeated episodes of segmental demyelination and remyelination. Collagen fibrils and fibroblasts become interspersed with layers of Schwann cells during remyelination, resulting in neural "hypertrophy." Frequently, nerves become palpable under the skin. Conduction studies show marked slowing in affected nerves. The *neuronal* form is less severe, and patients have faster nerve conduction velocities than patients with the hypertrophic form. Currently, the hypertrophic and neuronal forms are classified as *hereditary sensory motor neuropathies,* types I and II, respectively. Numerous other types exist, including *Dejerine-Sottas disease* (type III), a severe infantile disorder, and *Refsum disease* (type IV), which is characterized by excess phytanic acid.

Symptoms of Charcot-Marie-Tooth disease begin in the first or second decade with gradual weakness in the legs and cavus deformities of the feet (Fig. 10.13). The high arch is initially flexible but later becomes rigid. Pes cavus results from the imbalance between weak peroneal muscles and relatively strong calf and in-trinsic muscles of the foot. As the disease progresses, the tibialis anterior and extensor digitorum longus also become weak, causing foot drop and claw toes. The legs typically resemble an inverted champagne bottle because of muscle atrophy below the knee. The disease can involve the upper limbs, especially the intrinsic muscles of the hand and extensor muscles of the forearm. Scoliosis affects approximately 10 percent of patients, and hip dysplasia is present in 10 percent.

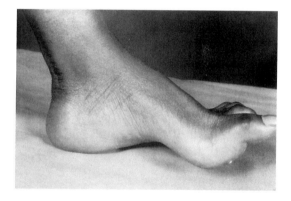

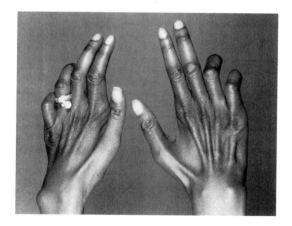

Figure 10.13   Charcot-Marie-Tooth disease. Note the high arch (cavus) and wasting of intrinsic muscles (interossei) in the hands.

Although the disease is primarily a peripheral neuropathy, changes also occur in the central nervous system. Autopsies have revealed degeneration of the dorsal columns and loss of anterior horn cells in the lumbar spinal cord, which account for the decrease in proprioception and vibration sense seen in some patients.

Most patients have a normal life expectancy with moderate disability. Scoliosis can usually be controlled with bracing. Bed rest and weight gain exacerbate the patient's difficulties and should be avoided. Orthotics may be sufficient for minimal foot deformities, but many patients need surgery. Heel cord lengthening is required for intractable equinus contractures; pain and fixed deformity in the hindfoot may necessitate triple arthrodesis, which fuses the talocalcaneal, calcaneocuboid, and talonavicular joints (Fig. 10.14). In recent years, clinicians have treated foot deformities at an earlier age, using plantar releases to avoid triple arthrodesis.

Muscular Dystrophy

Duchenne Muscular Dystrophy

Muscular dystrophy encompasses a group of hereditary disorders of muscle, characterized by progressive muscular weakness, atrophy, and contractures. Many different diseases are included under this heading. The most common is *Duchenne muscular dystrophy,* which occurs once in every 3500 live male births. It is one of the most severe forms of muscular dystrophy; patients suffer profound weakness, scoliosis, and early death. Aggressive orthopaedic treatment can improve the quality of life and sometimes increase life span.

Duchenne dystrophy is inherited as an X-

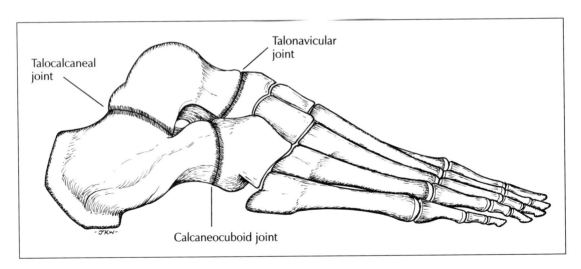

Figure 10.14 Triple arthrodesis. By fusing the talocalcaneal (subtalar), calcaneocuboid, and talonavicular joints, painful hindfoot deformities can be corrected.

linked recessive trait mapping to the P21 locus. The defective gene codes for dystrophin, a component of the cell membrane and cyto-skeleton of muscles. The function of this pro-tein is not yet completely understood. In Duch-enne dystrophy, a mutation causes an unstable, truncated protein to be made; levels of dystro-phin are extremely low or absent.

Females are carriers of the mutation and oc-casionally have mild clinical manifestations of the disorder. Males, by contrast, are severely affected. Diagnosis at an early age is unusual,

since weakness does not become apparent until 50 to 70 percent of the muscle mass is lost. At birth, the total muscle mass is near normal; however, degeneration and necrosis have al-ready begun (Fig. 10.15). By 18 months, most victims show subtle signs of impairment, such as toe walking or delayed running. If a child has not walked by this age, he should be tested for creatinine phosphokinase (see below). By 3 years, weakness has become apparent in run-ning, climbing stairs, and keeping up with peers. Initially, proximal muscles are affected

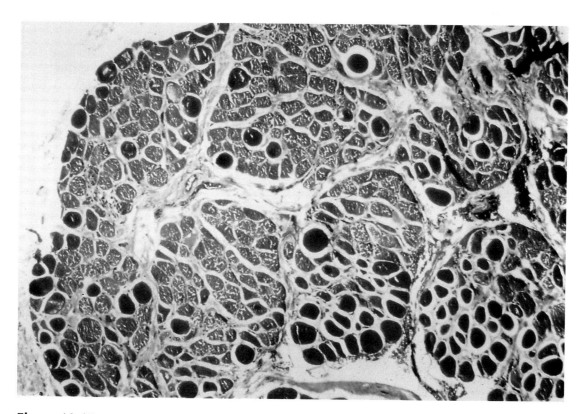

Figure 10.15   Duchenne muscular dystrophy. Note the patchy necrosis of muscle fibers.

more than distal muscles, but nearly all skeletal muscles will eventually be involved except, curiously, extraocular muscles.

Gower's sign illustrates the proximal muscular weakness (Fig. 10.16). To rise to a standing position from a sitting position on the floor, the child must use his arms to assist the quadriceps and gluteus maximus to extend the knees and hips. Another classic sign is a standing posture in which the trunk leans backward and the lumbar spine arches in hyperlordosis because of hip extensor weakness and flexion

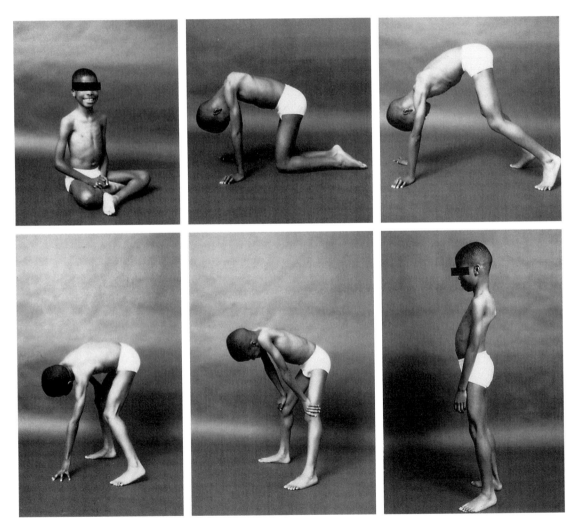

Figure 10.16   Duchenne muscular dystrophy. Gower's sign reflects proximal weakness of leg muscles. Patients must use their arms to assist the quadriceps and gluteus maximus when rising from a seated position on the floor. Note increased lumbar lordosis in the erect position.

contractures. Other deformities develop as muscles are replaced with fibrofatty tissue. Equinovarus contracture of the foot is common. Pseudohypertrophy of the calves, a result of fibrofatty infiltration, belies underlying weakness of leg muscles.

Many organ systems may be affected by the disease. Involvement of cardiac muscle leads to sinus tachycardia, right ventricular hypertrophy, and, in up to 10 percent of patients, life-threatening arrhythmias. Involvement of smooth muscles results in poor gastric motility. A static encephalopathy is sometimes present, causing diminished intelligence. The average IQ of patients is 85.

When the patient becomes wheelchair-bound, a progressive decline is inevitable. The transition from standing to sitting occurs at about 10 years of age, often accompanied by a fulminant scoliosis. Sitting reverses the normal lumbar lordosis to kyphosis, which unlocks the posterior elements and destabilizes the spine. Thoracic scoliosis is a devastating deformity, since it diminishes pulmonary reserve and hastens recumbency. Once bedridden, the patient is quickly overtaken. The combination of a weak diaphragm and diminished inspiration leads to pneumonia or respiratory failure, the usual causes of demise.

The traditional test for Duchenne muscular dystrophy has been serum creatinine phosphokinase (CPK), which is released from degenerating muscles. The enzyme level is markedly elevated in the first years of life, when it may reach 200 to 300 times normal. Later in the course of the disease, as muscle mass diminishes, the level of the enzyme decreases. The absolute level of CPK does not correlate with severity of the disease or progression. Female carriers of Duchenne muscular dystrophy may have slight to moderate elevation of CPK

levels. Other positive serum tests include elevation of serum lactic dehydrogenase, aldolase, and glutamic-oxaloacetic transaminase, all of which are enzymes liberated by dying muscle cells.

With the advent of molecular genetics and the isolation of the dystrophin gene, more sophisticated and definitive tests have become available for diagnosis. Muscle biopsy allows quantification of dystrophin levels and detection of mutations, which are analyzed by polymerase chain reaction (PCR) and Southern blotting (Fig. 10.16). These tests allow differentiation of Duchenne muscular dystrophy from other related diseases, most notably Becker muscular dystrophy (see below).

Treatment of Duchenne muscular dystrophy is difficult and controversial. Preservation of ambulation delays the onset of scoliosis and promotes good pulmonary toilet, but the best means to preserve it is debated. Agreement has not been reached on the role of bracing and the proper timing of surgery. Braces can be heavy and cumbersome, placing extra demands on weakened muscles, and they are not effective for scoliosis. Surgery, on the other hand, may further weaken muscles, especially if it involves tenotomies to correct flexion contractures.

Several schools of thought exist regarding the timing of surgery. Some advocate early intervention, while patients are fully ambulatory; others advise intervention just before patients become wheelchair-bound; still others believe that operations should be performed just after patients lose the ability to ambulate. Since none of these approaches yields consistently superior results, surgery should be tailored to individual needs. Regardless of timing, parents must be advised that the goals of surgery are limited. The ability to ambulate can be extended at most by only 1 to 3 years. Nevertheless, in the patient's brief life span, this interval may be extremely valuable.

Spinal surgery for scoliosis poses significant risks, especially if cardiopulmonary function is diminished. It should be performed while the curve is less than 40° and the cardiopulmonary system is still able to tolerate the procedure. Stabilization of scoliosis improves sitting posture and lengthens the time a patient is able to sit in a wheelchair. Surgery does not usually improve respiratory function, which declines more from weak respiratory muscles than from skeletal deformity.

Becker Muscular Dystrophy

Becker muscular dystrophy is closely related to Duchenne muscular dystrophy but is less debilitating. Like Duchenne dystrophy, Becker muscular dystrophy is caused by abnormalities in the dystrophin gene. There are numerous variants of the disease, probably stemming from different mutations in the gene, which produces a spectrum of severity. The levels of

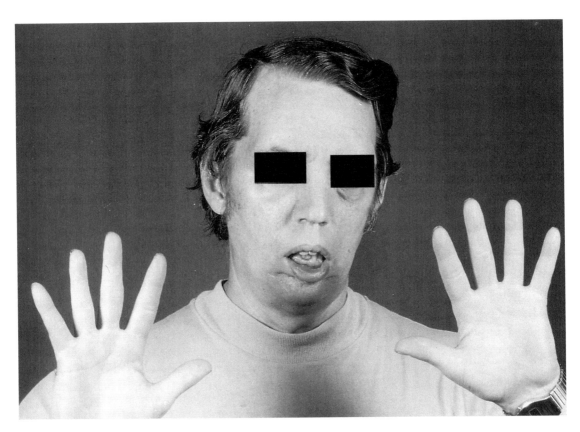

Figure 10.17   Myotonic dystrophy. Note the typical facies with temporal wasting, expressionless affect, and ptosis. Atrophy of intrinsic muscles of the hand is also characteristic.

dystrophin are generally higher than the levels found in Duchenne muscular dystrophy.

Becker dystrophy is not common, occurring approximately once in every 30,000 births. The prognosis is variable, but most patients survive well into adulthood. Since the disease is inherited as an X-linked recessive trait, males are affected and females are carriers. The diagnostic workup is similar to that for Duchenne muscular dystrophy, as is the management. Treatment again should be individualized. Heel cord lengthening usually improves ambulation if equinus contractures cause toe walking. In the more aggressive variants, scoliosis is common. Spinal fusion may be beneficial in this group, especially if the patient is not ambulatory.

Myotonic Dystrophy

Myotonic dystrophy is a slowly progressive disorder characterized by *myotonia* (failure of a muscle to relax) and weakness of limb and facial muscles (Fig. 10.17). It is relatively common, with an incidence of 1 in 8000, and is inherited as an autosomal dominant disorder linked to chromosome 19q. Myotonic dystrophy begins in adolescence or young adulthood, often with the inability to release a handshake. Dysarthria, ptosis, and weakness of facial and distal limb muscles soon follow. In addition to neuromuscular involvement, patients display mental retardation, frontal baldness, cataracts, glaucoma, testicular atrophy, and cardiac disease, which can lead to arrhythmias and heart failure in some older patients. Electromyographic findings are impressive. Insertion of the recording electrode into the muscle elicits a characteristic "dive bomber" sound, which reflects increased insertional activity, and trains of positive sharp waves that gradually wane.

This disorder is usually compatible with a normal life span; patients do not become totally incapacitated. Operative treatment may be required for such deformities as hallux valgus, talipes equinovarus, hip dysplasia, and scoliosis. Because of coexisting cardiac problems, surgical patients should have preoperative electrocardiograms (ECGs) and pulmonary function tests.

REGIONAL DISORDERS OF THE NEUROMUSCULAR SYSTEM

Traumatic Disorders

Injuries of the Spinal Cord

The spinal cord may be damaged by direct penetrating injury or by the indirect effects of trauma, which include compression, edema, vasospasm, hemorrhage, and hypoxia. Injuries to spinal roots behave as injuries to peripheral nerves. The chances for at least partial recovery are good if the root is still in continuity; if it is avulsed or completely severed, the root will not recover. Avulsion of a nerve root is rare and usually associated with injuries to the brachial plexus.

The level of injury is defined by the last functioning spinal cord level (Tables 10.1 and 10.2). Injuries are *complete* if no sensation or voluntary motor activity is present below the level of injury. If perianal sensation remains or the anal sphincter continues to function, the injury is an *incomplete* lesion. The distinction between complete and incomplete injuries is important, since improvement in complete lesions after 48 h does not occur, while incomplete lesions may recover.

In the acute setting, it is important to deter-

Table 10.1   Functional Level of Quadriplegia

Level	Muscle(s) Present	Function
C3+	Facial	Respirator-dependent; electric wheelchair; sip-and-puff controls
C4	Diaphragm, some neck muscles	Electric wheelchair; chin, mouth, or sip-and-puff controls
C5	Deltoid, partial biceps/brachialis	Electric wheelchair with hand controls; limited hand use with orthosis (e.g., ratchet)
C6	Biceps/brachialis, wrist dorsiflexors	Limited grasp with more advanced orthosis
C7	Triceps, wrist palmar flexors, finger extensors	Manual wheelchair propulsion (triceps); independent wheelchair transfers; hand orthosis for finger flexion
C8	Finger flexors, intrinsics	Same as C7; better hand control and function

Table 10.2   Functional Level of Paraplegia

Level	Muscle(s) Present	Function
L1+	Abdominal, paraspinal	Wheelchair (adults); crutch ambulation with HKAFO or reciprocating gait orthosis (children)
L2	Iliopsoas	KAFO (with drop-lock knee hinges); ambulation possible with crutches but usually limited
L3	Partial quadriceps	AFO; ambulation possible
L4	Quadriceps, tibialis anterior	AFO; ambulation likely
L5	Partial ankle plantar flexors, partial hip abductors	Foot orthosis; community ambulator

HKAFO = hip-knee-ankle-foot orthosis; KAFO = knee-ankle-foot orthosis; AFO = ankle-foot orthosis.

mine if the *bulbocavernosus reflex* is present. Pulling on an inserted Foley catheter should cause a contraction of the anal sphincter. If the reflex is absent, *spinal shock* may be present, which precludes determination of the injury level. Spinal shock usually lasts less than 24 h, with its end being heralded by return of the bulbocavernosus reflex.

Since the location and extent of injury varies from patient to patient, the clinical manifestations of incomplete cord injuries are also varied. Nevertheless, it is useful to think of patterns of injury as determined by the primary site of involvement. Damage may be concentrated in the anterior or posterior portion, the right or left half, or the central portion of the cord.

The most common pattern of injury is the *central cord syndrome,* which damages primarily the central gray matter of the cord. Patients who may appear initially to be quadriplegic have distal sparing of perianal sensation, which predicts early return of bowel and bladder control. The likelihood of partial motor recovery is about 75 percent. Recovery begins distally and proceeds proximally. Return of function in the upper limb is usually limited.

The *anterior cord syndrome,* characterized by injury to the anterior portion of the cord, can occur after burst fractures with retropulsion of vertebral fragments (Fig. 10.18). In the upper lumbar spine, however, where most burst fractures occur, the spinal canal is filled with the cauda equina rather than the spinal cord, and the anterior cord syndrome does not

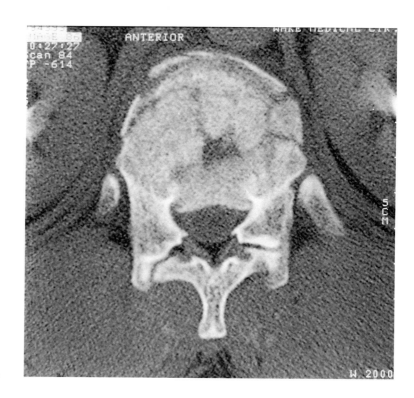

Figure 10.18 Burst fracture of the thoracic spine. There is retropulsion of bony fragments into the spinal canal, which can impinge on the spinal cord.

result. The posterior columns are spared in pa-tients with anterior cord syndrome, leaving proprioception and appreciation of vibration and deep pressure intact. Motor function is lost, since the motor neurons are located in the ventral gray matter. Appreciation of pain and light touch is likewise absent. The probability of recovery is approximately 10 percent.

In the rare *posterior cord syndrome,* the posterior columns are affected, while motor function and sharp pain are spared. Loss of proprioception produces a foot-slap gait simi-lar to that seen in tabes dorsalis.

The *Brown-Séquard syndrome* involves in-jury to the right or left side of the cord. The hallmark of the syndrome is ipsilateral paral-ysis and loss of position sense with contralat-eral loss of pain and temperature sensation. Chances for recovery are good; many patients regain bowel and bladder control and the abil-ity to walk.

Optimal treatment of spinal cord injuries in-volves a multidisciplinary approach, ideally in a spinal cord injury center. Often, patients are the victims of multiple trauma, and physicians must address concomitant surgical, medical, and emotional issues. With a high-level cord injury, neurogenic shock may develop. The sympathetic chain originates from T1 to L2, and cervical injuries may disrupt the sympa-thetic outflow, causing widespread vasodila-tion. Lumbar injuries do not cause neurogenic shock, so if hypoperfusion is present, other causes must be sought.

In the acute setting, patients should receive high doses of steroids. The secondary effects of acute trauma are partially reversible in the first 8 h, and steroids may mitigate cord dam-age. The need for decompressive surgery is best decided in conjunction with an orthopae-dist or neurosurgeon. An incomplete, progres-sive neurologic lesion is an indication for emergent decompression, whereas a complete neurologic lesion does not benefit from de-compression after 48 h. There is controversy over the indications for decompressive surgery in incomplete, nonprogressive injuries and complete lesions less than 48 h old.

Injuries of the Brachial Plexus

In the past, brachial plexus injuries were usu-ally the result of obstetric trauma, but such in-juries have become less frequent in modern obstetric practice. Current estimates of the in-cidence of neonatal brachial plexus palsy range from 0.3 to 2.5 per 1000 live births. Pen-etrating and nonpenetrating trauma is now a more frequent cause of brachial plexus inju-ries. The single most common form of trauma is a traction injury from sudden widening of the head-shoulder interval, which can occur during delivery but more often follows a blow to the top of the shoulder or side of the head (Fig. 10.19).

The brachial plexus is derived from nerve roots C5 to T1 and innervates the shoulder and arm (Fig. 10.20). Although injury can occur anywhere along the plexus, the most severe form of injury is avulsion of nerve roots from the spinal cord, which precludes both natural regeneration and surgical repair.

Erb palsy affects nerve roots C5, C6, and sometimes C7. Weakness is proximal, affect-ing especially the deltoid and rotator cuff, which are responsible for abduction and exter-nal rotation of the shoulder (Fig. 10.21). A weakened biceps reduces strength in flexion of the elbow and supination of the forearm. If contractures develop, the arm assumes the *"waiter's tip"* position (Fig. 10.22). Sensation is diminished over the lateral aspect of the shoulder, arm, forearm, and hand. Persistent

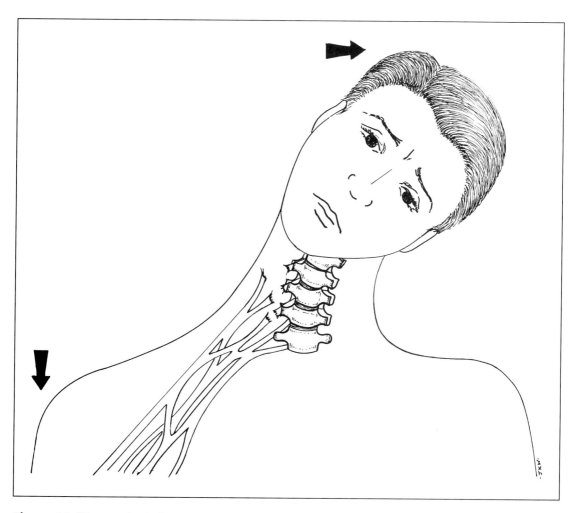

Figure 10.19   Brachial plexus injury. The mechanism usually involves
traction, which can result from violent depression of the shoulder or lateral
flexion of the neck, either of which produces widening of the head-
shoulder interval.

absence of sensation in the thumb, index finger, and long finger severely limits function of
the hand, regardless of motor function. The
prognosis for Erb palsy in the neonate is good,
with spontaneous recovery expected in 75 percent of cases.

Klumpke palsy affects C8 and T1, the lower

nerve roots of the brachial plexus. Weakness
is manifest in the intrinsic musculature of the
hand. If C7 is also affected, there is weakness
of the triceps and pronator teres, with the elbow postured in flexion and the forearm in
supination. Sensation is lost over the ulnar
portion of the hand and forearm. During

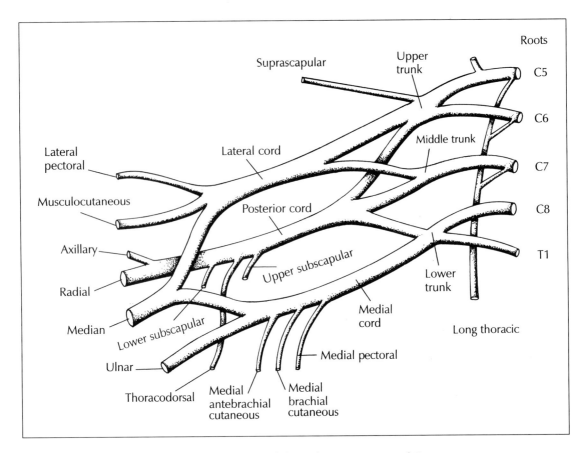

Figure 10.20   The brachial plexus is derived from the nerve roots of C5 to T1.

childbirth, a Klumpke palsy may result if the arm is vigorously pulled over the head of the infant. Obstetric causes are less common than for an Erb palsy.

Often, palsies are mixed, so it is important to document the full extent of motor and sensory deficits. Electromyography (EMG) and assessment of motor units are often useful in identifying affected nerves, and follow-up studies can be used to monitor the progress of recovery. In addition, it is essential to determine whether nerve root avulsion has oc-

curred, which forecasts a grim prognosis for recovery. While paralysis of the serratus anterior, levator scapulae, and rhomboids suggests nerve root avulsion, nerve conduction studies of the proximal portions of the plexus may be necessary for diagnostic certainty. In addition, myelography 6 to 12 weeks after injury may demonstrate pseudomeningocoeles at the sites of avulsion.

Careful, frequent examinations are essential to optimal management. If new motor units and signs of nerve recovery appear, continued

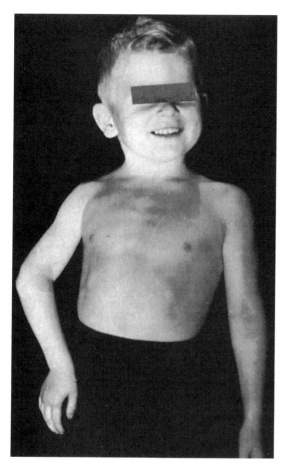

Figure 10.21   Erb palsy. Note atrophy of the shoulder and biceps muscles. The shoulder is internally rotated and forearm pronated. (Reprinted with permission from Brashear HR Jr, Raney RB: *Handbook of Orthopaedic Surgery,* 10th ed. St Louis, Mosby, 1986, p 222.)

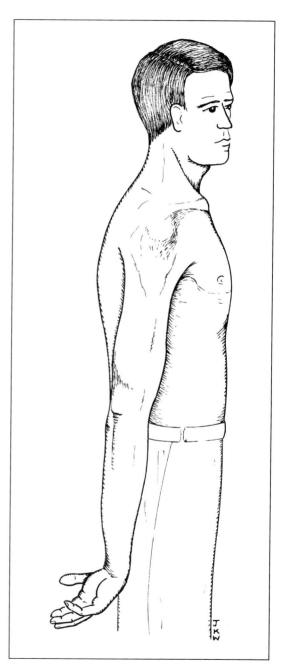

Figure 10.22   The "waiter's tip" position is characteristic of long-standing upper brachial plexus injury.

nonoperative therapy is warranted. During the period of observation, range-of-motion exercises are important, and splinting may be needed to minimize contractures.

If no recovery occurs, consideration must be given to surgery. In the early part of the twentieth century, there was great enthusiasm for exploration of plexus injuries, but the paucity of good results led most surgeons to shun surgical repair; however, recent advances in microsurgical techniques have led to a resurgence of interest in early repair of the plexus. There is evidence that results are better when surgery is performed less than 6 months after injury, especially if physical division of the plexus has occurred. The alternative to direct repair of the plexus is transfer of musculotendinous units, which utilizes nearby functional muscles as substitutes for paralyzed muscles.

Patients with nerve root avulsion are more difficult to treat. Experimental surgical procedures include "neurotization" of costal nerves, in which an upper thoracic nerve is rerouted to the brachial plexus, occasionally leading to a gain in function of the elbow. Salvage procedures include tendon transfers, arthrodesis, and, in rare cases, amputations for flail, insensate limbs.

Injuries of Peripheral Nerves

Injuries of peripheral nerves result from either blunt or penetrating trauma and are often associated with fractures or dislocations. The classification of peripheral nerve injuries most commonly used involves three grades of injury: neuropraxia, axonotmesis, and neurotmesis (see above). With neurotmesis or complete division of the nerve, surgical repair is indicated. When a deep laceration is located directly over a nerve, and there is complete nerve palsy distal to the laceration, surgical exploration should be performed promptly and not delayed for preoperative nerve conduction studies or EMGs. Complete absence of sensation is rare except in autonomous zones, because of overlapping areas of cutaneous innervation. Definitive nerve repair may be performed if the wound is clean and healthy; a contaminated wound should be debrided and nerve repair deferred until signs of infection are absent.

Nerve injuries that follow blunt trauma, such as a closed fracture, usually do not cause physical division of the nerves. Approximately 80 percent of neural injuries associated with fractures occur in the upper limbs. The radial nerve is especially vulnerable, being affected in approximately 10 percent of humeral fractures, especially those near the junction of the middle and distal thirds of the shaft. Most radial nerve palsies (90 percent) recover spontaneously within a few weeks or months, indicating a neuropraxia. Rarely, the nerve is lacerated, interposed between fracture fragments or trapped in callus.

If neural injury is suspected, a baseline EMG should be obtained 14 to 21 days after the injury. Performing the studies earlier may provide misleading information. As nerves regenerate, proximal muscles are reinnervated first, followed by distal muscles, and, finally, by the recovery of distal sensation. During the period of recovery, passive range-of-motion exercises are important to prevent joint contractures.

If no clinical improvement occurs, EMGs and nerve-conduction tests are repeated 2 to 3 months later, with emphasis on proximal muscles, which, if denervated, show fibrillation potentials and positive sharp waves (Fig. 10.23). Motor-unit assessment can be performed to determine the integrity of a nerve. Surgical exploration should be considered between 3 and 6 months following injury if there is no clinical evidence of recovery and no new motor units are being activated. The results of surgical repair are less satisfactory after 9 months. During the period of neural recovery,

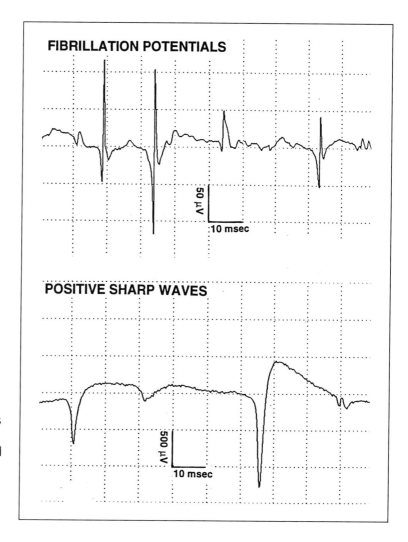

Figure 10.23 Muscle paralysis. Electromyograms show fibrillation potentials and positive sharp waves, which are abnormal findings in resting muscle. Positive sharp waves are broader and much larger in amplitude than fibrillation potentials (note the difference in gain on the tracings).

it is essential that motion be maintained in all joints. If recovery is absent or incomplete, musculotendinous transfers may provide useful compensation for lost functions. These operations, however, are contraindicated in a stiff limb with fixed contractures.

"Saturday night palsy" is a palsy of the radial nerve that arises from prolonged pressure on the arm. Patients typically awaken with a wrist drop after falling asleep in an awkward position. The deficit is usually a neuropraxia, lasting only a few days or weeks. Nevertheless, it is important to provide a cock-up wrist splint to improve grasp and avoid flexion contractures. The patient should also carry out passive extension exercises of the wrist and fingers.

Crutch palsy arises from incorrect use of crutches. Patients are often deceived by the padded appearance of the top of crutches and rest their axillae on the pads, or they use crutches that are too long and extend into the axillae. Pressure on the brachial plexus causes a neuropraxia, which can affect the musculocutaneous, median, radial, and/or ulnar nerves.

Traumatic Neuroma

A traumatic neuroma (or *amputation neuroma*) most often results from surgery. Frequently injured nerves include the saphenous nerve (during harvest of the saphenous vein) and the infrapatellar branch of the saphenous nerve (during knee surgery). Amputations of digits and limbs require division of nerves. Following section of a nerve, the body attempts to regenerate the nerve. If the neurites from the proximal stump cannot find the distal stump, a tangled mass of exquisitely sensitive free nerve endings (neuroma) develops, producing burning pain at the affected site that is made worse with light touch or pressure. *Tinel's sign* is positive at the nerve stump.

Prevention is the best treatment. If nerves must be sacrificed, as in amputations, the nerve ends should be buried deeply in soft tissue. A free nerve end near the surface of the skin is much more likely to be symptomatic. Treatment of established traumatic neuromas involves surgical excision, followed by placement of the nerve end into a bed of fat or soft tissue.

Entrapment Neuropathies

Entrapment neuropathies are common but often difficult to diagnose. Many patients have puzzling pain and paresthesias without obvious cause. To make the diagnosis, the possibility of entrapment must be entertained. Nearly every major nerve has the potential for compression in a confined space. When the compression is of sufficient duration and severity, a neuropathy results. The varied causes for entrapment include anomalous anatomic structures, degenerative changes, inflammation, new growths, and adhesions. Common areas for entrapment include the carpal tunnel (median nerve), the cubital tunnel (ulnar nerve), and Guyon's canal in the hand (ulnar nerve).

Grossly, the affected nerve is pale and attenuated beneath the compression and enlarged proximally as a result of congestion and edema. Microscopically, areas of demyelination and remyelination are seen at the site of compression, with loss of large myelinated fibers and axonal degeneration.

In a reliable patient, a careful history and physical examination allow identification of the affected nerve. Pain, paresthesias, and weakness are localized to an anatomic distribution. There are specific motor and sensory deficits, occasional muscle atrophy, and often a positive Tinel's test, in which light percussion of the affected nerve produces distal paresthesias. Some nerves, such as the suprascapular nerve, that lie beneath heavy muscles are difficult to percuss.

Occasionally the diagnosis is confounded by the potential for secondary gain. Both the history and examination become ambiguous, since they rely on honest and accurate responses from the patient. If a patient is unreliable or the physical examination equivocal, nerve conduction tests and EMGs are indicated.

Treatment of entrapment neuropathies begins with elimination of underlying causes. Activities that elicit or exacerbate symptoms should be avoided. Injections of corticosteroids decrease inflammation and swelling in surrounding tissues, which reduces pressure on the nerve. Rest and oral anti-inflammatory agents work in a similar fashion. If nonoperative treatment fails or if muscle weakness is apparent, surgical release should be performed before permanent paralysis occurs.

Carpal Tunnel Syndrome

Compression of the median nerve in the carpal canal (carpal tunnel syndrome) is the most common entrapment neuropathy. It predilects pregnant and middle-aged women, with a prevalence of approximately 50 to 100 per 100,000 and a male-to-female ratio of 1:3.

The carpal tunnel is an enclosed, unyielding space bounded by the proximal carpal row and the inelastic transverse carpal ligament (Fig. 10.24). Any condition that reduces the size or enlarges the contents of the tunnel can cause compression of the median nerve. Tumors, ganglia, and, more commonly, tenosynovitis of the flexor tendons (idiopathic, traumatic or rheumatoid), can reduce space in the carpal tunnel, thereby increasing pressure on the median nerve. Edema, which exacerbates compression, is often secondary to general medical problems, such as thyroid dysfunction and amyloidosis.

Complaints include paresthesias and pain in the distribution of the median nerve, which supplies sensation to the volar thumb, index and long fingers, and half of the ring finger. Sensation in the thenar area is intact, since it is supplied by a branch of the median nerve that arises proximal to the wrist. Patients may complain of clumsiness in the hand if the thenar muscles are affected. Symptoms are aggravated by activity, which increases inflammation and edema in the hand. Often they are worse at night because of sleeping on the wrist or maintaining it in palmar flexion, which presses the stout proximal edge of the trans-

verse carpal ligament against the median nerve.

Examination begins with close inspection of the hand for thenar atrophy, which is uncommon but important, since it is usually irreversible. Weakness of the thenar muscles can be detected by loss of strength in thumb abduction, opposition, and pinch. Patients with true weakness have a consistent, reproducible maximal grip strength, whereas malingerers exhibit an erratic pattern of maximal grip strength.

Sensation can be tested by assessing appreciation of light touch and pinprick as well as two-point discrimination (normally 3 to 5 mm in the fingertips). In mild or moderate cases, all of these parameters may be normal. Provocative tests include *Tinel's test,* performed by tapping over the median nerve at the wrist, and *Phalen's test* (Fig. 10.25). Distal median paresthesias constitute a positive test in both cases. The value of these tests is limited, since they are positive in 20 and 46 percent, respectively, of the normal population.

Electrophysiologic tests provide objective data that should support but not supplant clinical findings. Nerve conduction tests show delays in motor and sensory conduction across the carpal canal (Fig. 10.26). Electromyography of the thenar muscles helps establish the presence or absence of axonal damage. Relevant laboratory tests include thyroid function tests and blood glucose level, since both thyroid disease and diabetes are associated with carpal tunnel syndrome.

Treatment of carpal tunnel syndrome depends on the severity of the disorder. Thenar atrophy is an indication for prompt carpal tunnel release, since it indicates severe, long-standing compression of the nerve and may be

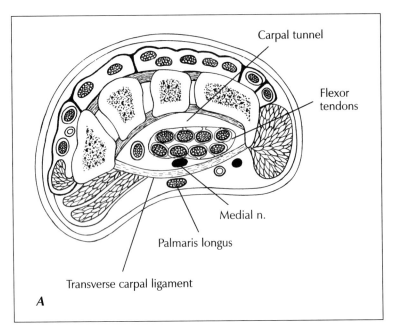

Figure 10.24   *A.* Carpal tunnel syndrome results from compression of the median nerve in the carpal tunnel, which can occur if the contents of the tunnel become enlarged (e.g., tenosynovitis of the flexor tendons). *B.* The median nerve provides branches to the thenar muscles as well as to digital sensory nerves that serve the thumb, the index and long fingers, and half of the ring finger. Note that the palmar cutaneous nerve arises before the median nerve enters the carpal tunnel.

irreversible. Severe, disabling pain is another indication for surgical release. In milder cases, a trial of nonoperative therapy is warranted. Underlying causes, such as rheumatoid arthritis, diabetes, and hypothyroidism should be addressed. Rest and avoidance of aggravating activities are the mainstays of nonoperative treatment and alleviate symptoms in many individuals. A wrist splint is worn at night if symptoms are particularly distressful during sleep. Nonsteroidal anti-inflammatory medications may be useful, but the benefit of steroid injections in the carpal tunnel is debated. If a patient fails nonoperative treatment, surgical release is performed. Recovery of grip strength after carpal tunnel release typically requires 3 to 6 weeks. The carpal tunnel syndrome of pregnancy usually terminates early in the postpartum period without surgical intervention.

Tarsal Tunnel Syndrome

An uncommon disorder similar to carpal tunnel syndrome occurs in the foot and causes similar symptoms of numbness, tingling, and

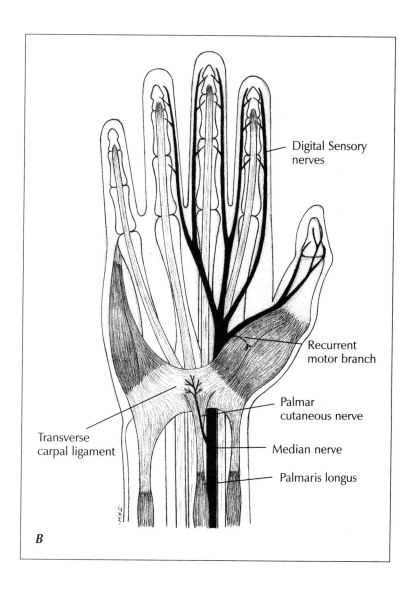

Digital Sensory
nerves

Recurrent
motor branch

Palmar
cutaneous nerve

Median nerve

Palmaris longus

Transverse
carpal ligament

B

Figure 10.24 Continued

burning pain. The tibial nerve is usually affected in its course posterior to the medial malleolus under the flexor retinaculum; rarely, the deep peroneal nerve is affected under the extensor retinaculum anteriorly. The cause is often related to trauma or tenosynovitis, and up to 5 percent of patients with rheumatoid arthritis are affected.

When the tibial nerve is affected, one or all of its three branches may be involved, including the calcaneal, medial plantar, and lateral plantar branches. Pain is typically in the sole of the foot and toes. The dorsum of the foot is spared. For unknown reasons, symptoms are often worse at night. In severe cases there may be atrophy of the intrinsic muscles and clawing

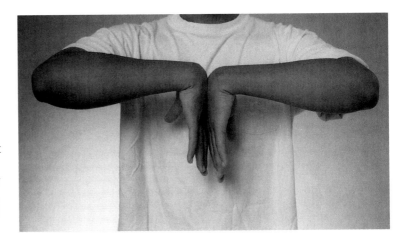

Figure 10.25 Phalen's test for carpal tunnel syndrome. When the wrist is maximally palmar-flexed for 30 to 60 s, numbness, paresthesias, and pain are reproduced.

of the toes. Tinel's sign is positive posteroinferiorly to the medial malleolus. Electrodiagnostic studies are helpful in establishing the diagnosis. Treatment is similar to that of carpal tunnel syndrome and includes rest, nonsteroidal anti-inflammatory medications, injection of steroids, and, in intractable cases, surgical release of the tarsal tunnel. Arch supports may be useful in patients with pronated feet.

Thoracic Outlet Syndrome

Prior to the 1950s, when the carpal tunnel syndrome became well known, the thoracic outlet syndrome was the favored diagnosis for patients with numbness and tingling in the hand. The symptoms were believed to result from compression of the neurovascular structures near the first rib. Most patients were probably misdiagnosed, and the disorder is now believed to be uncommon.

Manifestations of the thoracic outlet syndrome may be primarily neurogenic or vascular. Like other entrapment neuropathies, the diagnosis is often difficult because it relies

more upon the accurate description of symptoms than upon pathognomonic signs or tests. Middle-aged women are most likely to develop the syndrome.

The neurogenic form involves primarily the medial cord of the brachial plexus (C8 and T1), which affects the ulnar, medial brachial, and medial antebrachial nerves. Findings include weakness of the intrinsics of the hand and paresthesias along the medial aspect of the arm, forearm, and hand. The large area of sensory involvement is an important diagnostic clue. Patients with entrapment of only the ulnar nerve have sensory loss confined to the ulnar border of the hand.

The vascular form of the disease involves compression of the subclavian artery. Complaints of pain and coldness in the arm are associated with pallor or cyanosis. Chronic compression of the subclavian artery leads to intimal damage, post-stenotic dilation, aneurysmal formation, and thrombosis, with gangrene involving the tips of the fingers. Diagnosis is usually not difficult.

Most often patients have symptoms without

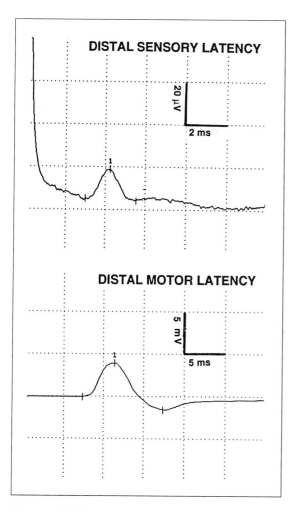

Figure 10.26 Nerve conduction studies in carpal tunnel syndrome. Note the increase in conduction times and decrease in wave amplitude. Distal sensory latency, which is measured at the peak of the waveform, is normally less than 2.2 ms, and amplitude should be greater than 40 μV (4.1 ms and 32 μV respectively, in this patient). Distal motor latency, which is measured at the onset of the waveform, is normally less than 4.2 ms (7.4 ms in this patient). The normal amplitude, which is dependent on the stimulus, should be greater than 5 mV (4 mV in this patient).

overt structural abnormalities, vascular lesions or neurologic deficits. Complaints of pain, tingling, or coldness are commonly associated with certain postures or positions.

Numerous structures may contribute to compression of the neurovascular bundle, including the scalenus anterior muscle, the first rib, a cervical rib, a long transverse process of C7, or an anomalous fibrous band, which connects the sternum to the end of the cervical rib or transverse process of C7 (Fig. 10.27). A short, incomplete cervical rib is more likely to cause neurologic symptoms, while a long, complete cervical rib is more apt to incite vascular problems, since the vascular bundle is situated more anteriorly than the brachial plexus. It has also been theorized that poor posture with ptosis or drooping of the shoulder girdle increases traction on the neurovascular bundle. Symptoms worsen with lifting of heavy objects and overhead activities, especially those involving extension and lateral rotation at the shoulder. Hairdressers, painters, and musicians, such as flutists and violinists, are especially likely to develop the disorder.

Objective clinical findings are elusive in the neurogenic form. Weakness may be demonstrable, but atrophy is rare. A number of provocative tests have been described. In *Adson's test*, there is a decrease in the radial pulse when the neck is extended and the head turned to the affected side (Fig. 10.28). The same effect may follow abduction and lateral rotation of the shoulder. Whichever variation is employed, it should be stressed that while a diminution of the pulse may be felt in normal subjects, reproduction of the patient's symptoms is a critical finding. Other tests include Tinel's test, in which light percussion of the supraclavicular area reproduces paresthesias. Auscul-

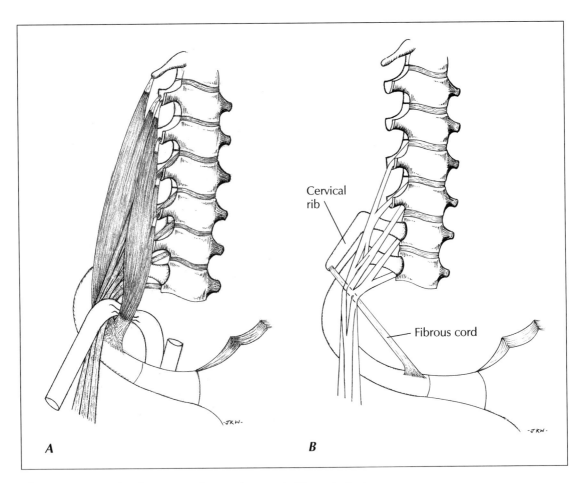

Figure 10.27   The thoracic outlet syndrome. *A.* The subclavian artery may
be compressed between the anterior and middle scalene muscles. *B.* The
brachial plexus may be compromised by a fibrous band that extends from
a cervical rib or a long transverse process of C7.

tation of the clavicular area may reveal a bruit
in vascular cases.

Electrophysiologic testing may be helpful
but is not diagnostic, since a negative test does
not exclude the thoracic outlet syndrome. Recording of somatosensory evoked potentials
has been successful in some patients. Arteri-
ography is not indicated unless a vascular
component to the symptoms is strongly sus-

pected. Important disorders to consider in the
differential diagnosis include cervical radiculopathy, the subclavian steal syndrome, and
other entrapment neuropathies.

Treatment of the thoracic outlet syndrome
begins with nonoperative measures, unless ar-
teriography has demonstrated an aneurysm or
other vascular lesion. Activities that exacerbate symptoms should be avoided and exer-

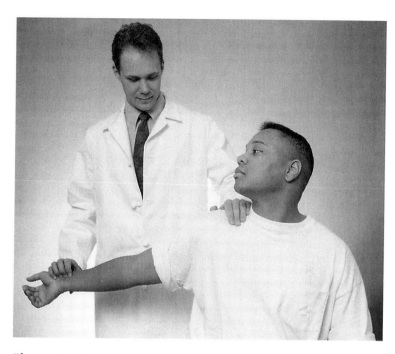

Figure 10.28   Adson's test for thoracic outlet syndrome. A decrease in the radial pulse can be felt when the neck is extended and the head turned to the affected side. Paresthesias, numbness, or pain that mimic the patient's complaints are also significant findings. A stethoscope placed over the subclavian artery during the maneuver may reveal a bruit.

cises to improve posture and diminish shoulder ptosis performed, with particular emphasis on strengthening of the trapezius and pectoralis major muscles. In selected patients who have failed nonoperative therapy, surgical resection of the cervical rib, constricting band, or first thoracic rib may be considered.

Charcot Joints

The development of a *neuropathic joint,* more commonly known as a Charcot joint, is the end result of numerous disparate disorders that cause a loss of sensation, especially pain, in joints. The condition was originally described in 1868 by Charcot in reference to tabes dorsalis. Since then, many other disorders have been noted to cause a similar picture, including diabetes mellitus, syringomyelia, leprosy, congenital absence of pain, and peripheral neuropathies, such as those caused by alcoholism and malnutrition. The Charcot joint is a particularly destructive arthropathy that is difficult to manage and often has devastating effects on the function of a limb. The pathogenesis is related to diminished proprioception and protective pain sensation. Repetitive injuries to the joint have an additive effect but are not rec-

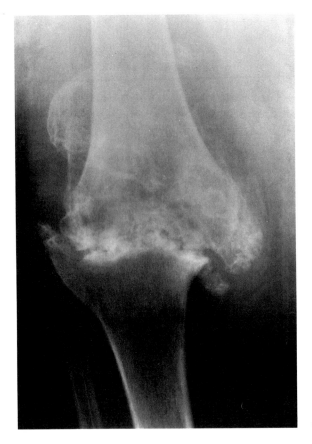

Figure 10.29   Charcot joint. Note the extensive destruction of the knee joint.

ognized by the patient. In addition, a hyperemic inflammatory response amplifies the destructive nature of the process. Cartilage, bone, ligaments, capsule, and soft tissue may all be involved by the inflammatory tissue.

It is important to note that the absence of pain need not be complete, and there is a popular misconception that Charcot joints are always painless. While the chief complaint in many patients is painless swelling, a substantial number of patients cite pain as their primary symptom. Other complaints include joint instability, weakness, numbness, and ulceration, which is especially common in the feet (Fig. 11.11). Most Charcot joints develop in middle-aged and elderly adults, and they most often involve the weight-bearing joints of the lower limbs. In the upper limbs, syringomyelia is a frequent cause of the disorder. When a Charcot joint is suspected, a careful search must be made for the underlying cause.

The radiographic appearance of an advanced Charcot joint is impressive (Fig. 10.29). Aside from neglected infections, few other disorders demonstrate such widespread destruction of the joint. The histologic appearance is likewise striking and characterized by bits of cartilage and dead bone interspersed through the deep layers of synovium and surrounding soft tissue.

Treatment of Charcot joints is challenging and often frustrating. When the condition is recognized at an early stage, protective measures such as bracing and crutch ambulation may slow down or even arrest the process. Neuropathic changes in the foot can sometimes be managed by customized hard orthotics and shoes. Exostectomy (the excision of a bony bump) may remove the inciting cause of an ulceration but can also be hazardous, since resection of bone may further destabilize the foot. Arthrodesis is sometimes attempted, but the rate of successful fusion is significantly less than that for other disorders, such as osteoarthritis. Replacement may benefit certain joints, such as the knee, but experience with this procedure for Charcot joints has been limited and not uniformly successful. Unfortunately, many patients still require amputation for definitive treatment.

SUGGESTED READINGS

BLECK EE: *Orthopaedic Management in Cerebral Palsy.* London, MacKeith Press, 1987.

BRACKEN MB, SHEPARD MJ, COLLINS WF, ET AL: A randomized, controlled trial of methylprednisolone or naloxone in the treatment of acute spinal-cord injury: Results of the Second National Acute Spinal Cord Injury Study. *N Engl J Med* 322:1405–1411, 1990.

BRADFORD DS, LONSTEIN JE, MOE JH, ET AL (EDS): *Moe's Textbook of Scoliosis and Other Spinal Deformities,* 2d ed. Philadelphia, Saunders, 1987.

BROOKE M: *A Clinician's View of Neuromuscular Diseases,* 2d ed. Baltimore, Williams & Wilkins, 1986.

DAWSON DM, HALLETT M, MILLENDER LH: *Entrapment Neuropathies.* Boston, Little Brown, 1990.

JACKSON ST, HOFFER MM, PARRISH N: Brachial plexus palsy in the newborn. *J Bone Joint Surg* 70A:1217–1220, 1988.

KUBAN KC, LEVITON A: Cerebral palsy. *N Engl J Med* 330:188–195, 1994.

KUSHNER SH, EBRAMZADEH E, JOHNSON D, ET AL: Tinel's sign and Phalen's test in carpal tunnel syndrome. *Orthopedics* 15:1297–1302, 1992.

NELSON KB, ELLENBERG JH: Antecedents of cerebral palsy: Multivariate analysis of risk. *N Engl J Med* 315:81–86, 1986.

PHALEN GS, KENDRICK JI: Compression neuropathy of the median nerve in the carpal tunnel. *JAMA* 164:524–530, 1957.

POLLOCK FH, DRAKE D, BOVILL EG, ET AL: Treatment of radial neuropathy associated with fractures of the humerus. *J Bone Joint Surg* 63A:243, 1981.

ROOS DB: Congenital anomalies associated with thoracic outlet syndrome. *Am J Surg* 132:771, 1976.

SHAPIRO F, SPECHT L: The diagnosis and orthopaedic treatment of childhood spinal muscular atrophy, peripheral neuropathy, Friedreich ataxia, and arthrogryposis. *J Bone Joint Surg* 75A:1699–1714, 1993.

SWASH M, SCHWARTZ MS: *Neuromuscular Diseases: A Practical Approach to Diagnosis and Management.* London, Springer-Verlag, 1988.

WILBOURN AJ, PORTER JM: Thoracic outlet syndrome. *Spine* 2:597, 1988.

Chapter 11

Infections

Patrick P. Lin, Gary D. Bos, and Frank C. Wilson

GENERAL ASPECTS
Microbiology

The ability of an organism to cause infection depends upon its virulence and the susceptibility of the host. Most musculoskeletal infections are caused by a small, select group of virulent bacteria. Among healthy adults, an alteration in susceptibility, such as that caused by local trauma, often predisposes to infection and gives bacteria the slight advantage they need to establish an infection. In debilitated patients, benign organisms may become pathogens, and weakened and immunocompromised hosts are also susceptible to infections with atypical organisms, such as mycobacteria and fungi.

Although bacteria are simple, unicellular organisms, they possess elaborate protective exteriors (Fig. 11.1). The *cell wall,* a rigid structure composed of sugars and peptides, surrounds the cell membrane and prevents the organism from swelling and bursting. Gram-positive bacteria have a thick, prominent cell wall, while gram-negative bacteria have a thin cell wall covered by an *outer membrane,* a phospholipid layer containing proteins and the lipopolysaccharide *endotoxin,* which can cause septic shock. The *capsule,* also known as the slime layer or *glycocalyx,* is a loose polysaccharide envelope around the cell wall of some bacteria (e.g., staphylococci) that provides a buffer zone for growth and protects the bacteria against harmful agents. *Pili* or fimbriae,

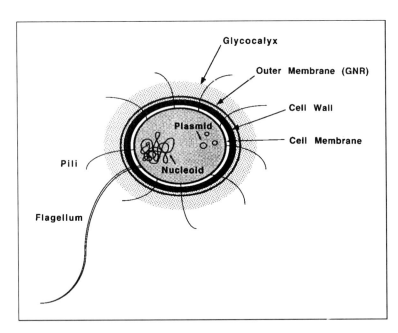

Figure 11.1   Bacterium. Some structures, such as the pili, flagellum and glycocalyx, are present only in certain organisms. The outer membrane is present on gram negative rods (GNR).

present in certain bacteria such as *Escherichia coli* and *Streptococcus pyogenes,* are extracellular structures involved in several functions, including exchange of genetic material and attachment to solids. Special receptors known as *adhesins* allow bacteria to identify and colonize sites that are most advantageous to their growth. Bacterial survival depends greatly upon adherence to a surface; once firmly anchored, bacteria can synthesize a glycocalyx, and their ability to withstand stress increases significantly.

Colonization of body surfaces is not the equivalent of infection; thousands of benign bacteria inhabit the skin and mucosal membranes. Virulent bacteria are characterized by their ability to penetrate and grow in normally sterile tissues. Virulence results from the elaboration of degradative enzymes, production of toxins, resistance to antibiotics, and mechanisms to elude the immune system. Antibiotic resistance may develop by means of chromosomal mutations or the acquisition of *transposons* (mobile genetic elements) and *plasmids* (self-replicating, circular DNA). Transposons and plasmids can code for multiple resistance genes and are readily exchanged between bacteria of the same species and sometimes bacteria of different species.

Staphylococcus aureus, a gram-positive organism, is the most common cause of musculoskeletal infections. The virulence of these bacteria, which are part of normal skin and nasal flora in 25 percent of the population, depends upon multiple factors, including the presence of adhesins that bind fibronectin, collagen, and other molecules in muculoskeletal tissues. Enzymes like *catalase* retard lysosomal killing and permit bacteria to survive in phagocytic cells. A number of different toxins have been isolated from various strains of

S. aureus, including α-hemolysin and leukocidin.

Other staphylococcal species also cause infections of the musculoskeletal system. These organisms differ from *S. aureus* by the absence of the enzyme *coagulase,* which causes plasma to clot. Among coagulase-negative staphylococci, *S. epidermidis* is a common pathogen. Although it is part of normal skin flora and less virulent than *S. aureus,* it has a prominent thick slime layer that adheres exceptionally well to inert substances, such as intravenous catheters and prosthetic implants.

Like staphylococci, streptococci are grampositive bacteria that often cause musculoskeletal infections. Many streptococcal species are part of the normal flora of the skin, respiratory tract, and digestive system. The most frequent pathogen, *S. pyogenes* (Group A streptococcus), produces numerous toxins, including streptolysin S and streptolysin O, which are cytotoxic, and streptokinase, which lyses fibrin clots. The M protein is a molecule on the cell wall of virulent strains that is associated with resistance to phagocytosis. *Enterococci* are a group of streptococcal species that normally reside in the intestines and are noteworthy for their exceptional resistance to antibiotics.

Gram-negative bacilli have become major pathogens in orthopaedic infections, especially those that involve chronic lesions, open wounds, and underlying debility. Among these organisms, *Pseudomonas aeruginosa* is the most frequent offender. Like *S. aureus,* its virulence arises from resistance to multiple antibiotics, production of proteolytic enzymes such as *collagenase* and *elastase,* and elaboration of toxins such as hemolysin, leukocidin, and exotoxin A, which inhibits protein synthesis in a manner similar to diphtheria toxin.

Immunology

Host defenses against bacterial infections involve both nonspecific and specific mechanisms. Nonspecific defenses include epithelial barriers, bactericidal enzymes, cytokines, and phagocytic cells. Specific mechanisms are mediated by antibodies and lymphocytes (see Chap. 15). Although the complete array of defenses is complicated, several components are especially important for protection against bacteria: antibodies, complement, and phagocytic cells.

Antibodies do not destroy bacteria directly but facilitate their elimination by opsonization, phagocytosis, and the activation of complement. Circulating antibodies against certain bacterial antigens are normally present in serum, allowing an immediate response to bacterial incursions. The production of most antibodies, however, depends upon an immune response involving both B lymphocytes, which develop into the plasma cells that synthesize the antibodies, and helper T lymphocytes, which stimulate the B lymphocytes.

Complement is a set of serum proteins that form lethal pores in bacteria and other target cells. Gram-negative bacteria are more susceptible to this mode of killing. An alternative method of killing, especially important in the elimination of gram-positive bacteria, involves phagocytosis of complement-coated particles. Two mechanisms activate the complement cascade. The classic pathway relies on antibodies bound to target cells; the alternative pathway is induced directly by certain antigens on the bacterial cell wall.

In an acute infection, neutrophils are the primary phagocytic cells that destroy bacteria. Lymphocytes and macrophages, which migrate more slowly but survive longer than neutrophils, become prominent later in the course of infection. Neutrophils ingest bacteria that are coated with immunoglobulin and complement. They also directly recognize the cell wall antigens of certain bacteria, including *E. coli* and *S. aureus.* After phagocytosis, neutrophils degranulate and fuse the lysosomal granules with the ingested bacteria. Although neutrophils are instrumental in killing bacteria, they are also responsible for much of the damage to host tissues. The by-products of neutrophils—neutral proteases, collagenases, and free radicals—degrade connective tissues and cause subsequent scarring and fibrosis.

Numerous nonspecific mechanisms are also vital to the defense against bacteria. *Lysozyme* is an enzyme in tissue fluids that directly lyses bacterial cell walls, especially of gram-negative bacteria. *Beta lysins* are serum proteins that have similar action against gram-positive organisms. *C-reactive protein* enhances phagocytosis of bacteria and may have direct bactericidal effects. *Histamine, bradykinin,* and other vasoactive molecules increase vascular permeability and produce local edema. Cytokines and growth factors amplify the inflammatory response. *Interleukin-1* and *tumor necrosis factor-α* produce fever and other clinical manifestations of sepsis.

Pharmacology of Antibiotics

Penicillins

Penicillin is the forerunner of many antibiotics (Fig. 11.2). Its action depends upon the *β-lactam ring,* which not only blocks cross-linking of the bacterial cell wall but also induces formation of bacterial lytic enzymes that destroy the cell wall. Resistance to penicillin may be acquired by action of the enzyme *β-lactamase*

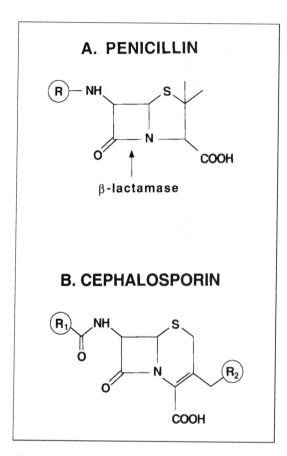

A. PENICILLIN

β-lactamase

B. CEPHALOSPORIN

Figure 11.2 Penicillins and cephalosporins. Note the similarities of chemical structures.

or by mutations of penicillin-binding protein, which transports penicillin into the bacterium. Most strains of *S. aureus* now possess plasmid-encoded β-lactamase.

The semisynthetic penicillins (e.g., oxacillin and dicloxacillin) are resistant to β-lactamase and are employed specifically for staphylococcal infections. Methicillin is used for laboratory testing but is not often used clinically because of nephrotoxicity. Most community-acquired staphylococcal infections respond to the semisynthetic penicillins,

but methicillin-resistant *S. aureus* (MRSA) strains, which are common in hospital-acquired infections, are not susceptible.

The ampicillin group of penicillins has greater activity against gram-negative bacteria, but they are vulnerable to inactivation by β-lactamase. Combination with a β-lactamase inhibitor, such as clavulanic acid or sulbactam, increases their coverage of *S. aureus*. Several of these penicillins (e.g., ticarcillin, carbenicillin, mezlocillin, azlocillin, piperacillin) are notable for their activity against *Pseudomonas*.

Cephalosporins

Cephalosporins are similar in action to penicillins and share a similar chemical structure (Fig. 11.2). Cephalosporins have variable susceptibilities to β-lactamase inactivation, since the active group includes a β-lactam ring. However, the antimicrobial activity of specific agents does not strictly correlate with resistance to β-lactamase. First-generation cephalosporins (e.g., cephalexin, cefazolin) have excellent activity against most β-lactamase-producing *S. aureus* strains, despite their susceptibility to β-lactamase. Second- and third-generation cephalosporins are less potent against gram-positive organisms but have broader coverage, especially of gram-negative bacteria and *Haemophilus influenzae;* and several third-generation drugs (e.g., ceftazidime, ceftriaxone) are active against *Pseudomonas aeruginosa.*

Vancomycin

Vancomycin is a small glycopeptide that is effective against nearly all gram-positive organisms; as such, it is the most widely used antibiotic for methicillin-resistant *S. aureus.* Vancomycin inhibits cell-wall synthesis and damages the cell membrane. Resistance emerges slowly, and there is no cross-resistance with other antibiotics. Hypersensitivity reactions, ototoxicity, and nephrotoxicity are uncommon. *Red man syndrome,* characterized by flushing, pruritus, tachycardia, hypotension, and a macular rash over the upper trunk, develops when the drug is given too rapidly and is not a true allergic reaction.

Aminoglycosides

Aminoglycosides bind ribosomes and irreversibly inhibit protein synthesis. They are used primarily for gram-negative infections but are also active against staphylococci. Streptococci, in contrast, are resistant. Anaerobic bacteria are also resistant, since the transport of aminoglycosides requires oxygen. Antibiotics that act at the cell wall enhance penetration of aminoglycosides and have a synergistic effect. Certain aminoglycosides (e.g., tobramycin and amikacin) are more active against *P. aeruginosa.* Hypersensitivity reactions are rare, but ototoxicity and nephrotoxicity occur with high doses and prolonged therapy. Resistance to one aminoglycoside does not necessarily produce cross-resistance to other aminoglycosides.

Other Antibiotics

Rifampin inhibits RNA polymerase and is active against staphylococci, including MRSA and *S. epidermidis.* It suffers from the rapid emergence of resistant strains, so the drug is used only in combination with other antibiotics for its synergistic effect.

Bacitracin, a group of polypeptides isolated from *Bacillus subtilis,* has strong activity against gram-positive organisms. Nephrotoxicity precludes systemic use, but topical use in ointments and irrigation solutions is safe, since absorption is negligible.

Clindamycin inhibits protein synthesis by binding to ribosomes and is effective against many gram-positive organisms, including MRSA. Resistance occasionally arises during treatment, and cross-resistance with erythromycin has been reported. Pseudomembranous colitis is a serious but uncommon complication.

Imipenem is a broad-spectrum agent with activity against *S. aureus* and *P. aeruginosa,* but not MRSA.

Ciprofloxacin is a quinolone that inhibits DNA gyrase. Oral dosing and a broad antimicrobial spectrum, including some MSRA and *P. aeruginosa,* have made it popular in the past, but resistant organisms have emerged, and resistance occasionally develops during treatment.

COMMON BACTERIAL INFECTIONS

Osteomyelitis

Infections of bone can be grouped into two broad categories: hematogenous and exogenous. Hematogenous osteomyelitis predilects the long bones of children. Exogenous osteomyelitis most often follows open fractures or surgery. A unique form of exogenous osteomyelitis is that associated with vascular insufficiency, as seen in diabetic foot infections. Each type of osteomyelitis has different pathophysiology and consequently requires a distinct approach to therapy.

Hematogenous

ACUTE HEMATOGENOUS OSTEOMYELITIS This infection predilects the distal femur, proximal tibia, and proximal femur of children. For unknown reasons, males are affected twice as often as females. The incidence of hematogenous osteomyelitis rises again among the elderly, but the majority of these infections involve the vertebrae and are discussed separately.

Occasionally, a distant site of infection, such as the ear with otitis media, can be identified, but a forgotten cut or abrasion usually provides the portal of entry for bacteria. Overall, *S. aureus* is the most common organism. Among neonates, group B streptococci and gram-negative bacilli are common, while *H. influenzae* is prominent in children between the ages of 1 and 4. Patients with sickle cell disease are particularly susceptible to *salmonella* infections.

The pathogenesis of hematogenous osteomyelitis is related to the unique vascular anatomy of growing bones. In children, metaphyseal vessels approach but do not cross the physis into the epiphysis; instead, they make a hairpin turn, causing sluggish blood flow, which favors bacterial lodgment (Fig. 11.3). In addition, fenestration of these blood vessels allows bacteria to escape into metaphyseal sinusoids.

When infection develops, an inflammatory reaction produces local hyperemia and edema, which eventually leads to death and resorption of bone. As purulent fluid expands inside the bone, pressure builds and forces pus through the porous metaphyseal cortex into the subperiosteal space, lifting the periosteum and creating a subperiosteal abscess. Metaphyseal bone is particularly vulnerable to necrosis, since it can lose both its endosteal and periosteal blood supplies. The physis, in contrast, remains viable because its blood supply is derived from epiphyseal vessels. The necrotic segment of bone is known as a *sequestrum*.

The periosteum, which is attached to overlying soft tissues, remains alive and often forms an envelope of new bone or *involucrum* around the infection.

Pain, erythema, and swelling are common, but drainage is rare in the acute phase. Fever and chills are variably present. The history can be misleading, since patients without fever and chills often ascribe their symptoms to a recent minor injury. Characteristic physical findings, such as bony tenderness and warmth, are less specific in infants, who may only limp, refuse to bear weight, or exhibit pseudoparalysis.

Helpful laboratory tests are the white blood cell count, which is elevated in most cases, and the erythrocyte sedimentation rate (ESR), which is more sensitive but not specific for infection. Blood cultures are positive in only half of all patients.

Radiographs are of little help early in the disease. The first radiographic findings are soft tissue swelling and obliteration of fat planes. Lytic areas in bone become visible 1 to 2 weeks after the onset of symptoms (Fig. 11.4). Mottling and osteopenia are followed in another week or so by new bone formation around the subperiosteal abscess. A sclerotic fragment of bone suggests a sequestrum.

A three-phase bone scan with technetium phosphate is 80 percent sensitive for infection but is not specific. Increased uptake occurs in areas of infection, neoplasia, osteophyte formation, and fracture. Decreased uptake, or a "cold spot," characterizes a sequestrum. The bone scan helps localize infection in infants or in difficult areas such as the spine. Other radioisotopic scans—gallium 67 citrate and indium-111 white cell scans—identify areas of inflammation but do not reflect bone turnover.

Aspiration of the subperiosteal abscess is the most important diagnostic test and does not

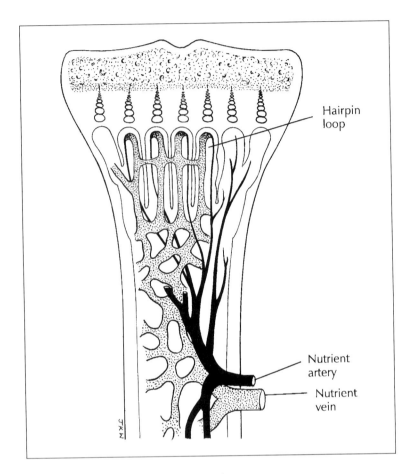

Hairpin loop

Nutrient artery

Nutrient vein

Figure 11.3 Vascular anatomy of acute hematogenous osteomyelitis. Hematogenous seeding occurs through the nutrient artery, which gives rise to the metaphyseal branch and the capillary. The hairpin loop at the physis is an area where blood flow is sluggish, and bacteria can establish infection. (Adapted from Hobo T: Zur pathogenese der akuten Haematogenen Osteomyelitis, mit Berücksichtigung der Vitalfärbungslehre. *Acta Scholae Med Univ Imp,* Kioto, 4:1–30, 1921.)

affect subsequent bone scans. If no pus is found, the needle should be advanced into metaphyseal bone with a trocar or stylet. Fluoroscopy may be needed to avoid the physis and ensure proper placement of the needle. If no fluid is recovered, nonbacteriostatic saline is injected into the suspect area, recovered, and sent for culture. Ultrasound may be useful to demonstrate a subperiosteal abscess in difficult cases. Blood cultures should be obtained in all patients, especially during a temperature spike.

Although controversy surrounds the management of acute hematogenous osteomyelitis,

the principles of treatment are similar to those for other infections. Antibiotics are the mainstay of treatment, but the bacteria must be sensitive to the medications, and they must be delivered to the site in sufficient concentration to eradicate the infection. In the early stages, osteomyelitis is similar to cellulitis. No pus is present, and antibiotics alone are usually sufficient. When an abscess or avascular sequestrum is present, effective delivery of antibiotics is compromised and surgical debridement becomes necessary. The importance of removing devitalized tissue cannot be overempha-

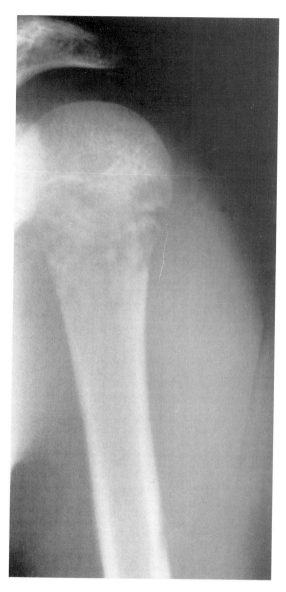

Figure 11.4   Acute hematogenous osteomyelitis of the proximal humerus. Mottling and patchy radiolucencies are present in the metaphyseal region.

sized, given the propensity of bone to chronic infection.

The optimal duration of antibiotic treatment is unknown. Although the clinical response is often rapid, microcolonies of bacteria often persist in segments of necrotic bone. Traditionally, 6 weeks of intravenous antibiotic therapy is recommended, with treatment extended if clinical, radiographic, or laboratory parameters remain abnormal. Recently, oral antibiotics have been substituted after 1 to 2 weeks of parenteral therapy, and the *serum bactericidal titer* used to monitor serum levels. The ratio of the bactericidal concentration to the actual serum concentration should not fall below 1 : 2.

NEONATAL OSTEOMYELITIS   Neonatal osteomyelitis is a potentially devastating disease. Often multifocal, it can also destroy the epiphysis, cause joint deformity, and arrest growth. The epiphysis is vulnerable because the physeal-blood barrier does not form until 12 months of age. Involvement of the epiphysis jeopardizes both the proliferating chondrocytes of the physis and the blood supply to the epiphysis. Early recognition, which may require extended observation of an immobile limb, is critical.

VERTEBRAL OSTEOMYELITIS   Vertebral osteomyelitis usually affects elderly, debilitated, or diabetic patients. *Staphylococcus aureus* is the most common pathogen, but one-third of these infections are due to gram-negative bacilli. Bacterial infections usually affect the lumbar vertebrae, while tuberculous infections (see below) favor the thoracic spine. The process tends to spread from one vertebral body across a disk to an adjacent body, sparing the pedicles and lamina; in contrast, neoplastic processes rarely cross the disk space. The clinical manifestations of vertebral infection vary markedly. If an epidural abscess develops, the disease may progress rapidly to paralysis. Most cases, however, have an insidious onset; back pain can be present for weeks or months before a physician is consulted. The most consistent finding is tenderness of the spine. Few patients have fever, limitation of motion, positive straight leg–raising tests, or neurologic deficits.

The white count is inconsistently elevated, but the ESR is usually abnormal. Blood cultures are positive in only one-fourth of cases. Radiographs demonstrate disk space narrowing, with erosive changes in adjacent vertebrae (Fig. 11.5). The bone scan is usually positive. Computed tomography (CT) scans are sensitive for bony changes and abscesses and help guide percutaneous aspirations. It is important to screen for mycobacteria and fungi as well as bacteria.

Surgery is indicated for an epidural abscess and/or neurologic deterioration, but paravertebral abscesses can often be drained percutaneously with CT guidance, and spinal instability can be managed by a brace until spontaneous spinal fusion occurs. Six weeks of parenteral antibiotics is recommended. The ESR is useful for monitoring disease activity and should fall to at least one-third of its initial value before therapy is discontinued.

DISCITIS   Discitis is a relatively benign infection of the disks and vertebral end plates in children. The disease is usually caused by *S. aureus.* The typical patient is a child 1 to 6 years old who appears well but complains of back pain and has difficulty walking. Spasm of paraspinous muscles and hyperlordosis of

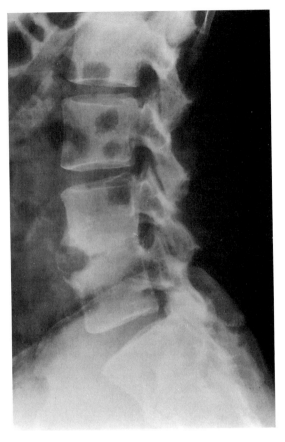

Figure 11.5   Vertebral osteomyelitis of the lumbar spine. Note involvement of two adjacent vertebrae (L4 and L5) and the intervening disk.

the lumbar spine occur, and a kyphotic arch fails to develop when the patient bends forward. The white count is characteristically normal, but the sedimentation rate is elevated. Lateral radiographs of the spine demonstrate irregularity of the vertebral end plates and narrowing of the disk space (Fig. 11.6). Bone scans are usually positive, but magnetic reso-

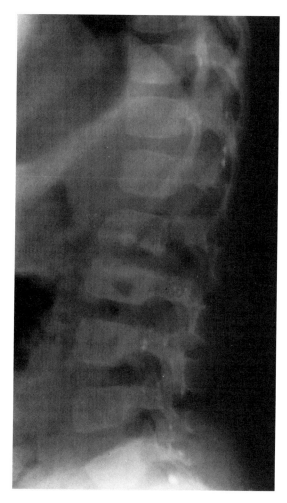

Figure 11.6 Discitis. Note the moth-eaten appearance of the vertebral end plates of two adjacent vertebra (L1 and L2).

nance imaging (MRI) scans are even more sensitive, especially early in the course of infection. Most patients respond rapidly to intravenous antibiotics directed against *S. aureus;* if not, aspiration is necessary to identify the organism. The duration of treatment is similar to that for hematogenous osteomyelitis. Brac-

ing or casting relieves pain but is not necessary for mild symptoms.

SUBACUTE HEMATOGENOUS OSTEOMYELITIS A primary subacute hematogenous osteomyelitis may occur, which has a more indolent course than acute hematogenous osteomyelitis. Symptoms are typically present for more than 2 weeks before patients seek medical attention. Involvement of the lower limbs does not preclude weight bearing and walking. Histologically, lesions are composed of granulation tissue without frank pus or sequestrum formation. The pathogenesis may be related to organisms of low virulence or to early administration of empiric antibiotics, which minimizes or suppresses the acute phase and results in sterile cultures. Among the 60 percent of patients with positive cultures, *S. aureus* and *S. epidermidis* are the usual pathogens.

The disorder is characterized radiographically by a radiolucent area and periosteal new bone formation. Since these changes cannot occur in a few days, they confirm the suspicion that the process has been present for 1 to several weeks. Periosteal reaction in the diaphysis usually leads to an *"onionskin"* appearance that simulates Ewing sarcoma (Fig. 11.7). A *Brodie abscess* is a well-contained infection in bone characterized radiographically by a small, lytic, round lesion surrounded by a sclerotic rim and no periosteal reaction (Fig. 11.8). Biopsy of the lesion reveals the granulation tissue characteristic of subacute osteomyelitis.

Laboratory findings, including the white blood cell count and ESR, are less markedly abnormal than in acute hematogenous osteomyelitis. Most patients respond to debridement and appropriate antibiotics. The length of

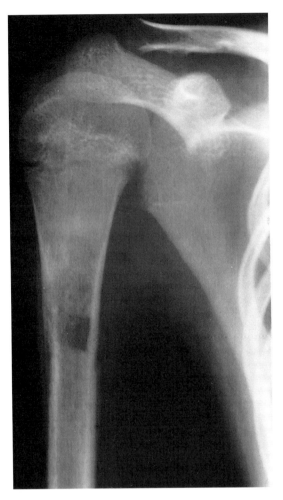

Figure 11.7 Subacute hematogenous osteomyelitis of the humerus. Note the "onion-skin" appearance and diaphyseal involvement reminiscent of Ewing sarcoma.

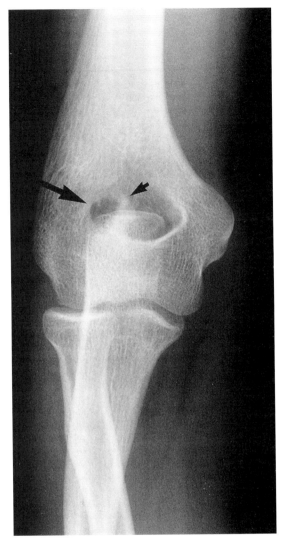

Figure 11.8 Brodie abscess. Note small radiolucent defect in bone *(large arrow)* surrounded by a sclerotic rim *(small arrow)*.

treatment is similar to that for acute osteomyelitis.

CHRONIC HEMATOGENOUS OSTEOMYELITIS Chronic hematogenous osteomyelitis is an infectious process that has been present for an extended period, usually longer than 3 months. The radiographic sine qua non is a sequestrum, a sclerotic fragment of dead bone, which portends periodic recurrence of active disease, since it harbors small foci of bacteria that are inaccessible to antibiotics (Fig. 11.9).

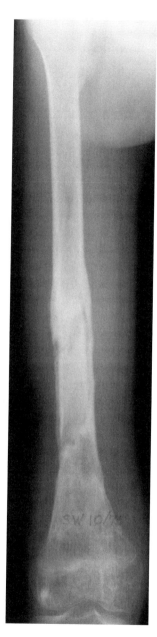

Figure 11.9 Chronic hematogenous osteomyelitis of the femur. Note the formation of an involucrum around a large sequestrum in the middle of the bone.

Other than pain and a draining *sinus,* which is a frequent finding, both systemic and local signs of infection are absent. Chronic osteomyelitis is a surgical disease. Sequestra and sinus tracts must be removed, along with as much infected bone and scar as possible. Local or free flaps of muscle and skin may be necessary to provide soft tissue coverage and blood flow to the region. Occasionally, the resection needed to effect a definitive cure is so extensive that it is preferable to treat the patient with intermittent or long-term antibiotics, which suppress clinical manifestations of the infection (Fig. 11.10).

Exogenous

Exogenous osteomyelitis may be defined as an infection in bone arising from direct contamination or a contiguous focus of infection. Most cases are related to open fractures or surgery. The causative bacteria differ from those associated with acute hematogenous osteomyelitis. While *S. aureus* is still a frequent pathogen, *S. epidermidis,* which adheres to foreign objects, is equally prominent; gram-negative organisms and polymicrobial infections also account for many infections.

The onset may be abrupt or insidious. Immediate postoperative infection may cause wound dehiscence; however, the presentation is usually less dramatic, with slowly progressive pain, swelling, erythema, and drainage. Patients with infected prosthetic joints typically have chronic pain without drainage. Infections in the setting of fractures often result in nonunions.

As in hematogenous osteomyelitis, the ESR is elevated. Radiographs and bone scans are more difficult to interpret because of traumatic and/or postsurgical changes. Direct culture of

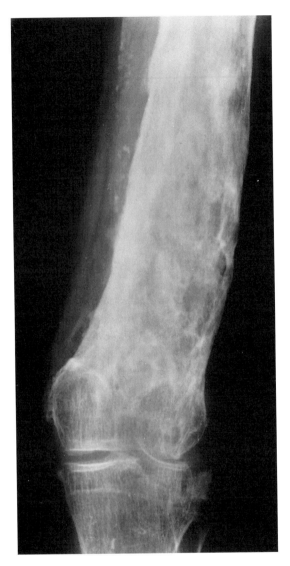

Figure 11.10 Chronic osteomyelitis of the femur. This indolent infection had been present for over fifty years.

though antibiotics are necessary, they usually do not effect a cure without surgical intervention. Treatment is similar to that of chronic hematogenous osteomyelitis, with debridement and soft tissue reconstruction. Removal of surgical implants may be required for cure; however, with rigidly fixed fractures, it is better to retain the hardware until the fracture unites, since it is easier to eradicate the infection once the fracture has healed. If infected prosthetic joints cannot be salvaged, removal of the components, debridement, and intravenous antibiotics (usually for 6 weeks) allow successful reinsertion of a prosthesis in some 80 percent of patients.

Patients with peripheral vascular insufficiency are vulnerable to infections, particularly in the feet, and may develop osteomyelitis either as a primary or, more commonly, as a secondary infection in the setting of chronic ulcers. Poor blood flow favors bacterial growth, compromises natural immune mechanisms, and retards healing.

Foot infections in diabetics pose special problems, since the foot is frequently insensate. These patients are at risk of developing a *Charcot foot* (see Chap. 10), characterized by disintegration and collapse of the bony architecture (Fig. 11.11). The diagnosis of osteomyelitis in this setting is often difficult. Underlying degenerative changes make interpretation of radiographs and bone scans uncertain. Surface swabs of the ulcer bed are rarely helpful because of the presence of contaminants. Ideally, cultures should be obtained from either deep purulent collections or biopsy specimens; these cultures typically grow *S. aureus, P. aeruginosa,* or multiple organisms.

Management of foot infections begins with prevention. Many infections result from a mechanical problem—an ingrown toenail, a bony

infected material is the best means of documenting infection.

The management of exogenous osteomyelitis varies according to the clinical setting. Al-

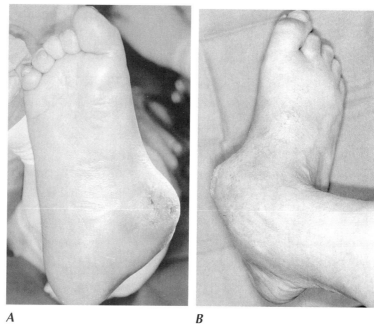

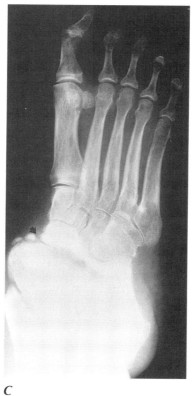

Figure 11.11 Charcot foot. *A* and *B.* Note the ulcer over the prominent talar head Radiographs reveal *(C, arrow)* collapse and disintegration of the talonavicular joint. The ulcer became infected, and the patient eventually required a below-the-knee amputation.

A

B

C

deformity, or poor shoe fit—which must be corrected or accommodated. Open wounds and ulcers demand meticulous care, however small or innocuous they seem, to avoid eventual infection of bone and other deep structures.

The role of antibiotics is limited. Unless an ulcer is associated with cellulitis or osteomyelitis, the patient can be treated without antibiotics. Total contact plaster casts are excellent means of treating clean, uninfected ulcers. If cellulitis is present, antibiotics are used to prevent spread of the infection. Chronic infections of bone may be suppressed by antibiotics but are difficult to cure with antibiotics alone. Such infections usually require debridement or amputation for definitive treatment. The underlying problem must also be addressed. The cause of the peripheral vascular insufficiency should be determined and consultation with appropriate specialists obtained in an effort to improve circulation.

Septic Arthritis

Pathophysiology

Septic arthritis usually arises from hematogenous spread of bacteria, typically from a cut in the skin or an infection elsewhere. Occasionally, penetrating trauma innoculates the joint directly, or an osteomyelitic focus spreads into the joint, especially where the physis is intra-articular, as in the shoulder and hip (Fig. 11.12). The most common causative organism is *S. aureus,* but other organisms are prominent at certain ages (Table 11.1). In newborns, group B streptococcus and gram-negative bacilli are frequent offenders. Among children aged 1 to 4 years, *H. influenzae* infections are especially common. In young, healthy adults, the predominant pathogen is *Neisseria gon-*

orrheoae, which is much more prevalent than *S. aureus.* In older patients, *S. aureus* emerges again as the most likely agent, but gram-negative bacilli are also common, especially *E. coli,* which is the most frequent cause of urinary tract infections.

Septic arthritis occurs in patients with preexisting joint disorders, such as rheumatoid arthritis and osteoarthritis, but it is curiously rare in gout and other forms of crystalline arthropathy. Septic arthritis also predilects patients with debilitating medical problems, including liver disease, renal disease, diabetes mellitus, malignancy, and alcoholism. Intravenous drug abusers are more likely to develop infection with virulent gram-negative organisms, such as *Pseudomonas.*

Clinical Features

The peak incidences of septic arthritis are in the young and the elderly; in some estimates, up to half of the patients are less than 2 years of age. Boys are affected twice as often as girls. The knee is the most commonly affected joint, followed by the hip, shoulder, and wrist.

Articular pain is a consistent finding. Passive movement produces a level of pain matched by few other disorders. The patient splints the joint in the most comfortable position, which in the hip and knee is usually one of slight flexion. Infants and small children refuse to bear weight and may exhibit pseudoparalysis. Erythema, warmth, and effusion are especially notable in superficial joints, such as the knee and elbow. Fever and chills are common.

Gonococcal infection often produces inflammation in multiple areas. Classically, tenosynovitis is followed by migratory polyarthritis and finally by oligoarthritis. Patients also develop conjunctivitis, urethritis, cervici-

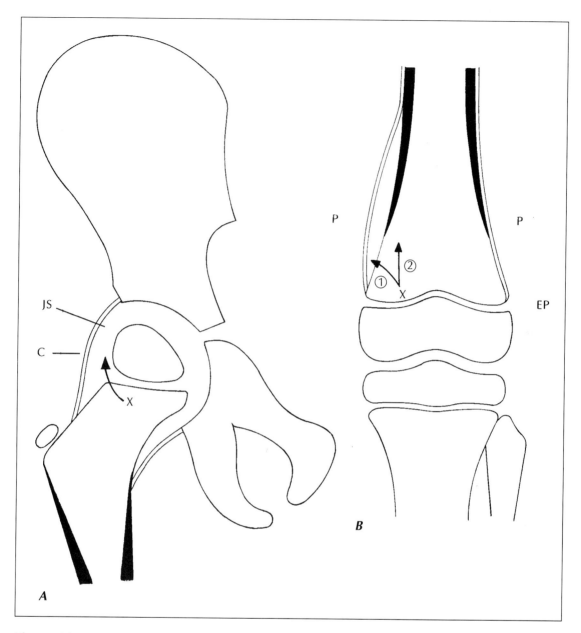

Figure 11.12 *A*. Relationship between osteomyelitis of the proximal femur (X) and secondary septic arthritis of the hip. Note seeding of the joint space (JS). The epiphysis is contained within the joint capsule (C). *B*. Osteomyelitis of the distal femur (X) may spread to the subperiosteal space (1) under the periosteum (P) or to the metaphyseal bone (2); however, it does not cross the epiphyseal plate (EP) and enter the knee joint. [Redrawn with permission from Brashear HR, Wilson FC: Infections of bones and joints, in Wilson FC (ed.): *The Musculoskeletal System: Basic Processes and Disorders,* 2d ed. Philadelphia, Lippincott, 1983, p 149.]

Table 11.1   Common Organisms in Septic Arthritis

Age	Organism	Initial Choice of Antibiotics
0–6 months	*S. aureus* Group B streptococcus Gram-negative bacilli	Semisynthetic penicillin or first-generation cephalosporin Aminoglycoside or third-generation cephalosporin
6 months–4 years	*S. aureus* Group A streptococcus *H. influenzae* *N. meningitides* *S. pneumoniae*	Second-generation cephalosporin (cefuroxime)
4 years–adolescence	*S. aureus*	Semisynthetic penicillin or first-generation cephalosporin
Adolescence-adulthood	*N. gonorrhoeae* *S. aureus*	Third-generation cephalosporin (ceftriaxone)
Elderly	*S. aureus*	Semisynthetic penicillin or first-generation cephalosporin
	Gram-negative bacilli	Aminoglycoside or third-generation cephalosporin

tis, proctitis, hepatitis, endocarditis, meningitis, and a vesiculopapular skin rash. Joint pain is less severe than in other forms of septic arthritis.

Diagnostic Studies

The most important diagnostic test is *arthrocentesis.* Large-bore needles should be used, since the pus may be very thick. The hip is probably best aspirated under fluoroscopy to assure correct positioning of the needle (Fig. 6.19). The aspirated fluid is sent immediately for laboratory studies and kept warm during transport. The laboratory should be informed of the possibility of *N. gonorrheoae* or *H. influenza,* which require special culture media. The white cell count in infected fluid, normally less than 200, is usually greater than 50,000/ mm^3 (less in gonococcal arthritis), of which over 75 percent are neutrophils. The glucose level is depressed, sometimes to less than 25 percent of serum levels, while lactic acid is increased. The presence of crystals makes infection unlikely but does not preclude septic arthritis, since it can cause crystals to leach out of synovium and cartilage.

Blood tests show a leukocytosis in only half of all cases. The ESR and C-reactive protein are more sensitive indicators of infection and are useful for monitoring treatment. Blood cultures are positive in 50 percent of cases and are important, since a significant percentage of joint fluid cultures are negative. When gonococcal arthritis is suspected, other body orifices should be cultured.

Plain radiographs should always be obtained and may show concurrent osteomyelitis or underlying joint disease. Bone scans are often positive but are not specific for septic arthritis.

Treatment

Initial therapy includes splinting and elevation, which decrease swelling and pain. After the joint has been aspirated but *not* prior to aspiration, broad-spectrum antibiotics should be started without awaiting results of cultures. The initial choice of antibiotics depends upon the clinical setting and the organisms most likely to be present (Table 11.1). Once culture results are available, broad-spectrum antibiotics can be changed to specific therapy. Although synovial fluid is quickly sterilized by intravenous antibiotics, a long period of treatment is necessary for bacteria that persist in the interstices of cartilage and synovium. After 1 to 2 weeks of parenteral administration, antibiotics are continued orally for another 3 or 4 weeks. Resolution is marked by the disappearance of pain and effusion, the presence of clear, scant, sterile joint fluid; and a normal ESR and C-reactive protein level.

Drainage of purulent fluid is important to minimize damage to the articular cartilage, which has limited potential for repair and regeneration. Although removing pus helps eradicate the infection, septic arthritis is not truly an abscess, and antibiotics penetrate the joint capsule and synovium well. The primary reason to evacuate the joint is to protect the cartilage. Purulent material, even if sterile by culture, is damaging because the neutrophils and inflammatory reaction destroy the cartilage matrix. An exception may be gonococcal infections, which produce a less intense inflammatory reaction.

Drainage of joints can often be accomplished with serial aspirations and limited irrigation through the same needle (or an intravenous catheter). Aspiration avoids surgical trauma, which may compound scarring and joint stiffness. In certain large joints, such as the knee, arthroscopy allows drainage and irrigation with minimal operative trauma. In less accessible joints, such as the sacroiliac joint, formal surgical arthrotomy may be required. If the infected fluid is thick and loculated, aspiration may be ineffective. Surgery is also recommended for young children, who tolerate repeated aspirations poorly.

The hip and shoulder require open arthrotomy because of the potential for avascular necrosis. Blood flow to the heads of the femur and humerus can be quickly compromised by increased pressure in the joint. If aspiration yields purulent material with a high neutrophil count or positive gram-stain for organisms, surgical decompression should be performed immediately without awaiting the results of cultures.

It is important to recall that numerous noninfectious disorders—including trauma, rheumatic fever, rheumatoid arthritis, and Legg-Calvé-Perthes disease—can also cause pain, inflammation, and synovitis in the hip. *Transient synovitis of the hip* (also known as *toxic synovitis of the hip*) is a self-limited, inflammatory condition that affects otherwise healthy children. This common cause of hip pain in pediatric patients is a diagnosis of exclusion.

There is recent evidence that beyond the first few days of treatment, early motion may reduce stiffness and scarring, which is one of the chief causes of late morbidity. On this basis, some have advocated continuous passive motion after pain subsides.

SPECIFIC INFECTIONS

Infections of the Hand

Bacterial infections of the hand require open drainage unless they are limited to cellulitis. Early recognition is the key to preservation of function. Most surgically drained wounds on the hand require 2 or 3 days of packing; healing occurs by secondary intention, and early motion reduces subsequent stiffness.

Paronychias and felons are the most common infections of fingertips. A *paronychia* involves the tissues around the fingernail, with a hangnail a frequent antecedent. Before an abscess develops, the process may be aborted by soaks and antibiotics; thereafter, incision adjacent to the nail is needed for drainage. If the abscess extends across the base of the nail, that area must also be elevated and drained. *Felons* are infections of the pulp of the finger tip (Fig. 11.13). Tenderness and swelling are prominent findings. If a felon is not adequately drained, skin necrosis and/or osteomyelitis may result. In general, incisions for drainage are placed longitudinally on the lateral aspect of the finger tip, with through-and-through incisions occasionally required for adequate drainage.

Deep bursal spaces in the hand may become

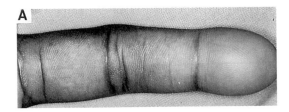

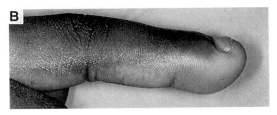

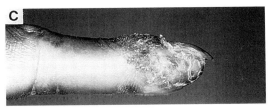

Figure 11.13   Felon. Note (*A* and *B*) the tense swelling in acute infection and *(C)* necrosis of the fingertip in a neglected infection.

infected after penetrating trauma or may spread from a more superficial infection. Careful palpation of the hand, especially on the palmar aspect, will elicit point tenderness over the infected area. Paradoxically, swelling and erythema are more prominent on the dorsum of the hand even though the infection is palmar, because the lymphatic drainage of the palm is dorsal and the skin more lax there. Prompt recognition and drainage are necessary to preserve hand function.

Pyogenic flexor tenosynovitis, or infection of a flexor tendon sheath, is manifest in its classical form by a flexed, enlarged, sausage-like digit that is exquisitely tender on its pal-

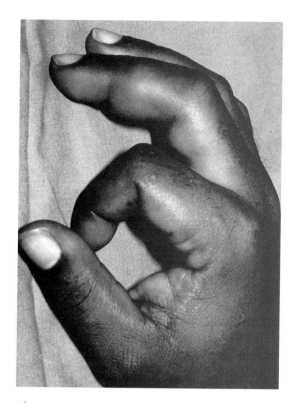

Figure 11.14   Pyogenic flexor tenosynovitis of the long finger. Note the flexed position and swollen, sausage-like appearance of the digit.

mar aspect and quite painful with passive extension (Fig. 11.14). Recent minor penetrating trauma is a usual antecedent, and *S. aureus* is typically the responsible organism. On rare occasions, if the infection is recognized at an early stage, it may be aborted by antibiotics alone; however, in most instances the infection demands immediate surgical irrigation and drainage to prevent scarring of the tendon sheath, destruction of the tendon, and, rarely, necrosis of the entire digit.

The herpetic *"whitlow"* is a viral infection of the fingers that should not be incised, since open debridement is ineffective and likely to accomplish nothing more than bacterial super-infection. Herpes simplex infections predilect dental personnel and children. A careful history and examination establishes the diagnosis. Pain precedes erythema and the formation of small vesicles, which may coalesce into bullae containing clear fluid. The lesions form a crust and usually involute spontaneously in 3 or 4 weeks. Antiherpetic creams and medications lessen the severity of symptoms.

Infections of the Foot

While most puncture wounds of the foot heal uneventfully, infection occasionally supervenes, often with *pseudomonas,* which tends to colonize shoes. Infected puncture wounds should be cleaned with soap after cultures are taken. Dead tissue and foreign bodies are removed and tetanus and antibiotic prophylaxis given. If the wound is seen late or persists in spite of treatment, osteomyelitis or septic arthritis must be suspected and surgical debridement performed, followed by appropriate antibiotics. Paronychias, felons, and deep-space infections of the feet are analogous to those in the hands and are treated in a similar manner. Foot infections associated with diabetes and vascular insufficiency are discussed above.

Human and Animal Bites

While patients bitten by animals give reliable histories, people who sustain human bites, especially those over the knuckles, are often disinclined to reveal the true cause of their injury. Any wound over a knuckle should be considered a human bite and treated as such until proven otherwise. Bite wounds should not be closed primarily, and cultures should be obtained at the time of debridement. Several unusual organisms are associated with bite wounds: *Eikenella corrodens,* an anaerobic species, has been cultured from human bites; and *Pasturella multocida* is encountered after animal bites or scratches, especially those inflicted by cats. These organisms and most other bacteria cultured from bites are sensitive to penicillin.

Postoperative Infections

The increased use of surgical implants has resulted in a rise in postoperative infections. Plastic and metal become coated with fibronectin and other connective tissue molecules, which are recognized by the adhesins on *S. aureus* and other bacteria. Once bacteria are bound to an implant, they multiply and form a protective slime coating (glycocalyx), which makes them difficult to eradicate without removing the foreign material. While two-thirds of postoperative infections are caused by staphylococcal and other gram-positive organisms, the incidence of gram-negative infections has also increased.

Prophylactic antibiotics reduce the rate of infection after surgery. The likelihood of infection is also lowered if antibiotics are administered promptly after open fractures. First-generation cephalosporins have been used most frequently for routine prophylaxis, since these antibiotics are well distributed in musculoskeletal tissues and have excellent gram-positive and limited gram-negative coverage. The most valuable time for administration of prophylactic antibiotics is just prior to surgery, with continuation for only 24 to 48 h after surgery, which minimizes side effects and the development of resistant organisms. A longer course of therapy does not enhance prophylactic activity.

Postoperative infections involving only soft tissues in immunologically competent hosts usually respond to appropriate drainage and antibiotics; however, if an implant or dead bone is left in the wound, bacteria may bind to the surface of the dead bone or foreign body and become difficult to eradicate (see "Exogenous osteomyelitis," above).

Necrotizing Infections of Soft Tissue

Many different organisms can cause severe, life-threatening infections that destroy soft tissues. In the past, infections were recognized and distinguished by various clinical criteria, but it has become increasingly clear that there is much overlap between the syndromes. The overall mortality rate is approximately 30 percent, and it is higher for patients with major medical problems, such as immunosuppression, diabetes, and peripheral vascular disease. Prompt recognition is vital and immediate surgical debridement essential. Many infections previously ascribed to a single organism are due to polymicrobial infections with both aerobic and anaerobic organisms, for which broad-spectrum antibiotics are necessary.

Clostridial Infections

Clostridial myonecrosis or *gas gangrene* is a potentially fatal condition that may develop insidiously, beginning with a low-grade fever and benign-appearing wound. The onset of acute, severe pain is the earliest sign of systemic involvement, which can progress in as little as 12 h to death. Other signs of sepsis include a rapid pulse, low blood pressure, confusion, and hemorrhagic blisters. Drainage from the wound is characteristically thin, brownish, and clear, with little odor. Careful examination reveals surrounding crepitus, and the presence of gas in the soft tissues can be confirmed by a plain radiograph; however, gas production may be a relatively late finding and should not be relied upon for early diagnosis. The offending organism is usually *Clostridium perfringens,* an anaerobic gram-positive bacillus that destroys muscles by the production of multiple toxins. Many other facultative organisms are also present that contribute to the anaerobic conditions necessary for clostridial growth. *Clostridium perfringens* is ubiquitous, occurring in dirt, dust, and normal bowel flora. In poorly vascularized or necrotic areas, lack of oxygen promotes the germination of clostridial spores and multiplication of bacteria. Once the condition is diagnosed, prompt surgical debridement of all necrotic muscle is essential; high doses of aqueous penicillin (or metronidazole in allergic patients) and extensive fluid replacement are important but cannot supplant debridement.

Not all clostridial infections produce gas gangrene; less serious infections, such as anaerobic cellulitis, generate a large amount of subcutaneous gas without systemic signs of sepsis. Conversely, organisms besides *C. perfringens* may produce anaerobic cellulitis and gas gangrene. Nonclostridial gas gangrene pre-

dilects the feet of diabetics with peripheral vascular disease.

Necrotizing Fasciitis

Necrotizing fasciitis usually affects patients who are systemically compromised, such as diabetics or those with human immunodeficiency virus (HIV) infections. The organisms may gain access to the fascia through a small, forgotten wound and spread rapidly through the fascia, causing severe pain. Strictly defined, necrotizing fasciitis involves only the fascial sheaths and spares the enclosed muscles; consequently, it is primarily the gray, necrotic fascia that must be debrided. These infections are polymicrobial, often involving anaerobes such as *Peptostreptococcus.* Perhaps more common than necrotizing fasciitis are posttraumatic streptococcal and staphylococcal infections that involve not only fascia but also muscle, skin, and subcutaneous tissues. The skin is mottled and dusky, and wounds are foul-smelling. Sharp debridement must often be repeated several times to obtain a healthy, granulating wound (Fig. 11.15). Because multiple organisms are common, broad-spectrum antibiotics are required.

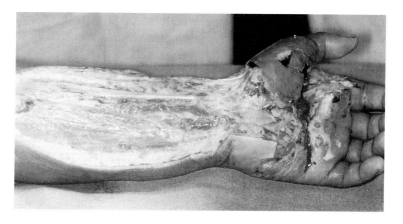

Fig. 11.15 Necrotizing fasciitis of the forearm. Overlying dead skin has been debrided. The process started with a wound on the dorsum of the hand.

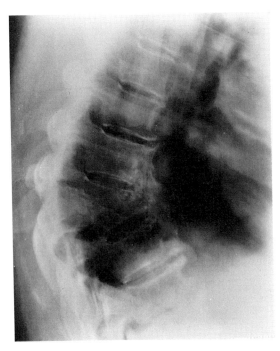

Fig. 11.16   Pott disease (tuberculosis of the spine). Note the gibbus (acute kyphotic deformity) and spread of the process across the disk space.

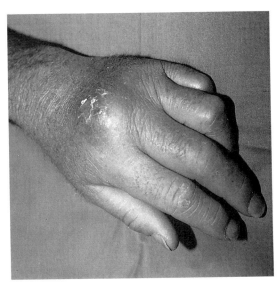

Fig. 11.17   *Mycobacterium marinum* infection of the dorsum of the hand and extensor tendons. Note the indolent, chronic appearance of the lesion.

Tuberculous Infections

Mycobacterial infections, after a period of relative dormancy, are again becoming a common clinical problem. Contributing to the increase in primary disease is the number of immunosuppressed and HIV patients. Musculoskeletal spread of the disease from the usual primary site in the lungs is generally to the thoracic spine (*Pott disease,* Fig. 11.16), followed by large joints such as the hips, knees, shoulders and ankles; however, any bone or joint may be involved. The predominant clinical features in tuberculous arthritis are chronic swelling and pain. Tuberculous infections in the spine are often followed by deformity and neurologic loss.

Mycobacterial diseases of the soft tissues usually result from direct innoculation through a scratch or other penetration of the skin. Development of these infections does not require an immunologically compromised host. The infection tends to be indolent and eventually produces a granulomatous lesion. *Mycobacterium marinum* infections are common on the hands of fishermen or others who work around boats and water (Fig. 11.17).

The diagnosis of tuberculous infection can be difficult. Laboratory studies are rarely helpful, and skin tests are not uniformly reliable, since they may be falsely negative in immunologically compromised patients. With bony involvement, radiographic studies early in the disease show periarticular osteopenia with preservation of the cartilage space; later, joint destruction becomes apparent. Imaging studies such as CT or MRI are useful to define the extent of the disease and identify abscesses. Histologic examination of infected tissue is usually the best means of diagnosis, often providing earlier confirmation of infection than mycobacterial culture, which may take up to 6 weeks.

Antituberculous drugs are the mainstay of treatment and should be started before results of cultures are known. Since resistant organisms are prevalent, multiple drugs are employed for prolonged periods. Surgery is indicated for diagnostic biopsy, drainage of large abscesses, and spinal decompression and stabilization. Arthrodesis is the classic treatment for tuberculous arthritis.

Fungal and Miscellaneous Infections

Nonbacterial organisms, such as fungi and protozoa, are rare causes of musculoskeletal infections (Fig. 11.18). The primary site of fungal infections is most frequently the lung, where inhalation of spores establishes the initial infection. The usual mode of spread to the musculoskeletal system is by way of the blood. Typically, the complaint is of a chronic nature, such as back pain; a progressively swollen, painful joint; or an ulcer over bone. This presentation should lead to a discussion of the patient's travel, activity, and work history. While individual fungi are indigenous to certain regions, they are not limited by geography. Frequently the patient is immunologically compromised by malignancy, diabetes, immunosuppressive therapy, or HIV infection. In these patients, there is a higher incidence of infection by direct inoculation through a break

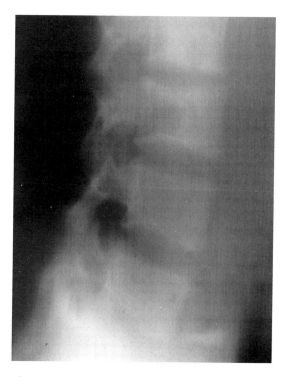

Fig. 11.18 Vertebral blastomycosis. The tomogram reveals a lytic lesion in the body of L3.

in the skin, often forgotten by the patient. The term *mycetoma* is applied to a fungal infection of soft tissue produced by direct inoculation.

There may be little systemic evidence of illness, and the ESR is sometimes normal; however, the chest should be examined carefully for primary infection. Cultures are better obtained from tissue than fluid, but results are usually unavailable for a month or longer. It is important to search the tissue microscopically, since organisms, if found, are diagnostic. A potassium hydroxide (KOH) preparation of the tissue may also reveal organisms. The reliability of immunohistochemical stains is improving and may eventually allow early diagnosis. It is essential that the laboratory be aware of the possibility of a fungal or uncommon bacterial infection so that appropriate special precautions and studies may be initiated. Unusual organisms that may cause musculoskeletal infections are listed in Table 11.2.

Treatment in most cases is surgical removal of all infected tissue, especially in the compromised host. Frequently, the surgery resembles an excision for tumor. The operative procedure is supplemented with antifungal agents, such as amphotericin B. Antibiotic treatment is prolonged and best monitored by a specialist in infectious diseases.

Human Immunodeficiency Virus

Patients with human immunodeficiency virus (HIV) infection do not have a markedly higher incidence of bacterial osteomyelitis or septic arthritis than the general population. However, among traumatized patients with open fractures, the incidence of wound infection and osteomyelitis is greater for HIV-positive patients, even if they have not progressed to the *acquired immunodeficiency syndrome* (AIDS). The appearance of an atypical musculoskeletal infection in an HIV-positive patient may herald the progression to full-blown AIDS.

The physician treating an HIV-positive patient must take precautions to avoid puncture with a needle or other sharp instruments that have been in contact with infected blood. It is estimated by the Centers for Disease Control and Prevention that 1 of 200 needle punctures from an HIV-positive patient will result in transfer of the virus. Inadvertent contact with infected blood must be reported to the local infection control group in the hospital and appropriate testing carried out.

Treatment of patients with HIV infection continues to be challenging. Most therapeutic interventions are directed toward specific infections, which often become life-threatening

Table 11.2   Unusual Infections of the Musculoskeletal System

Disorder	Characteristic Features
Bacteria	
Brucella	Infected milk in third world. Prominent bone and joint symptoms. Granulomatous lesions.
T. pallidum (syphilis); *T. pertenue* (yaws)	Periostitis, arthritis, osteomyelitis, and tenosynovitis common in secondary stage.
Actinomyces	Branching, filamentous bacteria in oral flora. Crosses tissue planes. Sensitive to penicillin.
Fungi	
Histoplasma	Growth in macrophages. Ohio and Mississippi river valleys. Bat and bird droppings.

Table 11.2   Unusual Infections of the Musculoskeletal System *(Continued)*

Disorder	Characteristic Features
Coccidioidomyces	Semiarid climates, southwestern United States. Large spherule with multiple organisms.
Blastomyces	Large round yeast forms with broad-based buds. Central and eastern United States.
Candida	Most common fungal infection. Immunocompromised host.
Cryptococcus	Thick cell wall, seen with India ink. Immunocompromised host.
Aspergillus	Ubiquitous; often a laboratory contaminant. Immunocompromised host.
Sporothrix	Ubiquitous, especially in soil, gardens, rose thorns. Occasional infection of multiple joints and bone.
Viruses	
Arthritis	Multiple organisms can cause synovitis, including varicella, Paramyxovirus (mumps), rubella, coxsackievirus, hepatitis.
Variola (smallpox)	Viral osteomyelitis in 2–5% of patients.
Rubella	Radiolucency, probable osteitis.
Cytomegalovirus	Osteomyelitis associated with HIV infection.
Epstein-Barr virus	Periostitis.
Protozoa and helminths	
Toxoplasma	Intracellular sporozoan. Bone and muscle lesions in congenital infection.
Trichinella	Nematode associated with uncooked pork. Larval cysts (sometimes calcified) in muscle.
Taenia solium	Pork and beef tapeworm. Cysticercus (larval cyst) in muscle and soft tissue.
Echinococcus	Canine tapeworm. Large, hydatid cysts with multiple organisms, usually in abdomen, rarely in bone and muscle.
Dracunculus	Tropical worm. Skin ulceration (escaping worm) leads to secondary bacterial infection.

and difficult to control. The treatment of the underlying disorder is even more problematic. Zidovudine (AZT) and similar agents suppress replication of the virus but do not effect cure. Much effort has been devoted to the development of newer therapeutic strategies, including immune modulators, vaccines, inhibitors of viral receptors, and drugs to attack viruses at different stages of growth.

SUGGESTED READINGS

DIRSCHL DR: Acute pyogenic osteomyelitis in children. *Orthop Rev* 23:305, 1994.

ESPINOZA L, GOLDENBERG DL, ARNETT FC, ALARCON GS (EDS): *Infections in the Rheumatic Diseases: A Comprehensive Review of Microbial Relations to Rheumatic Disorders.* Orlando, FL, Grune & Stratton, 1988.

ESTERHAI JL, GRISTINA AG, POSS R (EDS): *Musculoskeletal Infection.* Park Ridge, IL, American Academy of Orthopaedic Surgeons, 1992.

GORBACH SL, BARTLETT JG, BLACKLOW NR (EDS): *Infectious Diseases.* Philadelphia, Saunders, 1992.

GREEN NE, EDWARDS K: Bone and joint infections in children. *Orthop Clin North Am* 18:555, 1987.

NORDEN C, GILLESPIE WJ, NADE S: *Infections in Bones and Joints.* Boston, Blackwell, 1994.

RYAN KJ (ED): *Sherris Medical Microbiology: An Introduction to Infectious Diseases.* New York, Elsevier, 1994.

WALDVOGEL FA, MEDOFF G, SWARTZ MN: Osteomyelitis: A review of clinical features, therapeutic considerations and unusual aspects. *N Engl J Med* 282:198, 1970.

Chapter 12

Tumors

Gary D. Bos and H. Robert Brashear

GENERAL ASPECTS

Benign tumors of bone and soft tissue are much more common than malignancies. Primary malignant tumors of bone are rare, with less than 2000 reported annually in the United States. Most of these tumors are sarcomas, which originate in mesodermal tissue and metastasize by the bloodstream to the lungs. Soft tissue sarcomas occur three times more often than primary malignancies of bone, and, in adults, metastatic carcinoma is more common than primary malignancy of bone.

The clinical features associated with musculoskeletal tumors include pain, a mass, impairment of function, and deformity. While some tumors of bone are more common in males, sex is of little diagnostic value. Age, however, is often of great help because of the predilection of certain tumors for specific age groups. An injury may call attention to a tumor, but only in very rare instances does trauma cause a tumor.

Malignant tumors of bone are usually associated with deep, aching pain, which, although not sharp or severe, is distressing because of its constancy. Pain that persists at night and is unrelieved by rest is suggestive of malignancy; however, certain benign tumors, such as osteoid osteoma, also cause nocturnal pain. Mild, dull, aching pain that suddenly becomes severe following minimal or no trauma suggests a pathologic fracture.

For some tumors, the primary complaint is a mass. If the mass is painful and attached to bone, it is likely to be malignant. Conversely, if the mass is attached to bone but painless, the lesion is more often benign unless it is a soft tissue tumor. Soft tissue sarcomas may become very large, especially in the groin and medial thigh, before they become painful. Because of the thinner soft tissue envelope, a small mass arising distally in a limb is easier to detect than a small mass in the medial thigh, which may explain why deeper, more proximally based tumors are not discovered until they are large and have a poorer prognosis.

Impaired function is occasionally the major complaint, especially if the tumor is near a joint. In addition to a feeling of tightness, nearby nerves may be compressed, causing weakness or loss of sensation distally. A painless limp must be investigated with the possibility of a neoplasm in mind.

The least desirable presentation of a tumor is a pathologic fracture, which suggests an aggressive tumor. Additionally, the fracture hematoma may spread tumor cells throughout the limb.

The history should include a search for such constitutional symptoms as fever, loss of appetite or weight, and previous malignancy, which suggest metastasis. A positive family history is common in patients with multiple enchondromas or osteochondromas.

The examination of the patient with a musculoskeletal tumor entails assessment of its dimensions, displacement of surrounding tissues, marginal contours, and fixation to adjacent tissues. Increased warmth points to a highly vascular lesion. A limp suggests pain, limited movement, or neurovascular compromise. Enlarged lymph nodes are sought in node-bearing regions, including the neck, axillae, epitrochlear areas, groin, and popliteal regions. The abdomen is examined for tenderness, masses, and organomegaly.

Diagnostic Modalities

Laboratory studies are of limited value in the diagnosis of musculoskeletal tumors. The *erythrocyte sedimentation rate* is most frequently elevated in metastatic and small round-cell tumors, such as Ewing sarcoma; however, it is also elevated in infection, which may mimic a bone tumor in other respects as well. Anemia is rarely present in the early stages of primary skeletal tumors but may occur with metastatic disease or myeloma. Serum calcium levels are rarely elevated except in the *brown tumor* of hyperparathyroidism. *Prostate-specific antigen* may be helpful in separating the causes of suspected metastatic disease in older males. The *alkaline phosphatase* is usually elevated when bone is being broken down and remodeled. Serum and urine *electrophoreses* are useful if myeloma is suspected.

For osseous neoplasms, the plain radiograph is the first and most essential diagnostic aid. Plain radiographs direct further study of osseous lesions and rule out osseous involvement by soft tissue neoplasms. In general, lesions involving cortical bone are best imaged by a computed tomography (CT), whereas marrow lesions, primary tumors of soft tissue, and soft tissue extensions of osseous tumors are better imaged by magnetic resonance imaging (MRI). In some cases, both modalities are indicated. Angiography is rarely used for the diagnosis of musculoskeletal neoplasms because of the excellent imaging supplied by MRI and contrast CT scans. Technetium bone scans and MRI are helpful in determining the extent of osseous involvement. The bone scan is a critical tool for detecting distant osseous metastases and periosteal involvement of contiguous soft tissue tumors.

Consultation from an orthopaedic oncologist should be sought early in the diagnostic evaluation to ensure that appropriate, cost-effective studies are employed in the evaluation of these patients.

Principles of Management

Management of musculoskeletal neoplasms begins with a biopsy, which must be carefully planned to avoid compromising definitive surgery. Most pathologists request a sizable piece of tissue, which allows special studies and reduces the possibility of sampling error in these frequently nonhomogeneous tumors.

The role of needle biopsy in limb lesions is limited. Often, inadequate tissue is obtained, and before the use of CT scans for guidance, falsely negative specimens were frequent. Finally, disappearance of the puncture site before definitive surgery may lead to failure to remove the biopsy tract, increasing the likelihood of recurrence.

Open incisional biopsy is preferred and should be performed by the surgeon who will carry out the resection. A frozen section at the time of biopsy is needed to confirm that tumor tissue has been obtained and that adequate material is available for special studies. The capsule of the tumor is closed tightly to prevent bleeding and local spread of the tumor.

There have been gratifying advances in the survival and limb salvage of patients with high-grade skeletal malignancies. Typically, patients are put on chemotherapy immediately after biopsy; a few months later definitive treatment is carried out, which includes limb salvage in over 75 percent of cases. Additional chemotherapy follows. With this program, 5-year survivals in excess of 60 percent can be expected for osteosarcoma and Ewing sarcoma.

Techniques for limb-salvage procedures have improved steadily. In the diaphyses of

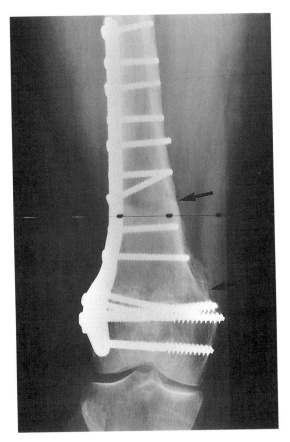

Figure 12.1 Femoral giant cell tumor 7 years after segmental replacement by a large frozen bone allograft. Arrows show the proximal and distal extent of the graft.

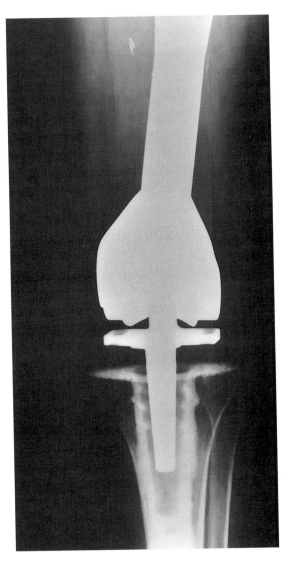

Figure 12.2 Custom prosthesis filling a 20-cm defect created by resection of a malignant tumor involving the distal femur and knee joint.

long bones, the use of massive bone allografts has led to high long-term success rates (Fig. 12.1). When a joint must be resected, either a bone allograft or a customized prosthesis is used to fill the defect. While these constructs cannot be expected to last the lifetime of a young patient, they usually provide reasonable function for many years (Fig. 12.2). Bone cement has been used to fill large cavitary defects in benign, aggressive tumors with good results

TUMORS OF BONE

Primary bone tumors are lesions that arise de novo from bone. Cellular elements that most frequently give rise to bone tumors are osteogenic, chondrogenic, or fibrohistiocytic in origin. Less commonly they arise from marrow elements, mononuclear phagocytic cells, and other tissues found in bone, such as endothelium, neural tissue, or fat. Benign and malignant forms of these tumors are listed in Table 12.1. The more common entities are discussed below.

Benign

Bone-Forming Tumors

Osteoid osteomas are painful lesions in which the pain is described as deep, boring, constant, nocturnal, and frequently relieved by aspirin or other nonsteroidal anti-inflammatory drugs. Children and adolescents are most frequently affected by this peculiar tumor, which may exist for many years without change. The lesion may occur in any bone but predilects the femur and tibia. In the spine, the lesion often causes a painful scoliosis. Radiographically, the lesion is an area of very dense bone surrounding a central lucent area or nidus that is less than 1.5 cm in diameter (Fig. 12.4). The reactive bone often has a fusiform pattern and may have a very fine, delicate onionskin appearance. If reactive bone obscures the nidus on plain radiographs, a CT scan may be necessary to disclose it. Histologically, the nidus consists of active osteoblasts, osteoclasts, and osteoid within a vascular connective tissue matrix containing unmyelinated nerve fibers. Initial treatment is with aspirin or other nonsteroidal anti-inflammatory medication. If these agents do

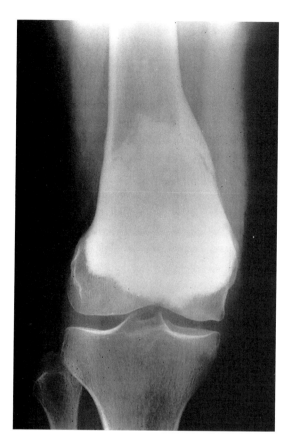

Figure 12.3 Giant cell tumor of the distal femur 2 years following resection and insertion of cement.

(Fig. 12.3). Smaller cavitary defects are often filled with allograft or synthetic bone-grafting materials rather than an autograft.

Soft tissue sarcomas have not shared the dramatic increase in survival rates achieved for osseous tumors. Soft tissue sarcomas are commonly treated with radiation therapy followed by local resection, with close clinical follow-up. The use of chemotherapy before and after resection has not as yet significantly improved survival.

Table 12.1   Partial List of Bone Tumors and Tumorlike Conditions

Tissue of Origin	Benign	Malignant

Cartilage	Osteochondroma
	Enchondroma
	Chondroblastoma
	Chondromyxoid fibroma
		Chondrosarcoma
		Variants of chondrosarcoma
		   Dedifferentiated
		   Clear cell
		   Mesenchymal

Bone	Osteoid osteoma
	Osteoblastoma
		Osteosarcoma
		Variants of osteosarcoma
		   Parosteal
		   Periosteal
		   Telangiectatic
		   Postradiation
		   Arising in Paget disease

Marrow elements	Eosinophilic granuloma	Ewing sarcoma Plasmacytoma Multiple myeloma Lymphoma of bone
Fibrous tissue and uncertain origin	Nonossifying fibroma Aneurysmal bone cyst Simple bone cyst Giant cell tumor Fibrous dysplasia Desmoplastic fibroma	Fibrosarcoma Malignant fibrous histiocytoma

not provide pain relief, surgical excision is indicated, although occasionally the lesion disappears spontaneously in 5 to 10 years.

Osteoblastoma, sometimes called *giant osteoid osteoma,* is a rare tumor that has a lytic nidus 2 cm or larger, with less surrounding reactive bone than an osteoid osteoma (Fig. 12.5). The spine is the most common location, but any bone may be affected. While the tumor is histologically similar to osteoid osteoma, relief of pain by aspirin is less likely, leaving surgical excision as the treatment of choice.

Cartilage-Forming Tumors

The *osteochondroma,* or cartilaginous *exostosis,* is one of the most common bone neoplasms. It is a cartilage-capped projection of bone from the metaphysis of a long bone near the growth plate. Any bone preformed in cartilage can be affected. The lesion has a cartilage cap that resembles a growth plate histologically and grows by enchondral ossification, which ceases at skeletal maturity. Clinically, the lesion is a hard, immovable, smooth mass that is firmly fixed to bone and

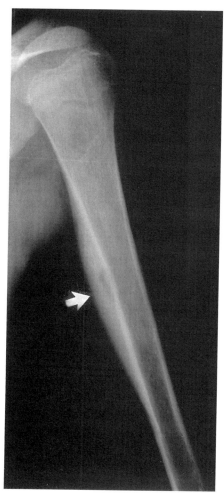

Figure 12.4   Osteoid osteoma of the humerus. The radiolucent nidus (arrow) is in the area of cortical thickening.

nearby joint (Fig. 12.6). The marrow cavity of the exostosis is continuous with the marrow cavity of the bone. The rounded cartilage cap on the protuberance is not seen on a plain radiograph, which explains why the lesion feels larger than it appears. The radiographic appearance of the lesion is diagnostic, but removal may not be necessary unless the lesion is painful or there is suspicion of malignancy, which develops in less than 1 percent of these tumors. Malignant change is heralded by growth or pain in a previously static osteochondroma. The presence of a cartilage cap thicker than 1 cm on a CT scan should arouse suspicion of malignant transformation, especially in a middle-aged patient with a lesion of the pelvis or shoulder girdle. An additional radiographic suggestion of malignancy is the development of lucencies in the bone of the cartilaginous cap (Fig. 12.7). Treatment of a symptomatic exostosis is surgical excision. Asymptomatic lesions require only observation.

Multiple hereditary exostoses are distinct from solitary exostoses, frequently cause growth disturbances and deformity, and are more often sessile than pedunculated (Fig. 12.8). The incidence of malignant change is probably similar for individual tumors, which places the patient with multiple lesions at a higher risk of developing this complication. Patients with multiple exostoses, which may be inherited in an autosomal dominant pattern, should have periodic radiographs of known, large pelvic and shoulder girdle lesions, since malignant change is more frequent in central tumors.

Enchondromas arise within the medullary cavity of bone, most frequently in the small tubular bones of the hands and feet, and are asymptomatic unless complicated by a patho-

nontender unless it has been traumatized. It is frequently discovered as an incidental finding on a radiograph taken for another reason. The usual radiographic appearance is a pedunculated bony protuberance from the metaphysis of a long bone that points away from the

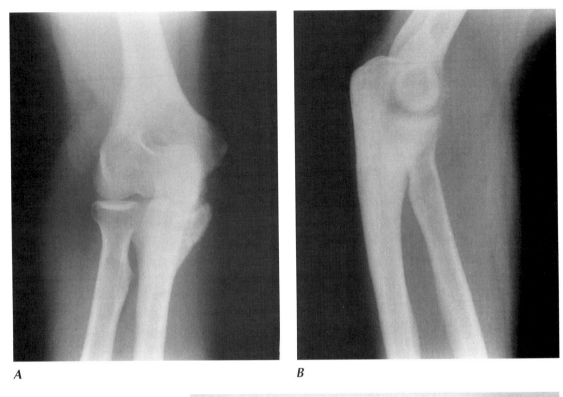

A

B

Figure 12.5
Osteoblastoma. Note (*A* and *B*) the expanded, sclerotic, coronoid process and (*C*) extensive uptake on a bone scan.

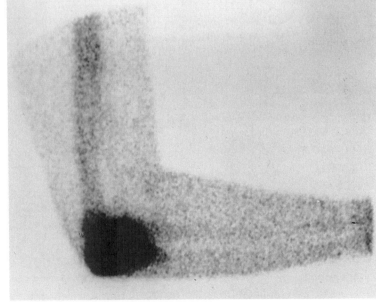

C

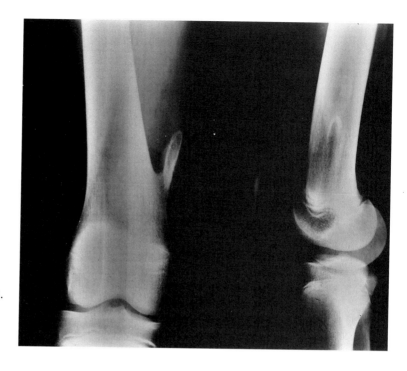

Figure 12.6
Osteochondroma. Note that it points away from the knee. On the lateral view, the lesion has a characteristic "teardrop" appearance.

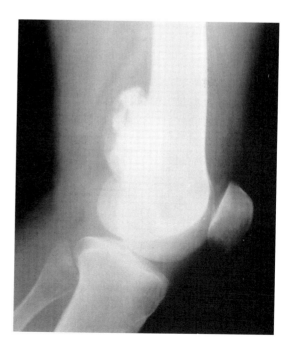

Figure 12.7 Osteochondroma. Note the lucencies in the bony cap. Histologically, this lesion showed atypical chondrocytes.

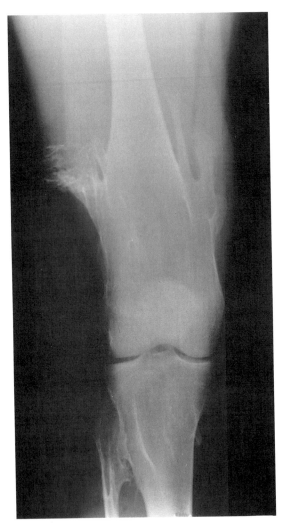

Figure 12.8 Multiple osteochondromas.

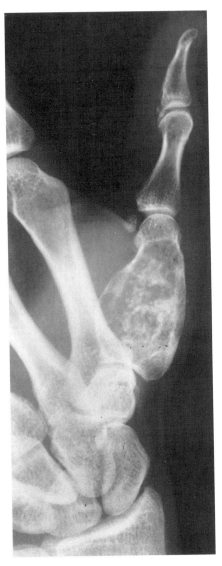

Figure 12.9 Large enchondroma of the thumb metacarpal. The tumor was asymptomatic until an injury.

logic fracture (Fig. 12.9). Enchondromas in larger bones, such as the femur and humerus, may produce dull, aching pain, although discovery of the lesion as an incidental osteolytic radiographic finding is common (Fig. 12.10). The lesion is usually discovered during the middle decades of life, but it may appear in childhood. Often calcification of the cartilage matrix gives it a characteristic speckled ap-

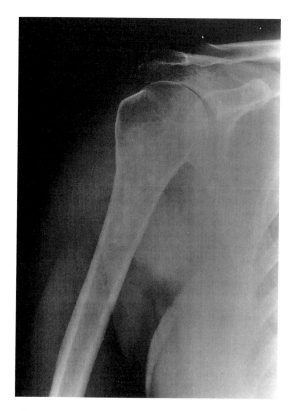

Figure 12.10 Humeral enchondroma. The lesion was discovered during evaluation for vague shoulder complaints. Note the speckled calcifications that do not involve the cortex.

since this behavior may forecast malignant transformation of the lesion. Malignant degeneration is unusual in patients under 20 years old and extremely rare in lesions of the hands and feet.

Multiple enchondromatosis or *Ollier disease* is a generalized osseous dysplasia in which numerous enchondromas are present. These patients have disfiguring bony deformities and a higher incidence of malignant transformation than patients with solitary lesions. Patients with multiple enchondromas and hemangiomas *(Maffucci syndrome)* should also be carefully observed for malignant change.

Chondroblastoma is a rare tumor of primitive cartilage cells that has a predilection for the epiphyses of long bones in children between the ages of 8 and skeletal maturity. Dull

pearance. Scalloping or thinning of the surrounding cortex is common and implies an active or growing lesion, which may rarely be associated with chondrosarcomatous transformation. Treatment is observation, with serial radiographs at 3- to 4-month intervals for asymptomatic lesions. If no growth is noted during the first year or two, the patient need return only if pain develops in the area. Painful lesions without cortical erosion should also be followed; if the lesion expands or becomes more painful, curettage should be carried out,

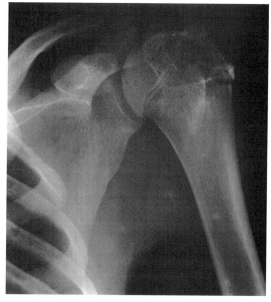

Figure 12.11 Chondroblastoma. Note the involvement of the epiphysis and faint calcifications within the lesion.

pain is the usual presenting complaint. Radiographically, the tumor appears as a lytic lesion in the epiphysis, occasionally with a thin, sclerotic border and faint, intralesional calcifications (Fig. 12.11). In spite of curettage and bone grafting, the tumor occasionally recurs, but sarcomatous change is rare.

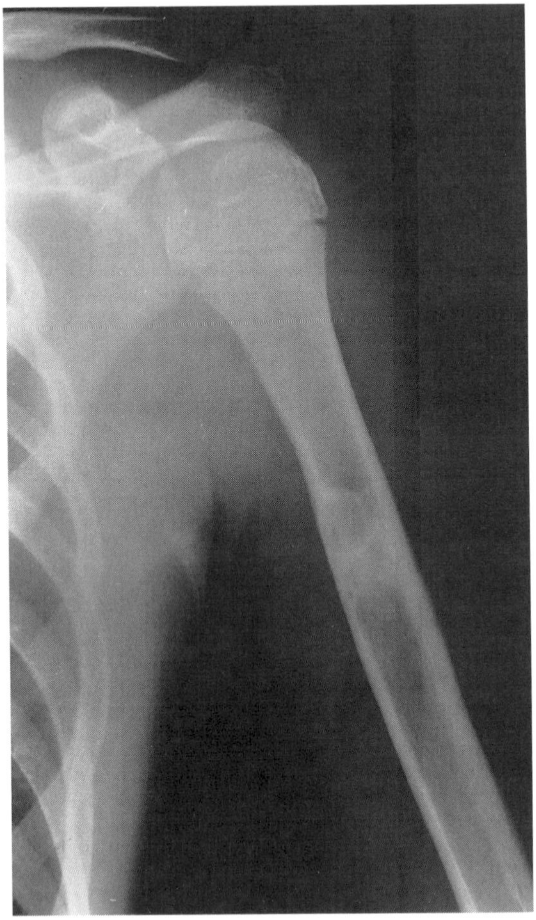

Chondromyxoid fibroma is an uncommon lesion containing cartilaginous, myxoid, and fibrous elements that is eccentrically located in the metaphyseal region of long bones, especially the tibia. Patients complain of pain and sometimes of a mass, since this tumor is known to expand the bony cortex. Radiographically, the lesion has a scalloped and often loculated appearance (Fig. 12.12). Since this rare lesion has a high recurrence rate, treatment is by en bloc excision. Recurrence, often of a more aggressive tumor, is frequent if excision is incomplete.

Figure 12.12 Chondromyxoid fibroma. Note the scalloping of the cortex and loculations. There had been a previous fracture that healed.

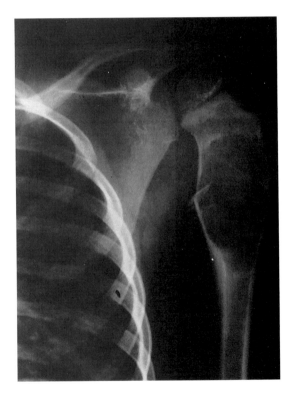

Figure 12.13 Unicameral bone cyst. Note the thinning of the cortex, expansion of the metaphysis, and recent fracture.

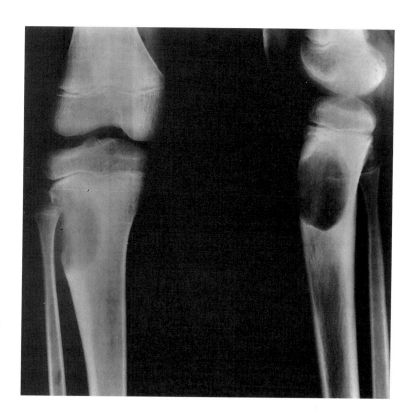

Figure 12.14 Aneurysmal bone cyst. Note the large lytic lesion with little reaction in the surrounding bone.

Other Benign Tumors and Tumorlike Conditions of Bone

Simple or unicameral bone cyst is a relatively common osteolytic lesion of the metaphysis in children that occurs most often in the proximal humerus or femur. It is usually asymptomatic until pathologic fracture occurs. Radiographs show a lytic, metaphyseal lesion that expands the bone and usually abuts the open growth plate (Fig. 12-13). The cortex is often eroded and thinned, with fine trabeculations and apparent septae in the lesion. The lesion contains clear yellow fluid and has a thin cellular lining of fibrous tissue containing scattered giant cells. Treatment is aspiration followed by injection of methylprednisolone under anesthe-

sia and fluouroscopic guidance. This procedure may be repeated at 3-month intervals if necessary until the cyst fills in with bone. If the bone has fractured, injection is delayed until the fracture has healed. Curettage and packing with bone graft is less often used and carries a significant risk of recurrence.

Aneurysmal bone cysts occur most frequently in children and young adults. Long bones and vertebrae are favored sites, although any bone can be involved. A painful, warm, fusiform swelling of a long bone is the common clinical presentation, while a very thin rim of reactive periosteal bone around an expansile, lytic lesion is the characteristic radiographic appearance (Fig. 12.14). These lesions

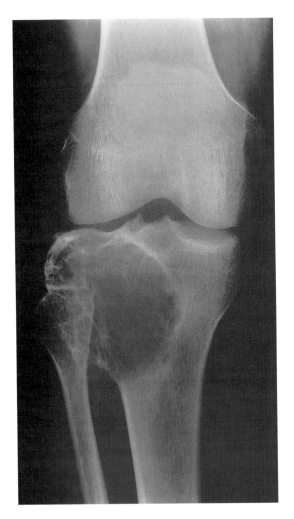

Figure 12.15 Giant cell tumor of the tibia. Note destruction of the subchondral bone by this eccentric epiphyseal lesion.

may grow very rapidly to large size. Treatment is curettage and removal of the tissue filling the cyst, including the lining.

Giant cell tumors occur in young to middle-aged adults. Typically, the tumor involves the epiphysis, metaphysis, and subchondral bone of the joint, which may necessitate complex reconstructive procedures. Radiographically, the tumor is a large, often eccentric lytic lesion that expands and thins the cortex (Fig. 12.15). The histologic hallmarks are plump, oval-shaped stromal cells and numerous giant cells that have the same type of nuclei as the stromal cells. Careful curettage of the lesion is the preferred treatment if there is enough cortical bone left to support the joint. The resulting cavity is often filled with bone cement for immediate stability and adjunctive therapy, since heat from curing of the cement may extend the margin of the resection. Recurrence, which is more frequent with giant cell tumors than with other benign bone tumors, entails en bloc excision. Approximately 1 percent of these tumors develop pulmonary metastases.

A *nonossifying fibroma* is a very common lesion of bone that is usually discovered incidentally in radiographs of a child or adolescent. It is most often metaphyseal, oriented to the long axis of the bone, and extends into the medullary canal. In at least one radiographic view, the lesion is eccentrically located, and there is usually a thin rim of sclerotic bone around the lesion (Fig. 12.16). Occasionally a pathologic fracture occurs through the lesion, but it is more commonly asymptomatic and may be followed with serial radiographs until it involutes, which is the natural history of the process. Smaller defects confined to the cortex are often referred to as *fibrous cortical defects*, but the lesions are histologically similar.

Fibrous dysplasia is a benign lytic lesion of bone, in which the central portion has the radiographic appearance of ground glass (Fig.

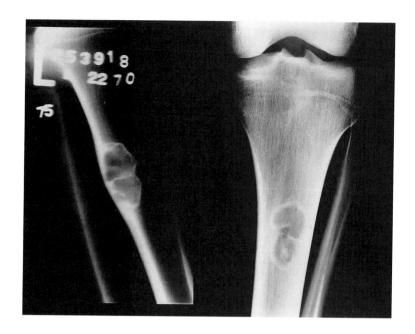

Figure 12.16
Nonossifying fibroma of the tibia. Note the sclerotic rim and eccentric location.

12.17). The femur, ribs, and tibia are preferred sites, but involvement of multiple bones, often limited to one side of the body, is an occasional occurrence. The bone lesions are filled with fibrous tissue containing immature dysplastic bone. Growth of the lesion usually stops at puberty, and it may disappear over the following few years. Stress fractures through the dysplastic bone occasionally lead to deformities, such as the "shepherd's crook" angulation of the proximal femur (Fig. 12.18). Surgery is often frustrating, since bone grafts are often resorbed and replaced by dysplastic bone. Fortunately, most lesions become dormant or resolve after growth is complete.

Eosinophilic granuloma, a part of the spectrum of *histiocytoses,* is usually manifest by local pain or a pathologic fracture. This lesion should be strongly considered in the differential diagnosis of any child with a lytic lesion in bone (Fig. 12.19). If a lateral radiograph of the skull shows another lytic lesion, the diagnosis of histiocytosis is confirmed, and biopsy is unnecessary. Some lesions are discovered in the healing phase, suggested by a sclerotic rim around the lesion, in which case no treatment beyond protection from full activity is necessary for the few weeks until the lesion heals spontaneously. Larger lesions in major weight-bearing bones should be casted until healing occurs. Occasionally curettage and grafting are required, although low-dose radiation is an alternative. While most children have a solitary lesion, others develop numerous lesions with associated endocrine involvement.

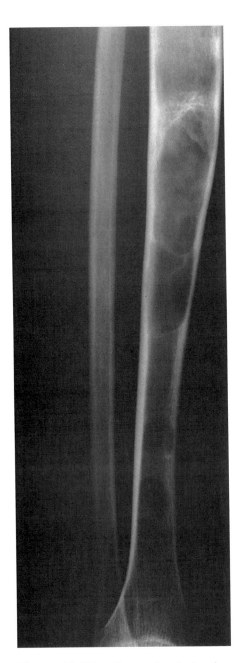

Figure 12.17 Fibrous dysplasia of the tibia. Note the "ground glass" appearance.

Malignant

Osteosarcoma

Osteosarcoma is the second most common primary malignant tumor found in bone. It favors the metaphyseal region of bones around the knee and the proximal humerus. The classic presentation of osteosarcoma in children and adolescents is that of deep, aching, persistent pain, with an enlarging mass fixed to the bone. Radiographs typically show a mixed osteolytic and osteoblastic lesion (Fig. 12.20) that often extends beyond the cortex and elevates the periosteum, creating a *Codman triangle* and/ or "sunburst" effect. Histologically, the tumor contains malignant spindle cells producing osteoid or tumor bone. Classic osteosarcoma and its high-grade variants, such as postradiation sarcoma and sarcoma arising in Paget disease, tend to metastasize to the lungs very early, often before the patient seeks medical attention. After staging of the primary tumor with imaging, a CT scan of the lungs, whole-body bone scan, and screening blood work, the lesion is biopsied; if the diagnosis is confirmed, chemotherapy is initiated. After three or four courses of chemotherapy, definitive surgery is carried out, usually in the form of a limb- salvage procedure, although in young children amputation is more frequently performed. Surgery is followed by further chemotherapy, with most treatment protocols taking about 1 year to complete. Five-year survival rates of 60 percent or more can be expected with these regimens. Low-grade variants of osteosarcoma, such as *periosteal* and *parosteal osteosarcomas,* which occur on the surface of bone, usually require only surgical excision (Fig. 12.21).

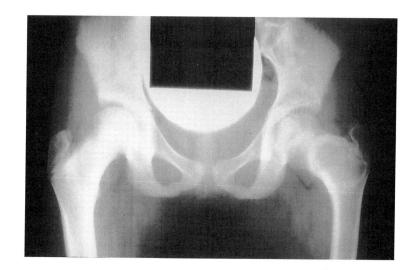

Figure 12.18 Fibrous dysplasia in the femoral neck. Note the developing varus ("shepherd's crook") deformity.

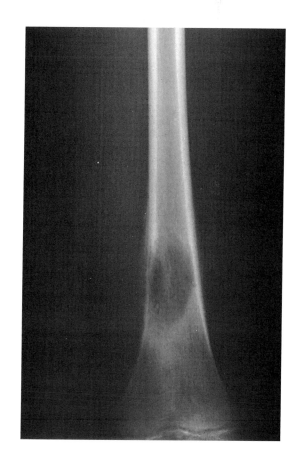

Figure 12.19 Eosinophilic granuloma of the femur. Note the periosteal reaction, which suggests early healing.

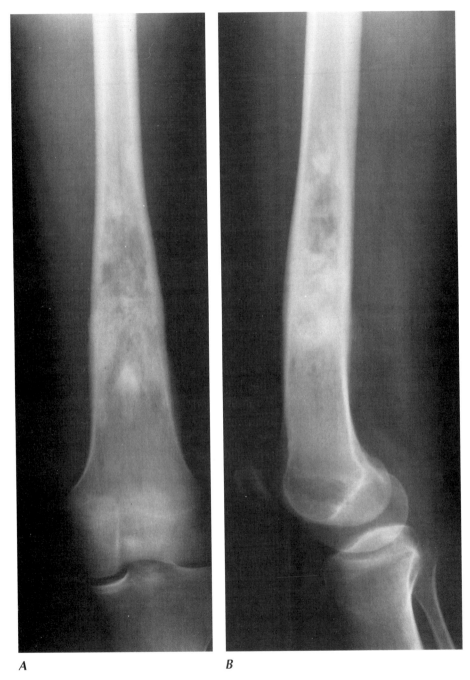

A   *B*

Figure 12.20   Osteogenic sarcoma of the distal femur. Anteroposterior
   A. and lateral *B.* X-rays show a mixed osteoblastic and lytic picture with
   subtle periosteal reaction.

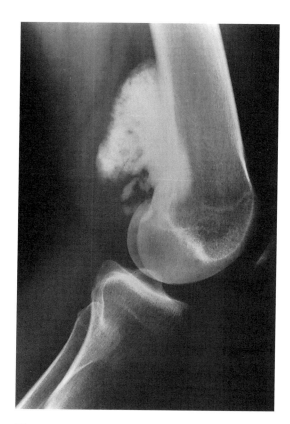

Figure 12.21   Parosteal osteosarcoma arising on the posterior aspect of the distal femur. Note extension of the highly calcified lesion into the popliteal soft tissues.

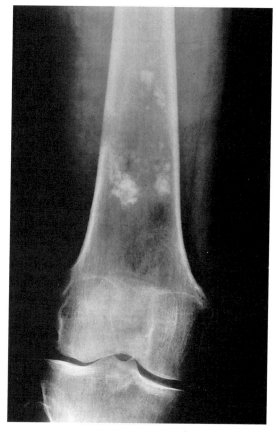

Figure 12.22   Chondrosarcoma. Note the speckled calcification and subtle cortical erosion.

Chondrosarcoma

Malignant tumors of cartilage, or chondrosarcomas, occur after skeletal maturity, with a peak incidence in the fifth and sixth decades. Tumors occurring in the third and fourth decades tend to develop in preexisting benign cartilaginous tumors such as enchondromas or ostoses, while chondrosarcomas in older patients are most commonly primary. The tumors often attain large size because they grow slowly and are not particularly painful. Lesions near the shoulder and pelvic girdles tend to be of higher-grade malignancy and larger at the time of discovery. Radiographically, the tumor extends beyond the bone and contains scattered "snowflake" calcifications (Fig. 12.22). Preferred treatment is wide surgical excision with limb salvage. Chondrosarcomas are unresponsive to chemotherapy or radiation, with the possible exception being a dediffer-

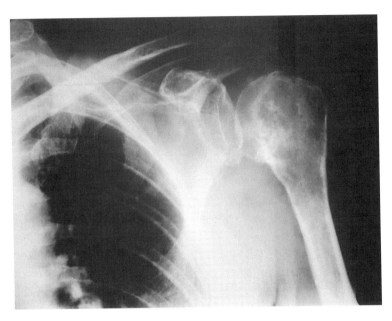

Figure 12.23
Dedifferentiated chondrosarcoma. Note the extensive lytic changes and cortical destruction of the proximal humerus. A few speckled calcifications are present.

entiated variant that occurs in about 10 percent of long-standing chondrosarcomas. This tumor is of very high grade malignancy and has a high mortality rate (Fig. 12.23).

Ewing Sarcoma

Ewing sarcoma is an uncommon, highly malignant tumor of neuroectodermal tissue that arises in bone or soft tissue. It occurs most often in the femur, ilium, or humerus of skeletally immature patients, but any bone can be involved. The usual local presentation is pain and a mass. Systemic manifestations include low-grade fever and elevation of the white count and sedimentation rate, which mimic infection. The radiographic appearance of mottled bone destruction and reactive "onion-skin" periosteal bone formation also simulates infection (Fig. 12.24). Histologically, the tumor contains sheets of round blue cells, slightly larger than lymphocytes, with large nuclei and little cytoplasm. Treatment with chemotherapy and surgery and/or radiation has raised survival rates to 60 or 70 percent.

Other Malignant Tumors of Bone

Multiple myeloma, a tumor of plasma cells, is the most common primary malignancy of bone. The lesions are predominantly lytic and occur most frequently in the skull, vertebrae, pelvis, and proximal long bones, although some patients manifest only diffuse osteopenia without discrete lesions (Fig. 12.25). This disease is notorious for having a normal bone scan. While the disease usually affects patients over age 60 in its multiple form, solitary myelomas *(plasmacytomas)* favor younger patients. Pathologic fractures are common in all phases of the disease. The solitary lesions generally respond to local radiation therapy, but a significant proportion of these patients

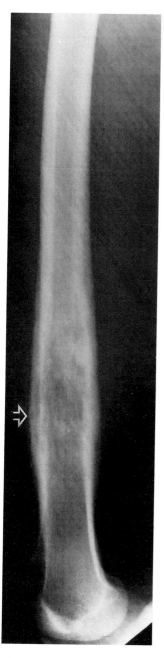

Figure 12.24   Ewing sarcoma of the femur. Onion-skinning and new periosteal bone formation are present (open arrow).

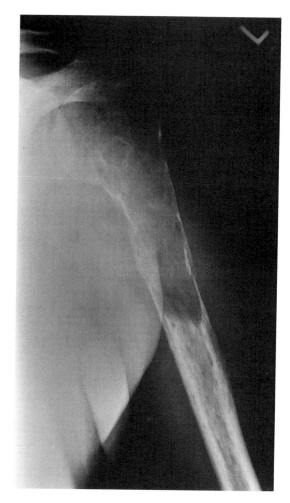

Figure 12.25   Multiple myeloma. Note the large lytic area and pathologic fracture.

later develop multiple myeloma. The multiple form responds temporarily to chemotherapy but usually takes the patient's life in a few years.

Large-cell or *B-cell lymphoma* of bone (formerly called *reticulum cell sarcoma*) often has the same clinical presentation as an osteosarcoma, although the patients are usually young

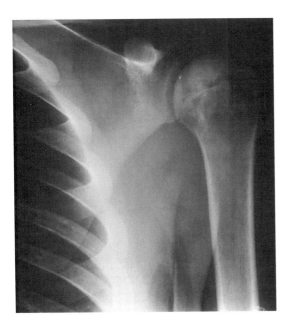

Figure 12.26   Large cell lymphoma in the humeral head. Note the numerous, small, lytic lesions creating a "moth eaten" appearance.

adults, and the radiographic appearance is almost entirely lytic (Fig. 12.26). Radiotherapy has been the traditional approach when the disease is localized to one bone; more recently, however, chemotherapy has been used. The long-term prognosis is generally better than for osteosarcoma, and surgery is rarely required.

Malignant fibrous histiocytoma (MFH) of bone can also resemble osteosarcoma in its presentation, although it favors middle-aged adults (Fig. 12.27). If osteoid is found in a bone tumor with the histologic appearance of malignant fibrous histiocytoma, the lesion is considered an osteogenic sarcoma. Most centers are treating MFH of bone and osteosarcomas in adults with pediatric osteosarcoma protocols, including limb salvage.

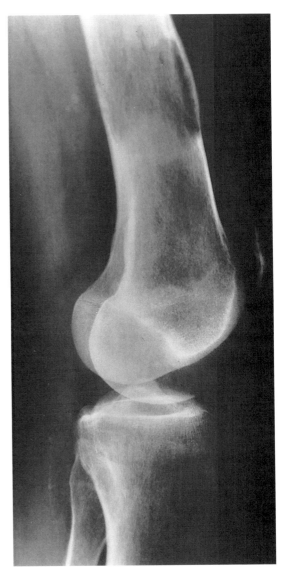

Figure 12.27   Malignant fibrous histiocytoma of the distal femur. Note the extensive destruction of cortical bone, with minimal reaction from the host bone.

TUMORS OF THE SOFT SOMATIC TISSUES

General Considerations

Benign and malignant tumors of the soft somatic tissues, which constitute 1 percent of all neoplasms, may arise in almost any tissue of the limbs. Among patients that seek medical attention, benign lesions outnumber malignant ones 100 to 1, although many additional benign lesions undoubtedly never come to medical attention. While only about 5000 soft tissue sarcomas are diagnosed annually in the United States, they account for 2 percent of the overall mortality from cancer. The possibility that any of the myriad soft tissue tumors can be malignant must be kept in mind.

Certain clinical behaviors are frequently associated with soft tissue malignancies; for example, tumors over 5 cm in diameter have a distinctly higher incidence of malignancy, as do tumors deep to the fascia and proximal lesions. Tumors fixed to surrounding tissues and rapidly growing tumors are also more likely to be malignant. Pain, however, is not a reliable symptom for prediction of malignancy, since many soft tissue sarcomas attain large size before becoming painful. Even with a large mass, "tightness" rather than pain is likely to be the primary complaint.

If a malignancy is feared, the evaluation should include routine hematologic evaluation and blood chemistries, a radiograph of the chest to rule out metastases, and imaging of the primary tumor. Plain radiographs show mass effects but lack diagnostic specificity. A CT scan does not provide adequate detail for soft tissue masses that have radiographic density similar to muscle. The preferred imaging modality for most soft tissue tumors is MRI, although edema around the tumor may cause it to appear larger than its actual size.

Because of histologic difficulties in distinguishing the many types of benign and malignant tumors of soft tissue, the biopsy must contain ample tissue for accurate identification and grading, since treatment often depends upon pathologic grade.

Benign Tumors

Lipomas, the most common soft tissue neoplasms, favor the subcutaneous tissues of the trunk or back. Their rubbery consistency resembles a cluster of grapes, which corresponds to the lobular nature of the neoplasm. If multiple masses are present, biopsy is usually unnecessary for diagnosis. Subfascial or intramuscular lipomas have a higher incidence of malignancy and should be removed.

Ganglia are even more common soft tissue masses but represent degenerative rather than neoplastic lesions. They contain a jellylike substance and are attached by a membranous stalk to a nearby joint or tendon sheath. Ganglia are especially common on the radial aspect of the wrist and dorsum of the foot (Fig. 12.28). Symptomatic or unsightly ganglia can sometimes be aspirated with a large-bore needle. If multiple punctures are made in the capsule of the cyst before all of the fluid is removed, the chance of recurrence is decreased. Care must be taken not to injure surrounding neurovascular structures, especially when aspirating a volar wrist ganglion.

The *angiomyoma,* or vascular leiomyoma, is a small subcutaneous tumor that has a predilection for the lower limbs of middle-aged persons. Tenderness or discomfort developing in a long-standing, small, mobile lesion typically brings the patient to medical attention. Simple excision is adequate treatment.

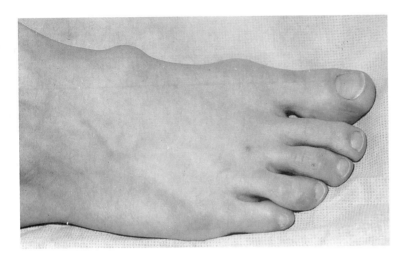

Figure 12.28   Ganglion on the dorsum of the foot.

The soft tissue neoplasm found most frequently in the hand is the *giant cell tumor of tendon sheath,* also known as *nodular tenosynovitis.* Middle-aged people are most often affected by this slowly growing lesion, which develops in close proximity to a tendon sheath in the hand or foot. Histologically, this lesion is closely related to *pigmented villonodular synovitis* (PVNS), which is a proliferation of synovium inside a joint. The PVNS tissue contains many giant cells, may destroy articular cartilage, and is more likely to recur after excision than a giant cell tumor of tendon sheath. Simple excision of the tendon sheath tumor is usually adequate.

Aggressive fibromatoses, or *desmoids,* are firm proliferations of fibrous tissue that cross fascial barriers anywhere in the body, predilecting persons between 10 and 30 years of age. The common presentations are pain and joint contracture. Recurrence is frequent following excision, in part because the borders of the lesion blend with surrounding tissues, making complete extirpation difficult. Radiation therapy reduces the rate of local recurrence but also makes subsequent surgery more difficult. Numerous medical therapies have been advanced, but none have been shown to be consistently effective.

Sarcomas

While there are many primary malignancies of soft tissue, most are sarcomas that are treated similarly. Table 12.2 lists the more common tumors and the typical ages of their occurrence. In general, soft tissue sarcomas are treated by surgical excision. If the tumor is large or lies close to critical neurovascular structures, preoperative radiation therapy is an advisable adjunct to surgery. There is no evidence that amputation or chemotherapy increases survival of patients with soft tissue sarcomas; therefore, patients are usually treated by wide local resection, with preservation of the limb. It is too early to know whether newer chemotherapeutic agents, such as ifosfamide and paclitaxel (Taxol), will improve survival beyond the 60 percent level attained by sur-

Table 12.2   Age Distribution of Soft Tissue Sarcomas

Tumor	Common Age of Incidence
Rhabdomyosarcoma	Birth–15
Synovial sarcoma	14–40
Fibrosarcoma	20–50
Liposarcoma	25–65
Malignant schwannoma	25–70
Malignant fibrous histiocytoma	40–80

gery alone in patients without metastatic disease. The improved imaging afforded by CT and MRI scans has increased surgical cure rates in patients without metastases.

Synovial sarcomas are painful tumors that commonly develop in close proximity to joints or tendon sheaths (Fig. 12.29). A mass or swelling is the usual mode of presentation, and many show small, focal calcifications on plain radiographs. This frequently aggressive tumor

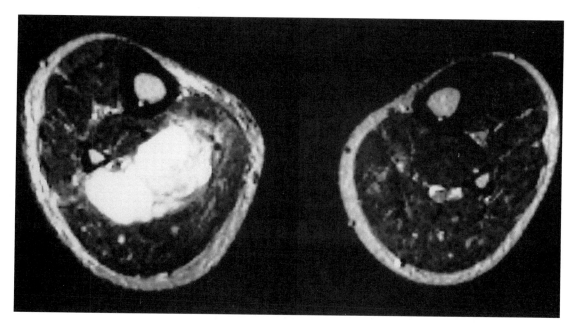

Figure 12.29   Synovial sarcoma of the calf. Note the high signal intensity on MRI, indicated by the white area.

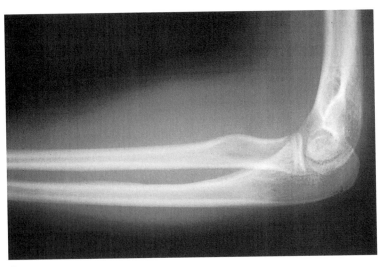

A

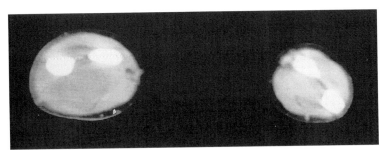

B

Figure 12.30
Rhabdomyosarcoma. *A.* Note the large soft tissue mass distal to the elbow. *B.* The CT scan reveals extension to both sides of the interosseous membrane.

most often affects younger patients. While en bloc excision remains the mainstay of treatment, there is evidence that long-term survival in synovial sarcoma may be improved by adjuvant chemotherapy.

Rhabdomyosarcomas, which are the most common soft tissue sarcomas in the limbs of children, are also common in the head and neck region (Fig. 12.30). This histologically diverse lesion is very responsive to chemotherapy and radiation; for this reason, surgery is used primarily to debulk large tumor masses in conjunction with chemotherapy and radia-

tion. A previously deadly sarcoma, it now has survival rates in the range of 60 to 70 percent, with most affected limbs being salvaged.

METASTASES TO BONE

Skeletal *metastases,* the most common osseous malignancies in the elderly, frequently cause severe pain and disability and are often the manifestation of neoplasia that leads a patient to be considered incurable. Unexplained pain in the limb of a patient with a history of carcinoma must be evaluated thoroughly; early discovery frequently enables prevention of pathologic fractures and other painful morbidities of end-stage disease (Fig. 12.31). Since the spine is the most common site for skeletal

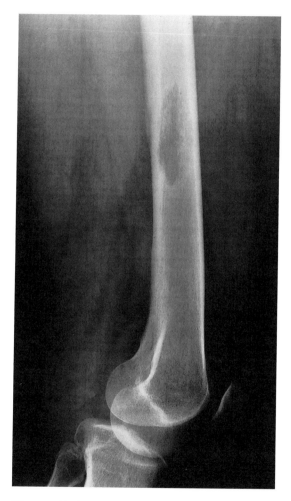

Figure 12.31 Metastatic breast cancer. After intramedullary nailing and 2 weeks of radiation therapy, the patient was able to walk without pain.

metastases, which have the potential for severe neurologic compromise, all complaints of back pain in at-risk patients must be investigated (Fig. 12.32).

For many patients skeletal metastasis is the initial sign of malignancy; in 10 percent of these patients, the primary site is not initially apparent.

The primary carcinomas that metastasize preferentially to bone are those of the prostate, breast, lung, kidney, and thyroid. Most metastases produce lytic changes in bone; prostatic and breast tumors may cause blastic, lytic, or mixed lesions. All metastases weaken bone and thus predispose to pathologic fracture. If a lesion involves over 50 percent of the width of a weight-bearing bone or occupies a section of cortical bone longer than twice the diameter of the bone, the risk of pathologic fracture is high, even if the lesion is treated with radiation therapy.

If the diagnosis of metastatic disease to bone is suspected, a needle biopsy often provides confirmation. The biopsy is done with CT or fluoroscopic guidance to avoid false-negative results. If a pathologist is present to confirm that adequate tissue has been obtained, the percentage of correct needle-biopsy results is increased.

The evaluation of a patient with metastases to bone is not complete until a bone scan has been obtained. If an asymptomatic lesion is discovered, treatment can be initiated early. While the spine and proximal bones of the limbs are most susceptible to metastases, the hands, feet, and soft tissues of the limbs are also affected, often with significant morbidity.

Treatment of skeletal metastases is aimed at relief of pain and preservation of function. The mainstay of treatment is radiation therapy.

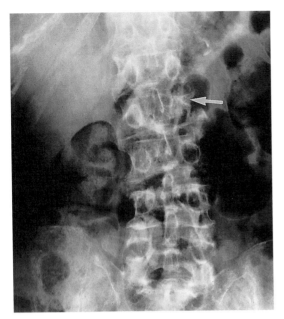

A

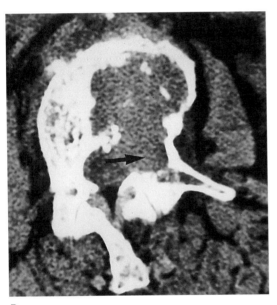

B

Figure 12.32 Metastatic disease to the lumbar spine. *A.* Note the absent pedicle (arrow), which proved to be a spinal metastasis. *B.* A CT scan of the lesion showing destruction of the vertebral body extending into the pedicle *(arrow).*

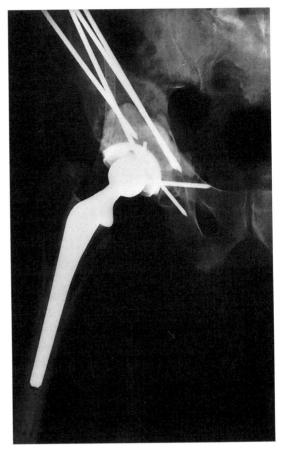

Figure 12.33 Pelvic radiograph of a man who underwent resection and reconstruction of the hip and acetabulum for prostatic cancer metastatic to the acetabulum.

324

Most carcinomas are responsive to radiation, and multiple sites can be treated simultaneously. Radiation therapy can usually be completed in 2 weeks, and bony reconstitution is common within 2 months. If a spinal lesion has led to neurologic compromise, steroids are added to radiotherapy.

Pathologic fractures in long bones should be considered for surgical stabilization if the patient has 6 weeks or more to live. Pelvic, acetabular, and spinal lesions are considered for reconstruction only if the patient has no or few other metastases, since stabilization of these areas is a major surgical undertaking (Fig. 12.33). After operative stabilization, radiotherapy is used to control residual tumor, which often dictates that the entire bone be radiated.

Follow-up of a patient with skeletal metastases entails regular examination and periodic bone scans. Every effort should be made to find disease before it causes structural compromise.

SUGGESTED READINGS

ENNEKING WF: *Musculoskeletal Tumor Surgery.* New York, Churchill Livingstone, 1983.

ENZINGER FM, WEISS SW: *Soft Tissue Tumors,* 3d ed. St Louis, Mosby, 1995.

MIRRA JM: *Bone Tumors.* Philadelphia, Lea & Febiger, 1989.

SIM FH: *Diagnosis and Management of Metastatic Bone Disease.* New York, Raven Press, 1988.

Chapter 13

Traumatic Disorders

Laurence E. Dahners, Louis C. Almekinders, and
Douglas R. Dirschl

Upper Limb
> *Clavicle; Acromioclavicular Joint; Scapula; Shoulder; Arm; Elbow; Forearm; Wrist; Hand*

Lower Limb
> *Pelvis; Hip; Thigh and Femur; Knee; Leg; Ankle; Hindfoot; Forefoot*

GENERAL ASPECTS

Causes

Trauma may be defined as mental or physical injury arising from any cause. As used in the surgical specialties, however, the term *trauma* refers to damage or disruption of tissue resulting from physical force. Most surgical trauma can be divided into three categories: blunt trauma, in which large objects strike the body causing disruptions of tissue, with or without piercing the skin; penetrating trauma, in which objects with a small cross-sectional area penetrate the skin; and thermal trauma.

Most musculoskeletal injuries arise from blunt trauma, especially that due to motor vehicle crashes, falls, or sports. Sports-related injuries are increasing with the number of participants, although less rapidly than one might expect because of improvements in equipment, rule changes to prevent injury, and better training regimens. Unfortunately, musculoskeletal injuries resulting from gunshot wounds are increasing. Except in the case of electrical injuries, where high voltages cause massive damage to the deep tissues in a limb, thermal injuries seldom result in musculoskeletal damage that is not overshadowed by damage to more superficial tissues.

The amount of tissue disruption produced by a traumatic event is proportional to the energy delivered to the tissue. The kinetic energy carried by an object that comes in contact with the human body is expressed by the formula $1/2\ mv^2$, or one-half the mass of the object times the square of its velocity. Since it is squared, velocity is more important than mass. Not all of the energy carried by an object is transmitted to adjacent tissues; some hard-point bullets produce only minimal injury as they pass through the body. The degree of injury caused by a fall varies with the distance fallen, because of the constant acceleration of a falling body. In sports, the mass is usually that of the participant and the velocity that of the athlete himself, so that sports-related injuries are rarely as devastating as vehicular injuries. It is important to recall the mv^2 phenomenon in managing a patient struck by a high-velocity bullet, as a seemingly innocuous wound may conceal massive tissue damage that requires extensive debridement and reconstructive surgery.

Of course the severity of a given injury is related also to the importance of the tissue (vessels, nerves, etc.) traumatized.

Societal Impact

It can be argued that trauma has a greater impact on society than any other major category of disease that affects humans. Cardiovascular disease and neoplasia have higher mortality rates than trauma; however, trauma is more common during the working years (ages 20 to 60). A recent statistic showed that while mortality from heart disease in the United States resulted in an annual loss of 1.4 million years of professional life (deaths under age 65) and cancer a loss of 1.9 million years, trauma resulted in the loss of 3.7 million years—a figure that does not include work loss from subsequent disability, which is more common following trauma than cardiovascular disease or cancer. Despite the enormous loss of productivity from trauma and the hidden costs of permanent impairment, society supports surprisingly little research into the prevention and treatment of injury.

The Systemic Response

Musculoskeletal trauma, especially when multiple, frequently produces systemic effects that can be more devastating than the injury itself.

Shock

The most obvious systemic effect of musculoskeletal trauma is shock, which usually results from the hemorrhage following fractures. Femoral fractures routinely cause blood loss in the range of 500 to 1500 mL. While loss of 500 mL of blood is not in itself life-threatening, superimposed blood loss from other sites can create a life-threatening problem. Fractures of the pelvis can be even more devastating, with some patients losing 10 to 15 L of blood into the retroperitoneal space. This insidious, persistent loss from the hematogenous marrow of the fracture surfaces and the veins of the presacral plexus results in the phenomenon of a patient in shock who responds rapidly to fluid resuscitation but deteriorates again

(often in transit to a tertiary care facility) because of continued bleeding.

The initial management of these patients requires recognition of the potential for extensive blood loss. The likelihood of significant bleeding increases with the size of the bone and displacement of the fracture, which disrupts surrounding soft tissues and prevents early tamponade. After achieving local hemostasis, venous access for fluid resuscitation should be secured and blood cross-matched for transfusion. Once the ability to replace lost blood is established, further control of bleeding is accomplished by reduction, immobilization, and tamponade. Reduction can be achieved by manipulation and/or traction. Splinting allows clots to form without disruption by motion at the fracture site. The application of traction to fractures of long bones produces a tamponade effect, and pneumatic antishock garments, by increasing pressure in the retroperitoneal space, have the same effect on fractures of the pelvis. Although a patient in shock has, through the sympathetic system, already benefited from the increased peripheral vascular resistance and autotransfusion from the lower limbs, most authorities agree that pneumatic garments further reduce blood loss from these fractures.

Fat Embolism

Another systemic effect of musculoskeletal injury is fat embolism, a phenomenon that usually occurs with fractures of major long bones. It is more common in patients who receive inadequate early fluid resuscitation. Within 12 to 72 h of injury, patients become confused and hypoxic as a result of fat emboli in the brain and lungs. It is unclear whether these emboli result from marrow fat forced into the vasculature at the fracture site or from the coalescence of lipids in the bloodstream. In any case, the lipids that embolize to the lung obstruct blood flow, and the products of their breakdown cause further pulmonary damage. The treatment of fat embolism is also controversial, but there is agreement that early fluid resuscitation plays an important role in minimizing its severity, and that patients who develop the syndrome require aggressive ventilatory support with oxygen and mechanical respirators. The value of steroids to diminish inflammation in the pulmonary parenchyma is debatable.

Respiratory Distress

Victims of multiple trauma may develop a type of respiratory failure known as *adult respiratory distress syndrome* (ARDS). Contributing factors include direct pulmonary contusion and the fat embolism syndrome. Even patients who do not develop the full-blown syndrome of fat embolism have emboli that contribute to the severity of other pulmonary complications. Pulmonary problems are further compounded by treatment that immobilizes the patient in a supine position. Early internal or external fixation of fractures to avoid prolonged recumbency is therefore advantageous.

The Local Response

The local response to injury may be divided into three phases: inflammation, during which necrotic tissue is removed; repair, when rapid synthesis of new matrix occurs; and maturation, wherein the poorly organized matrix laid down in the repair phase is remodeled into a compact and functionally efficient structure.

These phases have considerable overlap in time.

Inflammation

The inflammatory phase is essentially a physiologic debridement of the wound carried out by the local soft tissues. Blood and necrotic soft tissue are removed, as well as foreign bodies and bacteria introduced by the injury. The mediators of this inflammatory response are histamine and serotonin, which are released from basophils, mast cells, and platelets. Chemotaxis attracts leukocytes, which release their own mediators, including prostaglandins and arachidonic acid. The leukocytes also release lysosomal enzymes, which break down tissue by macromolecular cleavage. This process, effective in removing small amounts of necrotic material and organic foreign bodies, is aided substantially by operative debridement.

Repair

In the repair phase, capillaries invade the traumatized area, and fibroblasts begin to lay down collagen in a random, disorganized manner. There are several growth factors important in this process, including *platelet derived growth factor* (PDGF) released by the hematoma. This growth factor is active not only in the chemotaxis of new cells into the area but also in cell replication and matrix synthesis. In bone, the repair phase goes beyond fibrous tissue to the formation of cartilage and eventually new (woven) bone. *Bone morphogenetic proteins* (BMPs) are contained in bone and are members of the *transforming growth factor beta* (TGF-β) family of growth factors. The release of BMPs from bone that is being resorbed is important in stimulating new bone formation.

Maturation

The phase of maturation begins about 2 weeks after injury and continues for months or years. The disorganized matrix from the repair phase is broken down, and new, better-organized collagen (or lamellar bone in the case of fracture healing) is laid down in place of the disorganized collagen (or woven bone).

Repair of Specific Musculoskeletal Tissues

Muscle

Muscle is a highly vascularized tissue that is frequently wounded by blunt or penetrating trauma. Its rich blood supply makes it resistant to infection and receptive to skin grafts; it can also be stretched over less well vascularized tissues for coverage, and it heals relatively well. Poorly vascularized muscle is subject to rapid necrosis because of its high metabolic demand, and subsequent scarring may lead to contracture and severe limb dysfunction. When ischemic and contaminated, muscle is an excellent culture medium and a potent source of infection. Muscle is, to a limited extent, capable of regeneration through formation of new myotubes, and the remaining muscle is capable of hypertrophy.

Sports-related injuries of muscle are commonly referred to as "pulled muscles," but the medical term for partial tearing of a muscle is *strain*. Strains usually occur at the musculotendinous junction, even though pain, swelling, and tenderness more often occur in the central portion of the muscle—a fact explained by the long taper of the tendon extending into the belly of the muscle. These injuries heal through a process in which damaged muscle cells are resorbed, new myotubes formed, and an almost normal musculotendinous junction reformed. Since immobilization has an adverse effect on healing, functional mobility should be restored to the limb as soon as possible, with care to avoid overloading, which can cause reinjury.

Tendon

Tendon is an exceptionally well organized structure consisting of collagen fibrils arranged in parallel, longitudinal fashion, an arrangement that imparts the enormous tensile strength necessary for its tendon function. Gliding, also required for normal function, is provided by a surrounding bed of loose areolar tissue. The most frequent injuries are lacerations, ruptures through degenerated areas (see Chap. 14), and avulsions from bone. Restoration of satisfactory function usually requires operative repair.

Because of its limited blood supply, the response of tendon to trauma is not robust. In large, open wounds that expose tendon, it remains viable if its well-vascularized surrounding synovial tissues remain intact. However, if these tissues are damaged or stripped away (sometimes iatrogenically by overly zealous debridement), the remaining tendon becomes desiccated and dies.

Even sharp lacerations that transect tendon with minimal damage to peritendinous tissues pose significant problems, not the least of which is the difficulty of creating a strong enough repair to keep the tendon ends from being pulled apart by the muscles attached to them. In addition, adhesions often form between injured tendons and other damaged tissues nearby, which limits excursion of the tendon. To avoid the resultant loss of joint movement, early repair and resumption of motion are important.

Ligament

Although ligaments have a dense longitudinal collagenous arrangement similar to that found in tendon, they function to constrain and stabilize a joint rather than to deliver its motive force. Thus, they are attached to bone on both ends, and, rather than gliding longitudinally through tissue, tend to slide transversely as the joint moves. Injuries to ligaments are designated *sprains* and occur most often during participation in sports. Ligamentous injuries are classically divided into three grades: Grade I is injury on a microscopic level that results in pain without instability; Grade II tearing indicates partial, gross disruption of the ligament; this results in minimal but clinically detectable instability, in which the intact part of the ligament limits abnormal movement. This firm "endpoint" distinguishes grade II from grade III injuries, which are complete tears, with gross instability and no endpoint. Because one cannot stress a completely torn ligament, there is often surprisingly little pain when a grade III tear is being tested. Traditionally, severe sprains have been treated by immobilization; however, immobilization, in addition to causing stiffness of the joint, results in a slower gain of strength in the healing ligament. For these reasons, controlled movement of the joint during healing is advisable. An important exception is the anterior cruciate ligament, which is an intrasynovial structure. The ends of this ligament tend to float apart in the synovial fluid and rarely heal, even when sutured, so that replacement rather than repair of the ligament is preferred.

Articular Cartilage

Articular cartilage is an unusual tissue made up of collagen and proteoglycans. Having little or no blood supply, its nutrition comes from synovial fluid, which is pumped in and out of the cartilage by joint motion. Injuries to cartilage that do not involve the underlying bone provoke minimal tissue response. Because there is no clot to release PDGF, no blood cells to release chemotactic factors, and no source of cells to migrate into the area of injury, lacerations of cartilage rarely heal. When the underlying bone is involved, however, a blood supply becomes available, and healing similar to that in other tissues occurs, except that fibrocartilage rather than normal hyaline cartilage is formed. However, fibrocartilage contains more dense collagen and less proteoglycan and is thus less well suited for bearing compressive loads. Joint motion during healing results in the production of a better grade of fibrocartilage.

In open wounds that expose cartilage or tendon, it is important to obtain early coverage, since desiccation will rapidly destroy the cartilage that was not damaged by the trauma itself. Closed fractures involving joint surfaces require early and accurate reduction (usually with internal fixation) to prevent a step-off in the joint surface, which will damage the cartilage on the opposite side of the joint. Early restoration of joint motion is desirable to prevent adhesions and promote the pumping of synovial fluid into the matrix.

Bone

Most bodily tissues heal by formation of a collagenous scar. Bone is an exception in that new bone is regenerated at the fracture site. When bone does heal by forming a collagenous scar, it is termed a *nonunion,* which generally produces an unsatisfactory result. Two types of healing occur: in fractures with little motion at the fracture site (either because the fracture is incomplete or because it is internally fixed with a rigid metal implant), *primary union* is the rule. Fractures that have more motion between them heal by *secondary union.* In primary union, little radiographic evidence of healing response is seen; rather, the fracture appears to be simply "remodeled away." The inflammatory and repair phases of wound healing are markedly diminished, and the osteoclasts that normally remodel bone work their way directly across the fracture site, removing old bone and laying down new osteons (lamellae) in their wake. In secondary union, the inflammatory phase is followed by a repair phase in which granulation tissue is formed at the fracture site, followed by metaplasia to fibrous tissue, cartilage, and, eventually, to a large quantity of woven bone—all of which are referred to as *callus.* As this large volume of disorganized tissue increases in stiffness, it gradually immobilizes the fracture site. In the maturation phase, woven bone is slowly remodeled into lamellar bone by the same process that takes place in primary union. Primary union occurs more slowly than that by callus formation, so that internal fixation devices must usually be left in place for at least a year for the bone to gain sufficient strength.

Nonunions are usually divided into *pseudarthroses* and fibrous nonunions. A true pseudarthrosis is a "false joint" in which a fibrous capsule surrounds bone ends covered with fibrocartilage and contains fluid resembling that in synovial fluid. These nonunions usually require operative treatment. Fibrous

nonunions may be divided into hypertrophic and atrophic types (Fig. 13.1). *Hypertrophic nonunions* are surrounded by cartilage and woven bone, but excessive motion prevents connection of the bone fragments. In *atrophic nonunions,* adjacent tissues make little or no attempt to achieve bone union. Hypertrophic nonunions commonly unite following rigid internal fixation alone; but atrophic nonunions usually require supplemental bone grafting to restart the healing process. This additional bone is rapidly broken down by osteoclasts, releasing bone morphogenetic proteins (BMPs), which stimulate conversion of osteoprogenitor cells into the osteoblasts that initiate bone formation.

Factors Influencing Repair

Many factors, both systemic and local, have profound effects on the healing of musculoskeletal tissues.

Systemic Factors

A well-nourished, healthy patient heals fractures and other wounds more quickly and solidly than a patient who is ill. The nutritional requisites for wound healing are an adequate caloric intake, which is higher than usual because of increased metabolic demands imposed by injury, and sufficient protein to build collagen. Vitamins, especially vitamin C, and minerals, especially zinc, have also been linked to wound healing.

Certain diseases, such as diabetes and rheumatoid arthritis, affect wound healing adversely, as do increased levels of circulating corticosteroids. Smoking also has an adverse effect on fracture healing. Control of these

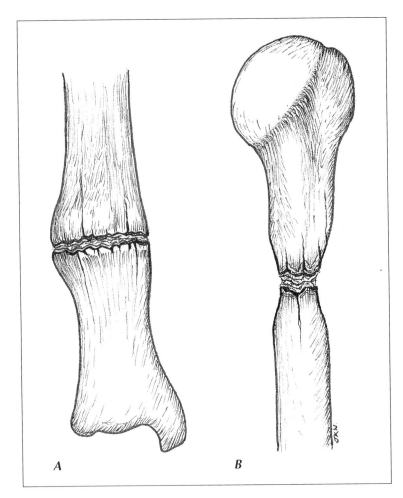

Figure 13.1 *A.* Hypertrophic nonunion with "elephant's foot" appearance. *B.* Atrophic nonunion with "penciled" bone ends.

conditions may be important in achieving the healing of fractures and other wounds.

Local Factors

Many local determinants of wound healing are under the control of the surgeon. One of the most important of these is infection, the risk of which is increased by necrotic tissue, foreign bodies, and bacterial contamination. Thorough irrigation and debridement are vital to reducing the risk of infection, as are both local and systemic antibiotics.

Drying of the wound is also to be avoided, as it contributes to tissue necrosis. Wet-to-dry dressings are often used in open, contaminated wounds, but these dressings should be employed judiciously. The gauze dries with time and adheres to underlying tissue. When the dressing is changed, it removes necrotic tissue and debrides the wound. Wet-to-dry dressings should not be used in wounds that do not have superficial layers of necrotic tissue to be debrided. As the drying itself can cause tissue necrosis, it is often better to keep the dressing moist. Certain tissues, such as bone and tendon, are especially susceptible to drying, so early efforts should be made to keep them moist and cover them with other soft tissues (usually muscle).

Other local prophylactic measures include elevation and gentle compression to minimize tissue edema, which promotes infection. However, occlusive dressings should be avoided, since they compromise blood flow and the delivery of oxygen, which is essential to wound healing.

Specific Types of Injury

Compartmental Syndromes

A compartmental syndrome can occur wherever soft tissues are surrounded by nondistensible fascia and/or bone. It is particularly common in the anterior leg and the volar forearm and can be functionally devastating. Compartmental syndromes occur less frequently in the hand, foot, thigh, arm, and buttock because the fascia is less constrictive in these areas. There is also evidence that *avascular necrosis* (AVN) of bone may be caused by a form of compartmental syndrome. In AVN, swelling of marrow elements from underlying disease within a nondistensible compartment (such as the femoral head) may cause bone infarction.

A compartmental syndrome results from swelling of the tissues within the compartment, which occurs most often after trauma. Edema and bleeding distend the compartment; when it cannot expand any farther, intracompartmental pressure begins to rise. When it rises to within 20 to 30 mmHg of the diastolic blood pressure, capillaries are closed off and compartmental tissues become ischemic. With higher pressures, a vicious cycle begins in which the veins are tamponaded, preventing egress of blood, but the arteries continue to pump blood in, which rapidly raises intracompartmental pressure. Once ischemia begins, there is a 6-h window during which the compartment may be decompressed prior to muscle necrosis and ischemic contracture.

Treatment begins with recognition of an injury that is likely to cause a compartmental syndrome, especially a crushing injury of a limb. The diagnosis is classically based on the "four Ps": pain, pallor, paresthesias, and pulselessness. It must be recognized that pallor, paresthesias, and pulselessness are late sequelae that follow occlusion of the arterial blood flow through the compartment, which does not occur until compartmental pressure exceeds systolic pressure. By that time, the muscle has usually been ischemic for hours. Thus, the clinician must rely on the pain of muscle ischemia, which can be difficult to differentiate from the pain of initial injury. If active muscle contraction or passive stretching causes severe muscle pain, the likelihood of a compartmental syndrome should be considered and pressure within the compartment measured with either a commercially available device or the Whitesides' technique (Fig. 13.2). If the pressure is within 20 to 30 mmHg of diastolic blood pressure, surgical release of the compartment is imperative.

Amputations and Near Amputations

Complete and near amputations (which leave the part physically attached but physiologically detached from the body) pose a significant challenge in management. Modern surgical technology allows replantation of these parts, but the part never functions as well as it did before injury. *Replantation* should be con-

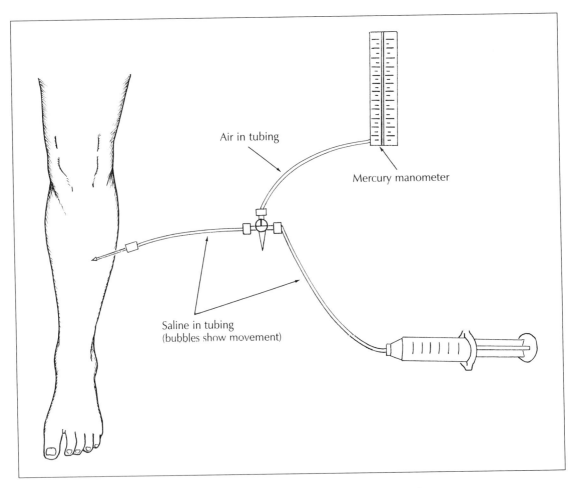

Figure 13.2   Whitesides' technique for measurement of compartmental pressure. The needle is in the anterior compartment of the leg. As the plunger of the syringe is depressed, saline is forced into the tubing and travels first toward the mercury manometer, elevating the column of mercury. Once the saline stops moving toward the manometer and begins moving toward the leg, the manometer pressure equals the compartmental pressure.

sidered in clean, sharp amputations of functionally important parts in young patients. Contaminated, crushed tissue does poorly following replantation, and older patients are much less capable of regenerating nerve fibers

into reattached parts. Replanted digits survive more often because they do not contain heavy musculature, which allows them to sustain ischemia for longer periods without major damage. Prolonged warm ischemic time is the major barrier to replantation. Any amputated part should be wrapped in a saline-moistened, sterile gauze, placed in a plastic bag, and kept on ice until a final decision is made regarding replantation. The part should never be disposed of prior to completion of the patient's operative procedure. Even parts that are not replanted can sometimes be used to provide skin, tendon, nerve, blood vessels, or bone for the remaining appendages.

Open Fractures

Open fractures, in which bone is exposed through a soft tissue wound, have a worse prognosis than closed fractures. They are classified according to Gustilo and Anderson into three categories: type I open fractures have a wound less than 1 cm in length; type II fractures have a wound up to 10 cm long; and type III fractures are those with wounds longer than 10 cm. Type III fractures are subdivided into subtypes A, B, and C depending upon the availability of soft tissue coverage (A, B) and vascular damage (C). At surgery, it is important to open even small wounds sufficiently to allow debridement of all devitalized and/or contaminated subcutaneous tissue and bone. Rapid immobilization of the fracture is important for soft tissue as well as bone healing. Because of associated vascular damage, grade IIIC open fractures of the tibia fare poorly and should be considered for immediate amputation.

Pathologic Fractures

Pathologic fractures are fractures that occur through bone weakened by an underlying disorder, such as *osteoporosis*. Fractures of the hip, spine, and distal radius are so common in older, osteoporotic women that they are seldom thought of as being pathologic. Other common causes are bone-destroying lesions, such as infection and neoplasia, both benign and malignant. It is particularly important to recognize "impending" pathologic fractures. One signal that a lesion has destroyed sufficient bone to put the patient at high risk for fracture is *crescendo pain,* i.e., increasing pain in the area of the pathologic lesion. Lesions that have destroyed 50 percent of the diameter of a bone are also at greater risk, especially if it is a weight-bearing bone. Unfortunately, many neoplastic and infectious processes destroy bone in a mottled or moth-eaten pattern, which defies radiographic determination of the amount of bone destroyed.

Stress Fractures

A stress fracture is a fracture occurring in normal bone that has been repeatedly stressed below its breaking point. The classic lesion is the *march fracture,* named for its occurrence in young military recruits taken from a sedentary lifestyle and subjected to long marches with heavy packs. Repetitive loading of the bone produces microscopic cracks, which eventually heal, with remodeling of the bone to accommodate the increased stress. However, if damage from repetitive stress exceeds the rate of remodeling, the fracture may suddenly become complete. The process is similar to what happens when a piece of wire is bent back and forth until it breaks.

The most important aspect of treatment for a stress fracture is recognition. Often the patient has recently begun an activity that produces repetitive stress, such as jogging. Although point tenderness is present initially, radiographs are frequently normal. The physician must suspect the diagnosis and instruct the patient to decrease his or her activity level. When radiographs are repeated several weeks later, callus is often seen, if not the fracture itself. The bone scan usually becomes positive 24 to 48 h after the onset of pain. Treatment involves decreasing the stressful activity or protecting the part in a cast until healing catches up with the microfractures. In some areas, most notably the femoral neck, the development of a complete fracture is so devastating that a case can be made for prophylactic internal fixation.

Child Abuse

The possibility of child abuse often creates an uncomfortable situation for the physician. Erroneous accusations can humiliate an innocent family, but the mortality rate in children sent home with abusive caretakers is alarmingly high. Most child abuse occurs in patients under 2 years of age. A fall from a sofa or table is commonly proposed as the mechanism of injury by the abuser, but in one study of nearly 800 patients less than 5 years of age who fell from such surfaces, there were only 7 fractures. In examining a suspected victim, the entire patient should be inspected, looking for ecchymoses, burns, welts, lacerations, scars, and evidence of old fractures. Suspicion may be confirmed by radiographic survey of the skeleton for evidence of old injuries. Although spiral fractures are highly suggestive of abuse (the twisting mechanism necessary to produce a spiral fracture is an uncommon natural cause of injury), most fractures caused by child abuse are transverse and/or involve a physis. The corner fracture, also known as a "chip" or *bucket-handle fracture,* is a subtle finding but is common in child abuse and should raise suspicion (Fig. 13.3). Multiple fractures of differing ages are also strongly suggestive of abuse.

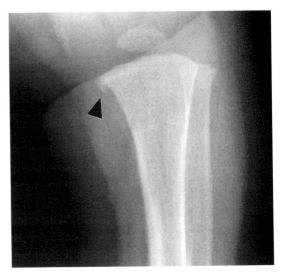

Figure 13.3   Bucket-handle ("chip" or "corner") fracture seen in child abuse. Note the metaphyseal fragment *(arrowhead).*

Reflex Sympathetic Dystrophy

The term *reflex sympathetic dystrophy (RSD)* refers to a number of poorly understood, painful conditions that often follow trauma. Patients complain of severe, burning dysesthesias that are usually out of proportion to the injury and often far removed from the site of injury. The exaggerated response to pain can assume extraordinary forms. Some patients must keep the affected part wrapped in moist towels; others cannot bear light touch with sheets, clothing, examiners, or even cool drafts; still others are affected simply by verbal suggestions. The full-blown disorder is striking; characteristic features include vasomotor disturbances, skin changes, and contractures. Initially, the affected extremity is hyperemic, erythematous, and warm; later it becomes pale, cool, clammy, or even cyanotic. Hair and skin creases disappear, imparting a glossy, tight appearance to the limb. Contractures develop with prolonged disuse (Fig. 13.4). The pathogenesis of RSD is obscure, but it is believed to involve dysfunction and overactivity of the sympathetic nervous system. Reflex sympathetic dystrophy is more likely to follow partial nerve injuries than complete nerve lacerations. Notably, crush injuries, which are frequently associated with RSD, do not sever nerves but impart considerable damage to them.

Because many different patterns and variants of RSD exist, the diagnosis can be difficult, especially early in the course of the disease; and it is often complicated by malingering and psychological abnormalities. Three-phase bone scans usually demonstrate diffuse uptake on delayed images, and plain radiographs may show localized osteopenia. *Sudeck atrophy* is a form of RSD characterized by patchy osteopenia on plain radiographs (Fig. 13.5). Vasomotor disturbances in the circulation of bone are presumably responsible for these positive imaging studies. *Transient osteoporosis of the hip* is a painful condition of the proximal femur occurring typically in young adults, who demonstrate osteopenia on radiographs and diffuse marrow changes on magnetic resonance imaging (MRI) (Fig. 6.9).

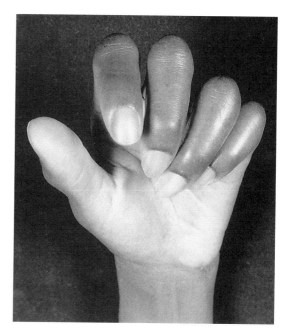

Figure 13.4   Reflex sympathetic dystrophy. Note the tight, shiny, glossy skin, fusiform atrophic digits, and flexion contractures.

The treatment of RSD is difficult. Approximately half of all patients can be managed nonoperatively. Desensitization measures include massage, electrical stimulation, and heat and ice treatments. Active range-of-motion ex-

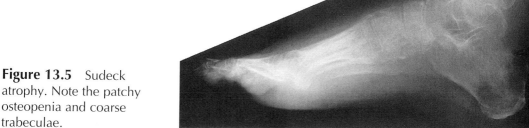

Figure 13.5   Sudeck atrophy. Note the patchy osteopenia and coarse trabeculae.

ercises should be encouraged, since disuse perpetuates the pain cycle; however, passive motion beyond the patient's tolerance may exacerbate the pain. Contractures may require dynamic splinting. Numerous medications have been used with variable success, including vasodilators, beta blockers, NSAIDs, sedatives, narcotics, and antidepressants. Sympathetic blockade is often beneficial, although several injections may be necessary to effect cure. In refractory cases, surgical sympathectomy can be performed.

Principles of Management

Since the time of Hugh Owen Thomas, a classic treatment of musculoskeletal injury has been rest and immobilization of the damaged part. Over the past several decades, however, it has been clearly shown that both bone and soft tissue heal better with "functional treatment," in which normal movement and function of the part are allowed, while abnormal movement is prevented. Immobilized fractures will heal, but the bone becomes osteoporotic—an event that may be prevented by compressive loading of the fracture as healing occurs. Cartilage heals better if the joint is allowed to move, which improves the nutrition of the cartilage by pumping synovial fluid in and out of it. Ligaments also heal better with normal movement, although they will heal in a lax state if abnormal movement is allowed. Tendons heal with fewer adhesions if they are allowed to glide gently through their beds after being sutured. Muscle also heals more quickly and strongly if an early return to light activity is allowed.

Fracture Immobilization

The objective of early fracture treatment is immobilization of the fracture fragments, simul-taneously allowing axial loading and movement of neighboring joints. Often the most effective means for accomplishing these goals is internal fixation; however, the risks and the costs of operative intervention make it unreasonable for fractures that can be treated satisfactorily with splints, casts, or braces.

Splints are made of a rigid material, usually plaster or fiberglass, applied on one or both sides of an injured part, and held in place with a wrap. Although usually employed as temporary measures, they are sometimes used for an entire course of treatment. Immediate splinting protects the injured part from further injury until complete radiographic evaluation has been obtained. After the fracture is evaluated and reduced, the reduction may be held securely with a molded splint, which allows swelling of the injured part without vascular compromise.

Casts, being circumferential and rigid, do not accommodate increased swelling and are therefore more safely applied after swelling subsides. When a carefully molded cast is necessary initially to maintain reduction, it may, if swelling becomes a problem, be "bivalved" by dividing it down to the skin on both sides and holding it in place with an elastic wrap. Inasmuch as *plaster* is less expensive and easier to mold to the injured part, it is preferred to fiberglass as a cast material during the early phase of healing; however, the durability of fiberglass makes it more attractive after early healing has stabilized the fracture. Carefully contoured *braces,* either plastic or metal, may be hinged to allow motion in joints neighboring partially healed fractures.

Reduction of a fracture entails reversal of the forces that caused the injury, which can often be determined from inspection of the original radiographs (Fig. 13.6*A* through *F*).

Splints and casts can be used to reverse

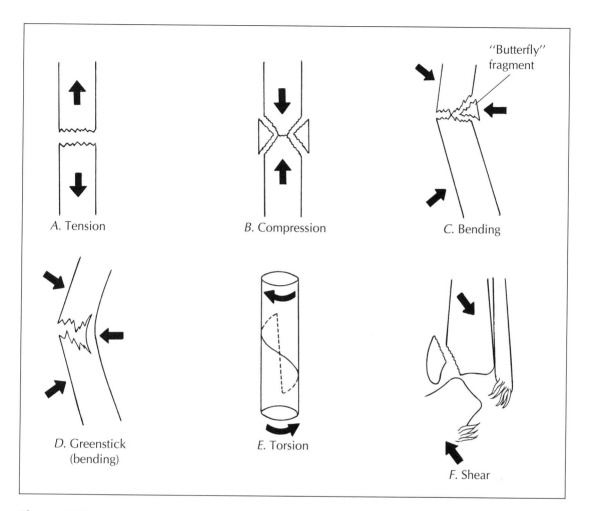

Figure 13.6 Fracture patterns in response to various types of loading.
A. Failure caused by tension forces produces a fracture line perpendicular
to the direction of the tensile load. *B.* Bone loaded in compression causes
fragmentation (comminution), with extrusion of bone fragments outward
("bursting"). *C.* Bone loaded in bending fails in tension on one side and
compression on the other side. The tension side fails transversely and the
compression side is comminuted, often producing a "butterfly fragment."
D. Under bending load, the greater elasticity of children's bone allows it to
fracture on the convex (tension) side only, producing a "greenstick"
fracture. *E.* Bone loaded in torsion fails in a spiral manner. *F.* Shear
loading is not common except in malleolar fractures; in this example, the
medial malleolus is forced proximally and fails in shear. The fracture line
tends to parallel the direction of the shear load.

bending forces (Fig. 13.7), and bone that has failed in tension due to a bending load can often be treated with a cast or splint (Fig. 13.8*A* and *B*). These devices cannot apply distraction, so a fracture shortened unacceptably by axial compression will likely require operative treatment.

Adequacy of Reduction

Appropriate treatment of fractures entails recognition of an adequate reduction, for which the following principles apply: (1) Fractures of the articular surfaces should be reduced anatomically to minimize the risk of arthritis. In children, these fractures usually involve the physis as well, and failure to reduce the growth plate precisely may result in bony bridging, with disturbance of growth. (2) Except for fractures that cross the physis (Fig. 13.9), less precision is required in the reduction of children's fractures because of their greater capacity for remodeling—rotational deformity ex-

cepted. (3) Shortening (caused by overriding, angulation, or compression) is better tolerated in the upper than the lower limb, since equal leg lengths are more important than equal arm lengths. (4) Reductions must be more precise in the diaphysis than in the metaphysis because healing is more problematic and residual deformity more visible in the diaphysis. (5) Angulation in the plane of joint motion is tolerated better than angulation out of that plane.

Reduction Techniques

Obtaining a satisfactory reduction requires adequate anesthesia. For outpatients, regional anesthesia is often sufficient, supplemented as needed by a sedative and a narcotic analgesic. Analgesics and sedatives are dangerous in children and the elderly and must be used cautiously in these age groups. Regional nerve blocks work well in the hand and foot; other fractures can be reduced with a *hematoma*

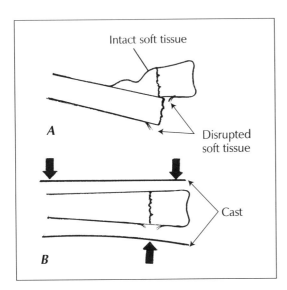

Figure 13.7   When a fracture results from a bending load, the soft tissue is disrupted on the tension side. The intact soft tissues on the compression side maintain the limb in a characteristic "bent" position (as it was broken). After reduction, a cast or splint that applies three-point bending forces *(large arrows)* can be used to maintain the reduction. The intact soft tissues on the previously concave side prevent overreduction.

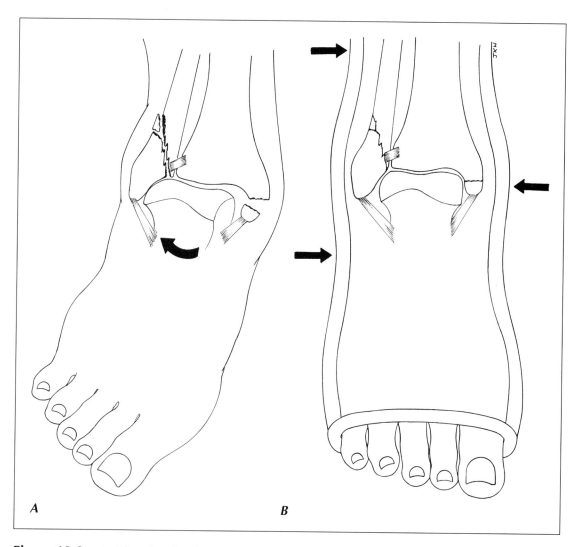

Figure 13.8   *A.* A bending load applied to the ankle *(large arrow)* has caused tension failure of the medial malleolus. *B.* A cast that applies three-point bending in the opposite direction reduces the malleolus.

block, in which a local anesthetic, such as lidocaine or bupivocaine, is injected into the hematoma (10 to 15 mL of 1% lidocaine for the distal radius).

In reducing fractures, it is important to understand the concept of "increasing the deformity," especially for those fractures that result from bending forces (Fig. 13-10A through *D).*

Restoration of Soft Tissue Function

After reduction of a fracture, those joints not immobilized should be allowed active move-

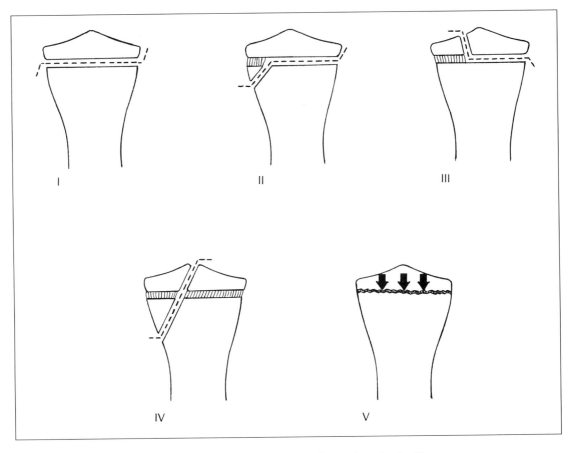

Figure 13.9   The Salter classification of fractures involving the physis. The dotted lines represent the paths of disruption. The higher numbers are associated with a greater risk of growth arrest.

ment, which reduces swelling, prevents adhesions, and lessens atrophy. Similarly, after dislocations, sprains, muscle injuries, or tendon lacerations, the limb should be mobilized using hinged braces or other devices to prevent abnormal motion. In the fingers or toes, this goal can be accomplished by "buddy-taping" the injured digit to an adjacent normal one, which allows the uninjured digit to serve as a hinged brace. The tape should not hinder movement in the interphalangeal joints.

REGIONAL FRACTURES AND DISLOCATIONS; SPORTS-RELATED INJURIES

Spine

Cervical

Injuries to the cervical spine can be devastating. They are more common than most physicians are aware, since many vehicular fatalities from upper cervical spine injuries never

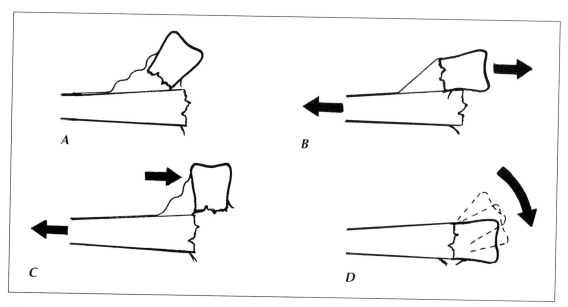

Figure 13.10   Fracture reduction. *A.* A fracture of the distal radius caused
by bending has intact soft tissues on the concave (dorsal) side. *B.* Simple
traction *(large arrows)* fails to reduce the fracture because the intact soft
tissue prevents reestablishment of sufficient length to obtain reduction.
C. "Increasing the deformity," followed by a "push" distally *(large arrows)*
allows reestablishment of length, leaving the intact soft tissues relatively
relaxed. The soft tissues on the volar side are disrupted and so do not
prevent the increase in deformity. *D.* Once length is reestablished, the
angular deformity can be reduced *(large arrow).*

reach the hospital. Although neurologic injury
is the most dreaded result, lesser injuries often
result in chronic disabling pain. Differentiating
unstable injuries, which may result in catastrophic neurologic compromise, from stable
injuries that are more likely to cause chronic
pain, and benign injuries that have a self-limited course is one of the most difficult tasks for
the clinician.

MUSCULAR INJURIES   Cervical pain is usually accompanied by spasm, which suggests
injury to muscle; however, a natural reaction
to any injury is "splinting" of the part by adjacent muscles. Thus, when a structure in the
cervical spine is injured, spasm of the overlying muscles is frequent; and after prolonged
contraction, the muscles themselves become a
source of pain, even if they are initially uninjured. Of course, primary strains do occur in
the neck, but whatever the cause, muscular
spasm is one of the more treatable sources of
pain resulting from injury to the neck. Muscle
does not contract well at higher temperatures,
so topical heat is an excellent relaxant. Most
pharmacologic "muscle relaxants" are actually
central nervous system depressants with great
potential for psychological if not physiologic

addiction. They should be avoided except for short-term use.

For a patient with a strain, a soft cervical collar allows relaxation of the muscles even when the patient is up and about. Further relaxation is obtained by rest in a supine or semireclining position.

FRACTURES   These injuries commonly result from axial loading and/or flexion and range in their effect from inconsequential to lethal. The complexity of treatment usually parallels the severity of injury, from simple immobilization to operative stabilization.

A fracture of the ring of C1 is also called a *Jefferson fracture.* The superior and inferior facets of C1 slant toward each other in the midline, so that an axial load applied to the skull (as in a diving accident) forces the occipital condyles toward the superior articular facets of C2, squeezing the lateral masses of C1 out from between them like watermelon seeds (Fig. 13.11*A* and *B*). Axial loading combined with hyperextension often fractures the pos-

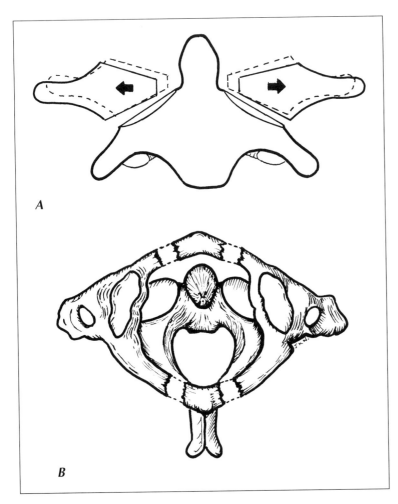

Figure 13.11   Fracture of the ring of C1. *A.* Axial loading extrudes the lateral masses of C1 outward. *B.* View from above, showing the actual pathology.

terior arch of C1; when combined with lateral bending, a comminuted fracture of one lateral mass is more likely, which may cause post-traumatic arthritis. The more common fractures of the ring are usually anterior or posterior to the lateral masses and are difficult to see on AP and lateral radiographs. The classic radiographic finding is enlargement of the ring of C1, which is most easily detected on the AP view of the C1 to 2 articulation ("open mouth" or "odontoid" view). On this view, the lateral masses of C1 overhang the lateral masses of C2, indicating expansion of the ring. Instability is suggested by a combined overhang of the C1 facets on C2 of more than 7 mm or by widening of the interval between the anterior portion of C1 and the odontoid process of more than 3 mm, which indicates rupture of the transverse ligament. Once suspected, a CT scan will demonstrate the fractures. Stable fractures can be treated with a hard cervical collar for 2 months, whereas unstable fractures generally require a halo orthosis. If healing does not occur, surgical fusion is indicated.

Fractures of the odontoid include three types (Fig. 13.12): type I is an avulsion through the superior tip of the odontoid; type II, the most common, occurs at the junction of the odontoid with the body; and type III fractures, which are rare, extend into the body of C2. Type I lesions are generally stable but may be associated with atlantooccipital instability. Type II injuries are stable if there is less than 5 mm of anterior or posterior displacement and less than 10° of angulation. All type III fractures should be considered unstable. In general, stable or minimally displaced fractures can be treated with immobilization in a hard collar or halo vest, while unstable fractures require operative stabilization.

A *fracture of the ring of C2* is also called a *hangman's fracture*. This fracture is actually a

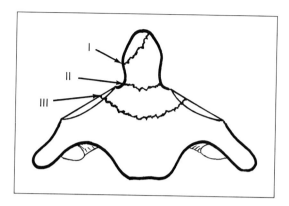

Figure 13.12   Three levels of fractures of the odontoid.

spondylolisthesis of C2, in which separation of the anterior and posterior elements allows the vertebral body to displace anteriorly (Fig. 13.13). They are best seen on the lateral radiograph, and, when there is less than 3 mm of displacement, can be treated by a hard cervical collar. With greater displacement, they should be managed in a halo vest. Occasionally, the facets dislocate, producing an extremely unstable injury that requires open reduction and internal fixation.

Fractures of C3 through C7 are considered together because of the similarity of the vertebrae and mechanism of injury in this region. They are usually caused by axial compression. If the spine is in neutral alignment, the entire vertebral body fails, often with the fragments extruding anteriorly and posteriorly, which can have devastating neurologic consequences (Fig. 13.14). With axial loading in slight flexion, only anterior failure occurs, causing a fracture of the anterosuperior aspect of the vertebral body or *teardrop fracture*. Since both of these injuries may be associated with posterior ligamentous disruptions, they are frequently unstable and should be treated either by trac-

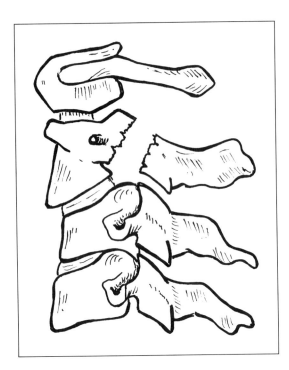

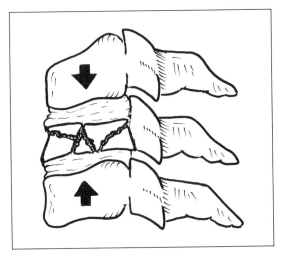

Figure 13.14   A "burst" fracture. Axial loading *(large arrows)* has caused comminution of the vertebral body.

Figure 13.13   C2 fracture ("hangman's fracture"). Note the anterior displacement (spondylolisthesis) of the body of C2. (Redrawn with permission from Levine AM, Edwards CC: Management of traumatic spondylolisthesis of the axis. *J Bone Joint Surg* 67A: 217–26, 1985.)

tion and operative stabilization or application of a halo vest.

Fractures of the spinous process (clay shoveler's fracture) of C6, C7, or T1 often follow repetitive, heavy, reciprocating motions of the shoulder girdle, such as shoveling, or they can be caused by a single, violent contraction of the muscles attaching to the spinous process. They are usually treated by rest and a cervical collar.

SPRAINS AND DISLOCATIONS   Many milder injuries of the cervical spine, such as those re-

sulting from *whiplash* mechanisms, represent partial ligamentous tears or sprains. These patients characteristically have nonfocal neck pain without neurologic changes. Radiographs are normal, and symptoms usually resolve spontaneously. Symptomatic treatment with a soft cervical collar and anti-inflammatory medication is sufficient. These injuries must be differentiated from the more severe ligamentous and bony injuries associated with instability and displacement, which have potentially catastrophic neurologic consequences.

Occiput-C1 dislocations are the cause of significant mortality in motor vehicular crashes; it is the rare patient who survives for treatment.

Rotatory subluxation of C1-C2 may follow injury or may occur spontaneously during upper respiratory infections in children. It is manifest clinically by acute torticollis. Radiographically, the diagnosis may be suspected when, on the open-mouth radiograph, the lat-

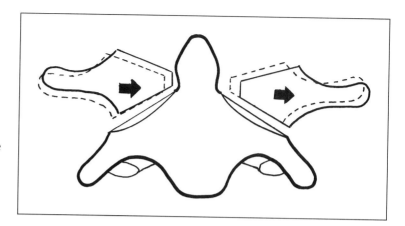

Figure 13.15 Rotatory subluxation of C1 on C2. There is displacement of one lateral mass toward the odontoid; the other lateral mass moves away from the odontoid.

eral masses of C1 are asymmetrical (one lateral and the other medial) in their relationship to the odontoid (Fig. 13.15). If, on the lateral view, the anterior arch of C1 is within 3 mm of the odontoid (*atlanto-dens interval,* or ADI), the injury is relatively stable and can be treated with gentle halter traction and stretching exercises, followed by a cervical collar after reduction occurs. Greater displacement indicates rupture of the transverse ligament and instability requiring surgical stabilization. In children, there is greater mobility of the cervical spine, and the ADI must be over 5 mm for a diagnosis of instability.

If no fracture is seen, the radiographs must be carefully studied for signs of instability between C2 and C7. These signs include (1) anterior or posterior translation of a vertebral body more than 3.5 mm on the lateral view; (2) disk or facet joint widening, or more than 11° angulation between adjacent segments on the lateral view; and (3) malalignment of the spinous processes on the AP view. Most commonly, unstable injuries result from flexion, with anterior displacement of a vertebra on the one beneath it. If the injury is associated with torsion, one facet may sublux or dislocate without displacement of the other. Unilateral

facet dislocation results in less than 25 percent anterior translation of the vertebral body, whereas bilateral facet dislocation produces at least 50 percent anterior displacement of the vertebral body (Fig. 13.16). Although some authors recommend that unstable injuries be treated with halo immobilization, most advise operative stabilization.

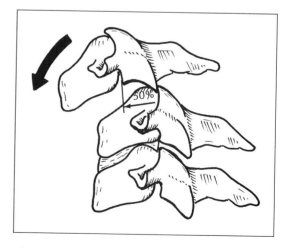

Figure 13.16 Dislocation of the cervical spine with "locked facets" from a flexion injury *(large arrow)*. Note that the vertebral body is displaced over 50 percent anteriorly on the body beneath it.

Thoracic and Lumbar

MUSCULAR INJURIES   Although *lumbar strain* is a common diagnosis in patients with acute posttraumatic low back pain (see Chap. 14), it is usually a diagnosis of exclusion. Muscular spasm, which accompanies most spinal injuries, is a nonspecific finding. Strain of the paraspinal muscles, evidenced by a palpable hematoma, should respond to rest and anti-inflammatory agents.

FRACTURES   Fractures of the thoracolumbar spine fall into two broad types. The first type, usually involving flexion-distraction and axial loading, occurs in young, healthy patients subjected to significant trauma, such as a fall or motor vehicular accident. Most of these fractures occur at the thoracolumbar junction, where displacement may cause serious neurologic consequences. The second major group are compression fractures, which often follow minimal trauma in elderly, osteoporotic patients. They occur typically in the kyphotic, upper portion of the thoracic spine. Displacement and neurologic sequelae are rare.

Burst fractures result from massive axial loading and may cause neurologic damage from fragments of the vertebral body retropulsed into the spinal canal. Young patients with over 20 percent loss of vertebral body height on the lateral radiograph should be evaluated with a CT scan to determine whether retropulsion of fragments has occurred. If less than 25 percent of the canal is compromised by a displaced fragment, application of an extension cast or brace after a brief period of bed rest usually suffices. With more extensive occlusion of the canal, extended bed rest is indicated; when a retropulsed fragment occludes over 50 percent of the canal or if there is an associated neurologic deficit, surgical decompression and stabilization should be considered.

Flexion-distraction injuries also predilect young patients and follow flexion of the spine around an external structure, such as a seat belt, which leads to anterior compression and posterior distraction forces on the spine. Some patients have compression of the anterior half of the vertebral body (anterior column), with the posterior half of the vertebral body (middle column) unaffected and the posterior elements of the spine (posterior column) distracted either by a posterior element fracture or facet subluxation. When the vertebral bodies are undisplaced and disruption of the posterior elements is mostly bony *(Chance fracture)*, these injuries can be adequately treated by an extension brace or cast. If the posterior injury is ligamentous, surgical treatment is needed to avoid chronic instability.

Fracture dislocations are extremely unstable injuries defined by translation of one vertebra on the other, in either the anteroposterior or mediolateral direction, associated with fracture of the posterior elements. They are usually neurologically devastating and require surgical treatment.

Osteoporotic compression fractures are frequently multiple. Classically, severe pain in the midback follows minor trauma, such as sitting down too hard. Radiographs show anterior wedging of one or more vertebral bodies. The possibility of the fracture occurring through a metastatic lesion must be ruled out by a directed history, examination of the breasts, and search of the radiographs for localized lytic lesions. Treatment entails early mobilization to avoid the complications of bed rest. Bracing is not used, since it limits excursion of the rib cage and potentiates pulmonary problems. A thoracolumbar corset with stays affords enough support for the patient to be up and about.

Upper Limb

Clavicle

The clavicle is the only bony connection between the scapula and the axial skeleton. Clavicular fractures are common and usually follow a direct blow or a fall onto the shoulder or outstretched hand. They occur most often at the junction of the middle and outer thirds of the bone, medial to the coracoclavicular ligaments. The distal portion of the fractured clavicle is pulled downward by the weight of the arm and the proximal portion upward by the sternocleidomastoid muscle. There are few indications for open reduction of a fractured clavicle, the most common being compromise of the subclavian vessels or brachial plexus by the fracture fragments.

Anatomic reduction of a displaced fracture is never achieved by closed means, but healing occurs almost invariably, even with overriding of the bone ends. Partial immobilization is accomplished with a *figure-of-eight dressing* or a simple sling. It is important, when applying a figure-of-eight dressing, to avoid axillary compression, which can compromise the axillary vessels and nerves (Fig. 13.17). Range-of-motion exercises are instituted as soon as tolerated. Immobilization is continued for 3 to 4 weeks in the younger child and for 6 weeks in the adult.

Complications of closed treatment are rare. The incidence of delayed union or nonunion is higher than is generally appreciated, but many nonunions are asymptomatic and do not require treatment. In adults, radiographic union

may not be apparent for 3 months following fracture.

Acromioclavicular Joint

The acromioclavicular (AC) joint is stabilized against anteroposterior displacement by the AC ligaments. The primary stabilizers of the AC joint, however, are the coracoclavicular (CC) ligaments. These stout ligaments (conoid and trapezoid), which suspend the upper limb from the clavicular "boom," extend from the coracoid process of the scapula to the undersurface of the distal clavicle. Only by rupture of the CC ligaments, with loss of their tethering effect on the clavicle, can a complete separation (dislocation) occur.

Acromioclavicular separations follow a fall or a blow on the point of the shoulder. The acromion and clavicle are driven downward until the clavicle encounters the resistance of the first rib, at which time part or all of first the AC and then the CC ligaments are torn. In some individuals, the ligamentous structures are so strong that the joint remains intact and a fracture of the distal clavicle occurs. These fractures are treated as AC dislocations.

Injuries of the AC joint are graded according to the degree of ligamentous injury (Fig. 13.18). A grade I AC injury is an incomplete tear of the AC ligaments without displacement of the joint. Pain and tenderness are present at the AC joint but there is no clinical deformity, and radiographs are normal. A grade II injury disrupts the entire AC ligamentous complex and often part of the CC ligaments, allowing partial separation (subluxation) of the joint. A grade III separation, or dislocation, results from complete disruption of the AC and CC ligaments. Obvious clinical deformity is present, and radiographs show no contact be-

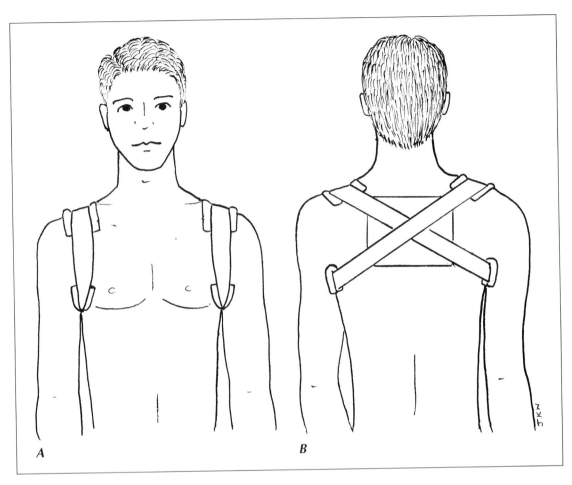

Figure 13.17 Figure-of-eight clavicular strap.

tween the articular surfaces of the clavicle and acromion.

It is possible to have a complete tear of the supporting ligamentous structures with normal radiographic findings if the arm is supported at the time of the examination; for this reason, radiographs should be taken (of both shoulders) with the patient standing, with and without weights suspended from the wrists.

Closed reduction of an incomplete separation is easy, but maintenance of the reduction is nearly impossible. Commercial devices, such as the Kenny-Howard splint, are uncomfortable and often do not maintain reduction any better than a sling.

Treatment of grade I and II injuries requires only support of the arm by a sling for comfort. Shoulder motion and a return to normal activities are allowed as symptoms subside. The distal clavicle may remain slightly prominent following this injury, and a small percentage of patients develop posttraumatic arthritis re-

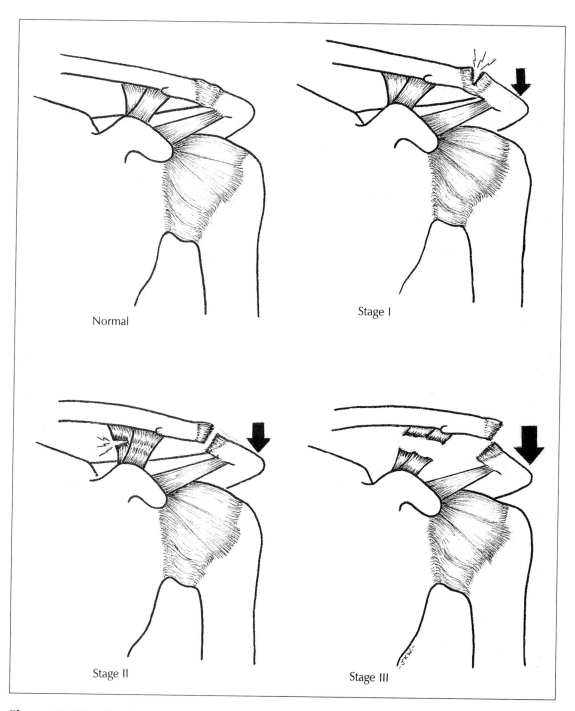

Figure 13.18   Classification of acromioclavicular separations.

quiring excision of the outer clavicle. In most cases, however, full, painless function may be anticipated within 4 to 6 weeks.

Treatment for grade III AC separations is controversial. Most orthopaedists recommend support in a sling for several weeks, acceptance of slight deformity, and early return to normal activities; others advocate open reduction and internal fixation.

Scapula

FRACTURES   Fractures of the scapula usually result from a direct blow or fall and are frequently associated with other injuries, such as clavicular and/or rib fractures, pneumothorax, or injury to the brachial plexus or subclavian artery. Fractures that do not involve the articular surface of the glenoid require little treatment beyond a sling. Displaced fractures of the surface of the glenoid, acromion, coracoid process, or glenoid neck and scapular fractures with associated fractures of the clavicle or disruptions of the AC joint should be considered for operative treatment.

Shoulder

INJURIES OF MUSCLE AND TENDON   *Acute rupture of the rotator cuff* is rare if the cuff is healthy. It is usually preceded by wear and thinning of the cuff from repeated compression between the humerus and acromion (see Chap.14). Physical findings include weakness and limitation of active abduction and external rotation proportional to the size of the tear. Passive motion is unrestricted. Tenderness is present at the insertion of the supraspinatus into the greater tuberosity, which is the usual site of rupture. The diagnosis may be confirmed by arthrogram, ultrasound, or MRI.

Rupture of the rotator cuff requires expert surgical management.

Rupture of the biceps tendon usually occurs in older patients with preexisting attritional changes in the tendon (see Chap. 14). The tendon of the long head of the biceps serves as a checkrein to cephalad excursion of the humeral head and has an active role in depressing the head of the humerus. In younger patients, a sudden overload can produce an acute rupture. Pain may be minimal, but "balling up" of the biceps with active flexion of the elbow is diagnostic. In less apparent cases, the *Speed test* elicits pain when the patient raises the extended, supinated forearm against resistance (Fig. 5.6).

In the young, active patient, early operative repair is preferred. For older, less physically active patients, a wait-and-see attitude is appropriate. Rest, anti-inflammatory medications, moist heat, and shoulder exercises are the cornerstones of nonoperative treatment. Although the contour of the arm improves little with time, pain subsides, and a return to normal activities is usually possible in 6 to 8 weeks.

FRACTURES   Fractures of the proximal humerus predilect older, osteopenic individuals and usually follow a fall onto the outstretched hand. The fractures are typically comminuted, with minimal displacement or loss of alignment (Fig. 13.19). Swelling and ecchymosis over the shoulder are characteristic. Radiographic examination should include AP, lateral scapular, and axillary views. The lateral radiograph is particularly important in order to exclude an associated dislocation of the glenohumeral joint.

Reduction of minimally displaced or im-

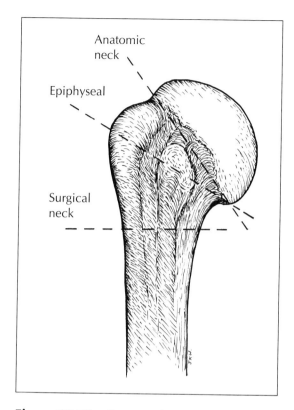

Figure 13.19   Common locations of proximal humeral fractures.

pacted fractures is unnecessary and unwise. Treatment consists of immobilization with a sling and swathe. Passive circumduction exercises in the sling may begin as soon as symptoms permit. The exercises are advanced and immobilization discontinued at approximately 4 weeks. Disability from this injury usually results not from the fracture itself, which heals readily, but from secondary stiffness in the shoulder.

If separation of the fragments exceeds 1 cm or angulation is greater than 45°, surgery is indicated. Fractures involving the articular surface of the humeral head or associated with dislocation of the glenohumeral joint and fractures of the greater tuberosity that are displaced more than 5 mm should also be strongly considered for operative treatment.

DISLOCATIONS   The lack of inherent bony stability and the wide range of motion permitted by loose ligaments and a redundant capsule account for the fact that dislocations of the glenohumeral joint represent almost 50 percent of all major joint dislocations. Over 95 percent of these dislocations are anterior; most of the remainder are posterior. Recurrence following anterior dislocation of the shoulder has been reported in 90 to 95 percent of those patients under the age of 20. With appropriate treatment, however, the recurrence rate can be reduced.

Anterior dislocations of the shoulder typically follow forcible external rotation and abduction of the arm, which levers the humeral head off the glenoid. As the humerus dislocates anteriorly, the labrum may be torn from its glenoidal attachment *(Bankart lesion),* the anterior lip of the glenoid may fracture, or a compression fracture may occur on the posterior aspect of the humeral head *(Hill-Sachs lesion).* Immediately following injury, the patient complains of severe shoulder pain and has difficulty internally rotating the arm and bringing it down to the thoracic wall. The humeral head may be palpable beneath the clavicle, and there may be an abnormal sulcus directly beneath the lateral acromion. The incidence of associated axillary nerve palsies is 5 to 14 percent, and associated fractures occur in approximately 40 percent of cases. A

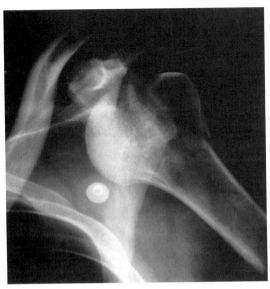

A

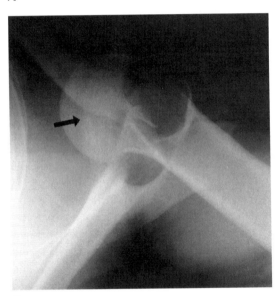

B

Figure 13.20 Anterior dislocation of the glenohumeral joint. *A.* Anteroposterior (AP) view. Note the associated fracture of the greater tuberosity. *B.* Axillary view. Note that the coracoid *(arrow)* points anteriorly.

displaced fracture of the greater tuberosity indicates a tear of the rotator cuff.

Anteroposterior and axillary or lateral scapular radiographs demonstrate the direction of the dislocation as well as the presence of associated bony injury (Fig. 13.20). Reduction of an acute anterior dislocation of the glenohumeral joint requires two basic elements: relief of muscle spasm and traction in the long axis of the arm. Following intravenous medication for sedation and muscle relaxation, steadily increasing longitudinal traction with gentle internal and external rotation of the arm will generally result in relocation. This modified Hippocratic maneuver may be accomplished by placing the unclad foot in the padded axilla of the supine patient and pulling the arm distally, using the pressure of the foot as countertraction and the breadth of the foot as a small lever to lift the shoulder into place (Fig. 13.21). If reduction cannot be obtained with reasonable ease, the patient should be taken to the operating room for reduction under general anesthesia.

Following reduction, the shoulder should be immobilized in a sling and swathe for 3 weeks, at which time gentle range-of-motion and strengthening exercises are begun.

Posterior dislocations of the shoulder result from a force directed posteriorly against the internally rotated arm, usually from a seizure or an electrical shock. The arm of a patient with a posterior dislocation lies in adduction and internal rotation; external rotation beyond neutral is impossible. The diagnosis is frequently missed on routine radiographs of the shoulder because the humeral head may not appear displaced. Often, however, a characteristic *light-bulb sign* is present (Fig. 13.22). A lateral scapular or axillary view discloses the

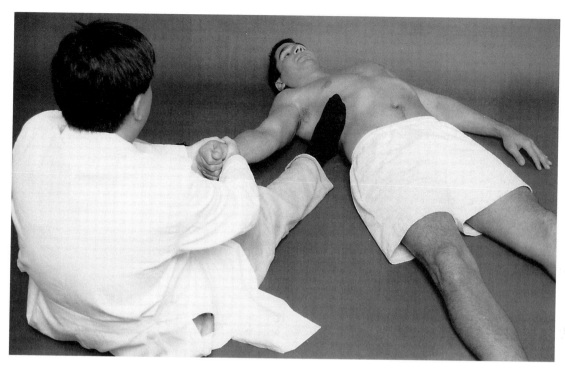

Figure 13.21   Reduction maneuver for anterior dislocation of the shoulder (Hippocratic).

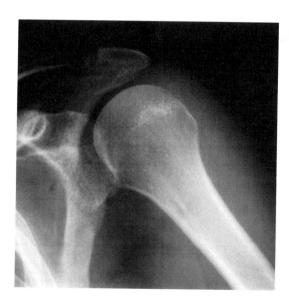

Figure 13.22   Posterior glenohumeral dislocation. Note the "light bulb" appearance (shape) of the internally rotated proximal humerus.

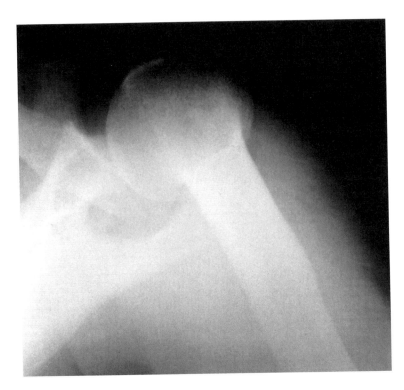

Figure 13.23   Posterior glenohumeral dislocation. The displacement is more apparent on the axillary view.

posterior displacement (Fig. 13.23). The principles underlying reduction of a posterior dislocation are similar to those for anterior dislocation. After adequate sedation and muscular relaxation, longitudinal traction combined with gentle external rotation of the humerus and anteriorly directed pressure on the humeral head will generally result in reduction. Immobilization in a sling for 4 to 6 weeks is recommended, followed by range-of-motion exercises and return to normal activities. Recurrence is relatively uncommon.

Because posterior dislocation is easily missed, the diagnosis is often delayed. If the dislocation is more than 2 weeks old, open reduction is usually required.

Arm

Injuries of muscle and tendon. Acute rupture of the biceps tendon at its insertion onto the radius occurs infrequently. If patients are significantly troubled by pain, weakness, or deformity, the tendon may be reattached surgically.

FRACTURES   *Fracture of the shaft of the humerus* is a common injury that follows twisting of the arm, a fall on the elbow, or a direct blow to the humeral shaft. The diagnosis is usually self-evident but should be confirmed by radiographs. Although the fracture may occur at any location in the diaphysis, the middle third is most commonly involved.

Physical examination includes careful evaluation of the limb's neurocirculatory status. Injury of the radial nerve is common, since the radial nerve is closely applied to the humerus at the junction of the middle and distal thirds. Injury of the nerve may occur at the time of fracture, during manipulation, or during fracture healing. Injury occurring at the time of fracture is usually a neuropraxia that recovers spontaneously. If loss of radial nerve function follows manipulation or immobilization of the arm, exploration of the nerve and fixation of the humeral fracture are indicated.

Fractures of the humeral shaft may be treated initially with a collar and cuff, plaster coaptation splints, or a Velpeau dressing. It is important for the elbow to hang free so that the weight of the limb may help maintain the reduction. When pain and swelling have lessened, functional bracing may be used to maintain alignment of the fracture fragments and allow motion of the elbow and shoulder. The brace is continued until solid union is obtained, which usually requires 8 to 12 weeks. Inability to attain or maintain alignment of a humeral fracture in less than 20° of varus is an indication for operative treatment.

Supracondylar fracture of the humerus, which occurs most often in children and the elderly, is produced by a fall onto the elbow or outstretched hand. In the young adult, this injury typically results from high-energy trauma, is comminuted intraarticularly, and usually requires operative reduction and stabilization.

In children, open epiphyseal plates may simulate fractures, so radiographs of the contralateral elbow for comparison are advisable. Since associated vascular and neurologic injuries are frequent, complete examination of the injured limb is essential. Immediate reduction is critical if vascular compromise is present. If distal pulses are not restored by this maneuver, surgical exploration of the vessels is necessary. Superior long-term results are best assured by pinning the fracture.

Elbow

FRACTURES   *Fractures of the olecranon* usually result from a fall onto the point of the flexed elbow. In nondisplaced fractures, the intact elbow extensor mechanism (triceps aponeurosis) makes subsequent displacement unlikely. These fractures may be treated by immobilization in a splint or cast, usually with the elbow in about 45° of flexion. Radiographs should be taken frequently during the first 2 weeks of treatment to confirm maintenance of the reduction. Displaced fractures require operative treatment to restore articular surfaces and function of the extensor mechanism.

Fractures of the radial head and neck commonly follow falls onto the outstretched hand with the elbow extended. Examination reveals tenderness over the radial head, localized swelling, and pain with rotation or flexion of the forearm. Radiographic examination should include AP and lateral views of the elbow (with comparison views of the contralateral elbow in children). Nondisplaced or minimally displaced fractures are treated in a posterior splint with the elbow flexed 90°. The splint is removed in a week and motion encouraged, with gradual return to normal activities as symptoms subside. Displaced (over 2 mm) or comminuted fractures in adults are usually treated by internal fixation or excision of the radial head.

In children, the same mechanism produces fractures of the radial neck rather than of the radial head. With less than 30° of angulation, these may be treated as nondisplaced fractures. With over 30° of angulation, reduction is indicated—closed if possible, open if not. The radial head should never be excised in a growing child.

In adults, fracture of the radial head is sometimes accompanied by disruption of the interosseous membrane and the distal radioulnar joint, the *Essex-Lopresti lesion.* For this reason, adults with radial head fractures should have clinical and radiographic examinations of the entire forearm. Patients with Essex-Lopresti injuries should be considered for operative treatment.

DISLOCATIONS   *Dislocations of the elbow* are usually posterior and result from a fall on the outstretched hand with the elbow extended. There is obvious deformity, but radiographs are needed to confirm the direction of the dislocation and to disclose any associated bony injuries. Fractures of the radial head and/or medial epicondyle of the humerus are often associated with dislocations of the elbow.

Reduction is accomplished by steady traction on the wrist with countertraction on the arm. Gentle extension of the elbow may first be necessary to unlock the coronoid process from behind the humerus. After reduction, the elbow is gently flexed and extended to assess stability. If the elbow is stable and there are no fractures on postreduction radiographs, the elbow should be mobilized as acute discomfort subsides. If subluxation recurs with extension, the elbow is maintained in flexion with a sling or collar and cuff for several weeks to allow ligamentous and capsular healing. Gentle exercises are then instituted. Immobilization of the elbow for more than 3 weeks often leads to significant stiffness.

Dislocation of the radial head is rare and commonly accompanies fracture of the proximal third of the ulna *(Monteggia fracture dislocation).* Closed reduction and immobilization in an above-elbow cast will usually suffice in children, but operative treatment is required in adults.

Pulled elbow or *"nursemaid's elbow"* describes a disorder in children under the age of 5 in which the head of the radius subluxates from beneath the annular ligament when the child is lifted by the wrist or hand. The child holds the forearm in slight flexion and pronation, and tenderness is present over the radial head. Radiographs are normal.

Reduction is accomplished by supination of the forearm and flexion of the elbow while continuous pressure is applied over the posterior aspect of the radial head. A palpable click often accompanies reduction. If the reduction is not this satisfying, immobilization of the arm in a posterior splint with the elbow flexed to 90° is usually followed by spontaneous reduction within a week. Continued pain or restricted motion after 1 week of immobilization should prompt further investigation.

Forearm

FRACTURES   *Fractures of the shafts of the radius and ulna in adults* usually result from high-energy trauma. Anatomic reduction is essential for full function of the forearm. Accurate reduction by closed means is difficult, and late displacement or angulation of the fracture is common. Thus, displaced fractures of one or both bones of the forearm in adults are generally treated by open reduction and internal fixation. Nondisplaced fractures may be treated in an above-elbow cast, but frequent radiographic follow-up is needed to ensure that late displacement has not occurred.

Fractures of the forearm in children differ from those in adults in that surgery is rarely necessary. Closed reduction is achieved by traction and manipulation of the distal fragments to align them with the uncontrollable proximal fragments; supination is also required when the radial fracture is proximal and pronation when it is distal. An above-elbow cast is applied and molded anteroposteriorly to "ovalize" the cast (Fig. 13.24). Slight overlapping of the bone ends is acceptable in young children if the alignment is satisfactory. The cast is continued for 8 to 12 weeks. Children should have weekly radiographs for the first 3 weeks, since displacement may occur as swelling subsides.

Greenstick fractures (Fig. 13.6*D*) are prone to late recurrence of angulation unless the fracture is overreduced, which entails intentional fracturing of the opposite cortex during reduction. An isolated fracture of the radius or ulna with plastic deformity of the other bone occurs occasionally in children and also has a propensity for recurrent deformity unless the plastically deformed bone is broken during the reduction maneuver.

Galeazzi fracture-dislocation is a fracture of the lower third of the radius associated with an injury to the distal radioulnar joint; it occurs almost exclusively in adults. The disruption of the distal radioulnar joint may not be seen on radiographs, but careful examination elicits tenderness, deformity, and painful motion at the joint. The injury is considered a "fracture of necessity," since open reduction and internal fixation of the radial fracture, with or without fixation of the radioulnar joint, are usually necessary. Failure to recognize injury to the distal radioulnar joint usually results in inadequate treatment.

Monteggia fracture dislocation is a fracture of the shaft of the ulna, with dislocation (usually anteriorly) of the radial head (Fig. 13.25). Since the results of closed treatment for this injury in adults are generally poor, operative treatment is recommended. In children, nonoperative treatment often suffices (see above).

Wrist

FRACTURES   *Fractures of the distal radius* are among the most common fractures encountered in practice. The *Colles fracture,* described by Abraham Colles in 1814, is a dorsally displaced fracture of the distal radius without involvement of the radiocarpal joint; however, the term *Colles fracture* is now applied to many fractures of the distal radius, a usage that, as shown in Table 13.1, is often incorrect.

Dorsally displaced fractures of the distal radius produce a *"dinner fork" deformity,* but local tenderness and pain with attempted movement may be the only signs of a nondisplaced fracture (Fig. 13.26). Function in the median nerve should be documented prior to treatment. Evaluation of the fracture is completed by AP and lateral radiographs of the wrist.

Intraarticular or volarly comminuted fractures of the distal radius often require surgical treatment, especially in young adults. Closed reduction of extraarticular fractures can usually be performed in the outpatient setting under hematoma block and/or intravenous sedation. Longitudinal traction is applied in the long axis of the forearm; as the fracture disimpacts and forearm musculature relaxes, the deformity is increased and pressure is applied to the dorsal aspect of the distal fragment with the operator's thumb (Fig. 13.10). The wrist and distal fragment are then flexed to hold the reduction. If reduction has been obtained, the

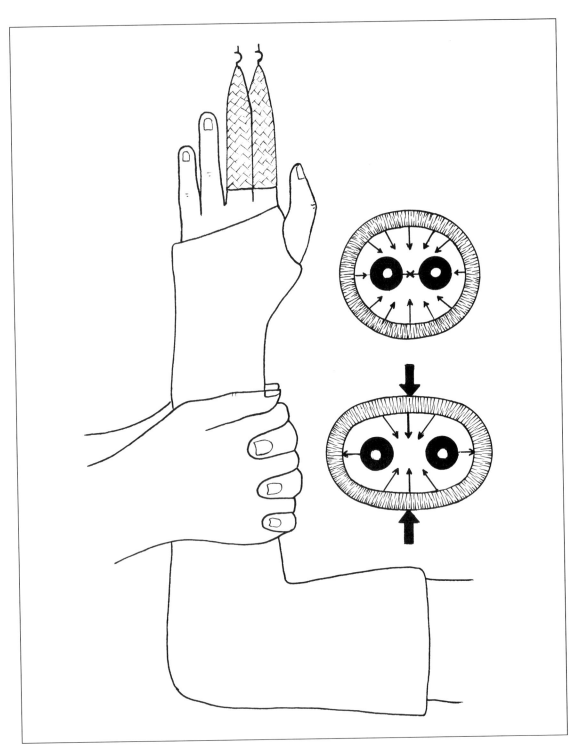

Figure 13.24 Volar and dorsal pressure results in ovalization of the cast, which increases the width of the interosseous space. (Redrawn with permission from Weber BG, Brunner C, Feuler F: *Treatment of Fractures in Children and Adolescents.* New York, Springer-Verlag, 1980.)

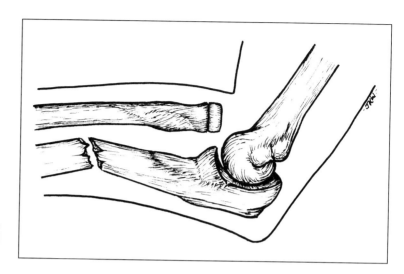

Figure 13.25 The Monteggia lesion. Note the fracture of the proximal ulna with dislocation of the radial head.

wrist will have been restored to its normal contour. The wrist should be splinted in flexion, ulnar deviation, and full pronation and radiographs obtained to document adequate align-

Table 13.1 Common Eponyms for Fractures of the Distal Radius

Eponym	Description
Colles fracture	Extraarticular fracture with dorsal displacement, dorsal angulation, and dorsal comminution
Smith fracture	Extraarticular fracture with volar displacement, volar angulation, and volar comminution
Barton fracture	Intraarticular fracture of the volar or dorsal lip, with displacement of the carpus with the articular fragment
Chauffeur fracture	Intraarticular, oblique fracture involving a triangular piece of bone that includes the radial styloid

ment. Inclusion of the elbow in the splint or cast helps maintain reduction (Fig. 13.27). Careful neurologic examination after reduction ensures that no compromise has occurred. The patient is converted to a below-elbow cast after 3 weeks, but immobilization of the wrist is continued for 6 weeks. Immediate active motion of the fingers and shoulder avoids stiffness in these joints.

The same force that causes a fracture of the distal radius in an adult typically produces a Salter II fracture of the distal radial epiphysis in a child, with the epiphysis displaced dorsally and radially. Gentle manipulative reduction is followed by casting for approximately 4 weeks.

Fractures of the scaphoid are associated with subtle radiographic findings and a high rate of complications. For these reasons, the probability of this injury should be entertained in patients with a painful wrist following a fall on the outstretched hand. The scaphoid serves as the link between the proximal and distal rows of the carpus, which accounts for the fact that it is the most frequently fractured carpal bone. Pain and tenderness are centered over the anatomic "snuff box." Multiple oblique radiographs may be required to demonstrate the fracture and should be taken before the injury is written off as "only a sprain."

Fractures of the scaphoid are prone to delayed union and/or nonunion because they are intraarticular (the fracture hematoma is washed out by synovial fluid) and difficult to immobilize. Since the blood supply to the proximal pole enters the bone distally and is usually disrupted by the fracture, avascular necrosis of the proximal fragment is a frequent complication.

Because of the infrequent occurrence of sprained wrists, pain following a fall on the outstretched hand should be treated as an undisplaced injury to the epiphyseal plate in a child and as a fracture of the scaphoid in an adult until proven otherwise. Adults with suspected fractures of the scaphoid should be immobilized in a cast that includes the MCP joint

of the thumb for 2 weeks, by which time resorption at the fracture site will usually render the fracture visible on radiographs. A minimum of 12 weeks' immobilization is usually required for healing.

DISLOCATIONS   A hard fall on the dorsiflexed wrist may displace the carpus dorsally, producing a *perilunate dislocation,* in which only the lunate remains in contact with the radius (Fig. 13.28). As the carpus snaps forward again, it may lever the lunate volarly out of position, producing a *dislocation of the lunate* (Fig. 13.29). These are severe injuries, readily evident on lateral radiographs of the wrist; they often require operative management. The interplay of bone and ligamentous damage in these injuries is complex and not within the scope of this text. It is important, however, for the physician to recognize these injuries early and to understand that ligamentous damage

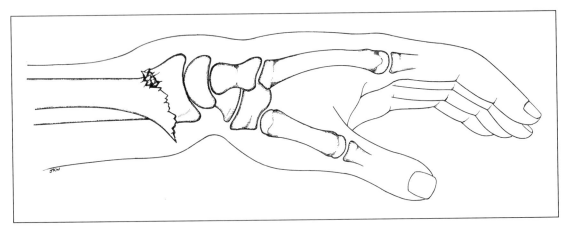

Figure 13.26   The characteristic "dinner fork" deformity seen with a Colles fracture of the distal radius and caused by dorsal and proximal displacement of the distal fragment.

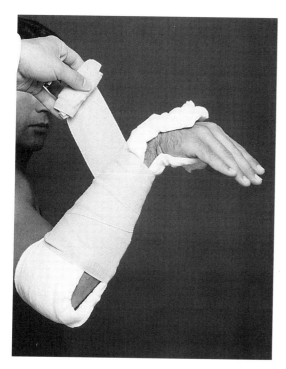

Figure 13.27   Sugar-tong splint for a distal radial fracture. Note the volar flexion and ulnar deviation. The metacarpophalangeal joints are left free to move.

may lead to carpal instability followed by degenerative changes and chronic wrist pain. The most common patterns are scapholunate dissociation, lunatotriquetral dissociation, and injury to the triangular fibrocartilage between the radius and ulna.

Hand

FRACTURES   *Fractures of the base of the thumb metacarpal* are classified as *Bennett* or *Rolando fractures* (Fig. 13.30A and B). The base of the first metacarpal is maintained in its position with respect to the trapezium by means of a constraining ligament. These frac-tures detach this ligament from the shaft, producing an unstable trapeziometacarpal joint that generally requires reduction and stabilization to reestablish congruence and stability of the joint.

Displaced fractures of the metacarpal shaft often require internal fixation to maintain reduction. Nondisplaced fractures may be immobilized in a splint and motion of the digit may be begun at 2 to 3 weeks. Union of the fracture is usually apparent at 5 to 6 weeks.

Boxer's fractures are fractures of the distal metaphysis of the fifth metacarpal that result from striking an object with a closed fist. When associated with lacerations of the overlying skin, they should be treated as open fractures. Up to 35° of dorsal angulation may be accepted with the expectation of excellent hand function. These fractures should be immobilized in an ulnar gutter splint extending from the forearm to the distal phalanx, with the wrist positioned in slight extension, the MCP joints of the ring and small fingers in approximately 90° flexion, and the PIP joints in full extension. Immobilization can usually be discontinued after 2 to 3 weeks and motion begun. Union may be expected in 5 to 6 weeks. Fractures with unacceptable angulation can be manipulated under local anesthesia and casted, but, if the reduction is unstable, pinning of the fracture fragments is advisable.

Fractures of the proximal phalanx, if displaced, are difficult to reduce. Nondisplaced fractures may be treated by splinting or buddy-taping the injured finger to an adjacent digit. Displaced fractures, fractures involving the joint surface, long oblique fractures, and comminuted fractures often require operative stabilization.

Fractures of the middle phalanx are usually nondisplaced. If volar angulation is present, re-

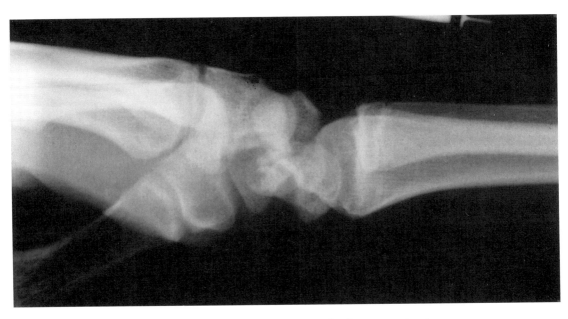

Figure 13.28   Dorsal perilunate dislocation. Note that the lunate retains its normal relationship to the distal radius.

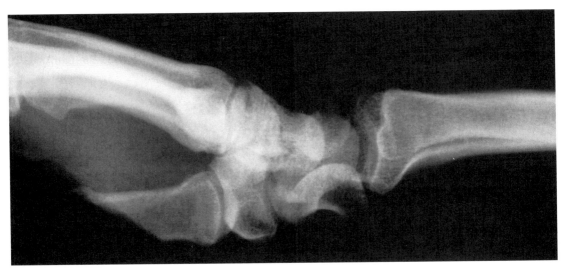

Figure 13.29   Volar dislocation of the lunate. Note that while the lunate is displaced volarly, the remainder of the carpus retains its normal relationship to the distal radius.

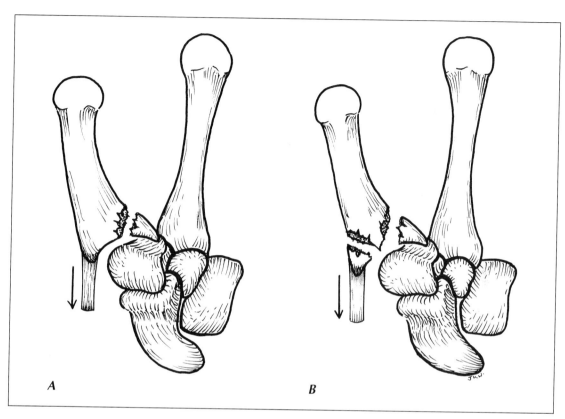

Figure 13.30 Intraarticular fractures of the base of the thumb metacarpal.
A. Bennett. *B.* Rolando. The abductor pollicis longus tendon exerts a
deforming force *(arrow).*

duction under digital block anesthesia may be
accomplished by gentle flexion. Immobilization in a dorsal aluminum splint is usually adequate. The splint may be removed after 2
weeks and gentle motion begun, with the finger buddy-taped to an adjacent digit.

Fractures of the distal phalanx are usually
the result of a crushing injury that produces
marked comminution. They almost always involve the nail bed, which lies directly on the
bone. Subungual hematomas should be evac-

uated; if the nail is disrupted or completely
loose, it should be removed, leaving a portion
of the nail or a splint beneath the nail fold to
ensure its patency. If the nail bed has been split
or lacerated, it should be repaired. Comminuted fractures of the distal phalanx do not require reduction; simple protective splinting of
the DIP joint affords adequate immobilization.

DISLOCATIONS *Dislocation of the metacarpophalangeal joint* is particularly common in

the thumb, where, if the ulnar collateral ligament has been torn, operative repair is recommended. Dorsal dislocations of the metacarpophalangeal joints are reduced by pushing the dorsally displaced proximal phalanx over the metacarpal head rather than by traction on the digit.

Dislocation of the proximal interphalangeal joint is the most common dislocation in the hand and may occur with minimal disruption of supporting structures. Reduction is accomplished by gentle traction and volarly directed pressure over the base of the middle phalanx. Immobilization is provided with a splint or, more frequently, by buddy-taping the finger to an adjacent digit. Volar dislocations and fracture dislocations often require surgical treatment.

Dislocation of the distal interphalangeal joint is rare, usually the result of violent trauma, and quite easily reduced. Splinting the joint in moderate flexion maintains the reduction.

OTHER INJURIES OF JOINTS   *Volar plate injuries,* sometimes called "jammed fingers," result from hyperextension and most often involve the proximal interphalangeal joint. Tearing of the fibrocartilaginous volar plate, which is the thickened volar portion of the joint capsule, causes pain and swelling. Radiographically, an avulsed speck of bone is sometimes visible at the base of the middle phalanx. Treatment by buddy-taping allows early, protected motion, which is important to prevent late stiffness.

Gamekeeper's thumb is an injury to the ulnar collateral ligament of the MCP joint of the thumb. Forced abduction of the thumb by a ski pole or similar object is the usual mechanism. Stable injuries can be treated with a thumb spica splint, but unstable injuries require surgical intervention.

TENDON INJURIES   *Extensor tendon injuries* are frequently caused by lacerations but can also result from avulsions. A *mallet finger* (inability to extend the DIP joint) is caused by avulsion of the insertion of the extensor tendon at the distal phalanx. A fragment of bone is often detached with the tendon. Acute injuries can be treated by splinting in extension unless the bone fragment involves over one-third of the articular surface, in which case surgery is indicated. Avulsions also occur at the insertion of the central slip into the middle phalanx, resulting in tenderness on the dorsum of the joint, with weakness of extension. Acute ruptures can be treated by splinting, but unrecognized injuries eventually result in a boutonnière deformity and require surgical reconstruction. When injuries to extensor tendons occur proximal to the MCP joint, it is important to test for the ability to extend this joint, since intrinsic muscles of the hand can extend the PIP and DIP joints but not the MCP joint. Lacerations of extensor tendons require prompt surgical repair.

Injuries of flexor tendons are usually the result of lacerations. A careful physical examination is essential to define the extent of injury. The function of both the superficialis and profundus tendons must be assessed (see Chap. 5). In addition, the digital nerves should be tested when the laceration is in the hand or fingers, since the digital nerves and arteries are closely applied to the flexor tendon sheath. Flexor tendon lacerations require early, metic-

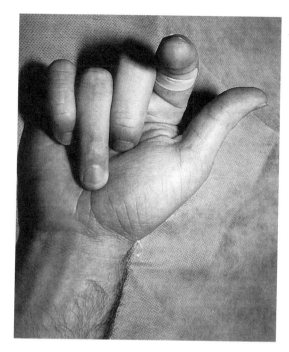

Figure 13.31 "Jersey finger" (flexor digitorum profundus avulsion of the ring finger). Note the inability to flex the DIP joint when the patient attempts to make a fist.

ulous surgical repair. Rehabilitation must be closely supervised to avoid rerupture as well as adhesions in the tendon sheath, which cause limited, painful movement. Failure to recognize acute injuries makes operative reconstruction difficult if not impossible.

Avulsion of the flexor digitorum profundus from the distal phalanx is a common injury and usually involves the ring finger. The rupture, evidenced by inability to flex the DIP joint, is also known as a *"jersey finger,"* since it often occurs when the flexed finger is caught and pulled forcefully by the jersey of a football player being tackled (Fig. 13.31). Treatment is

operative, and rehabilitation is similar to that for other flexor tendon repairs.

Lower Limb

Pelvis

FRACTURES *Fractures of the pelvis* are usually the result of high-velocity trauma. They are notorious for causing massive internal bleeding and disruption of urologic structures and frequently require surgical stabilization.

Fractures of the pubic rami may follow relatively minor injuries in osteoporotic patients (Fig. 13.32). In spite of minimal displacement, these fractures cause significant pain, especially in the groin. They may be difficult to distinguish clinically from impacted or nondisplaced femoral neck fractures, but radiographs of the pelvis and hip usually clarify the diagnosis. If any question remains, a bone scan will show increased uptake, usually within 48 h, in the area of the fracture. Treatment of these fractures is largely symptomatic, with analgesics and weight-bearing as tolerated. Healing may be expected in 6 to 8 weeks.

Stress fractures of the pelvis are most often overuse injuries. They commonly affect the pubic rami and predilect amenorrheic female athletes with associated osteoporosis. Pain is usually in the symphyseal area and responds to rest and analgesics.

INJURIES TO THE PELVIC JOINTS As with fractures of the pelvic ring, injuries of the sacroiliac and symphyseal joints are relatively uncommon. Dislocations of these joints result from high-energy trauma and are usually associated with other breaks in the pelvic ring

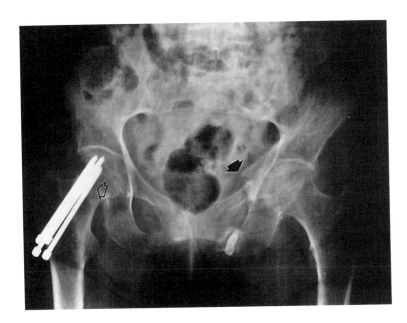

Figure 13.32   Pubic rami fractures *(closed arrow)*, with internal fixation for a previous femoral neck fracture *(open arrow).*

that require operative reduction and stabilization.

Hip

FRACTURES OF THE HIP   *Fractures of the hip* represent a major health problem in our society. Elderly patients affected by osteoporosis often sustain hip fractures from minor falls, which are common in this age group because of visual disturbances, syncope, thromboembolic events, unsteadiness, and the use of medications.

Most commonly, fractures of the hip occur in the femoral neck, which is particularly susceptible to twisting injury, or the intertrochanteric area, which is more commonly fractured by a direct fall onto the greater trochanter (Fig. 13.33*A* and *B*).

Patients with displaced fractures are unable to bear weight on the affected limb. Pain is usually localized to the groin, with occasional referral to the knee. The limb is shortened, externally rotated, and cannot be raised off the bed. Patients with nondisplaced or impacted fractures may be able to lift and bear partial weight on the involved limb.

Treatment of a fracture of the hip depends largely on its location and displacement and on the general health of the patient. Although impacted fractures of the femoral neck can be treated with bed rest and limited weight-bearing, pinning is preferred to avoid the 20 percent risk of displacement with nonoperative treatment (Fig. 13.32). Even with operative stabilization, displaced fractures of the femoral neck are complicated by nonunion and/or avascular necrosis of the femoral head in 40 to 50 percent of cases. Because of these risks, displaced fractures are often treated by prosthetic replacement of the femoral head. Internal fixation or prosthetic replacement allows early mobilization, which minimizes compli-

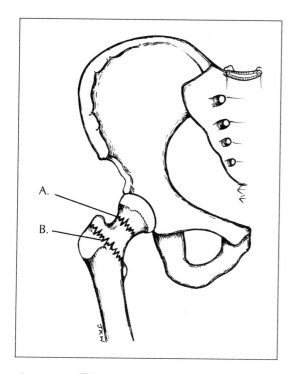

Figure 13.33 Levels of *(A)* femoral neck and *(B)* intertrochanteric fractures of the hip.

cations resulting from stasis of body fluids, such as thromboembolism and infections of the lungs and urinary tract.

DISLOCATIONS OF THE HIP JOINT Due to the protective effect of strong ligaments and muscles around the hip and the ball-and-socket configuration of the joint itself, dislocation of the hip requires high-energy trauma, such as a motor vehicle accident, for its production. Posterior dislocations are most common and result in a limb that is flexed, internally rotated, and adducted. Associated stretching or tearing of the capsule may impair the blood supply to the femoral head, causing avascular necrosis, a complication that can be minimized by prompt reduction.

OVERUSE INJURIES ABOUT THE HIP *Incomplete* or *stress fractures of the femoral neck* may result from repetitive impact exercises, such as running. Pain in the groin and an antalgic limp are the predominant clinical findings. It is imperative that the diagnosis be made by radiographs or bone scan, since completion and displacement of the fracture may result in avascular necrosis and subsequent osteoarthritis. Healing usually follows protected weight-bearing, but many surgeons recommend prophylactic internal fixation.

Trochanteric bursitis is caused by excessive friction of the iliotibial band over the trochanter (see Chap. 14). The greater trochanter is separated from the iliotibial band by bursal tissue. If the band is excessively tight, popping may occur as it snaps back and forth over the greater trochanter during flexion and extension of the hip. This *"snapping hip"* syndrome is usually relieved by exercises that stretch the iliotibial band.

Thigh and Femur

FRACTURES OF THE FEMORAL SHAFT These fractures typically follow vehicular trauma or falls from a height. Most are closed injuries, since the femur is circumferentially well protected by a thick layer of muscle. Because of the excellent blood supply to this area and the lack of limiting fascial compartments, these fractures are usually associated with significant blood loss into the soft tissues. For this reason, patients with confirmed or suspected fractures of the femoral shaft should be traction-splinted and transferred emergently to a trauma facility for further care. The standard of care in otherwise healthy patients is reduction and internal fixation to mini-

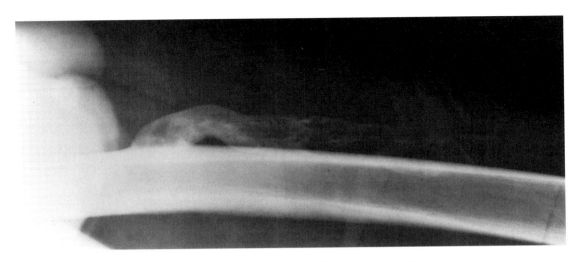

Figure 13.34 Myositis ossificans following a direct blow to the quadriceps muscle. A lateral view of the femur and thigh is shown.

mize the ill effects of prolonged immobilization.

INJURIES OF MUSCLE AND TENDON A large part of the thigh is made up of muscles and tendons. Injuries to these large musculotendinous units occur from direct impact or from a sudden stretch while the muscle is contracting. Direct impact injuries are most common in the quadriceps during participation in contact sports. A contusion of the quadriceps results in immediate pain and swelling from partial disruption of the muscle (strain) and hematoma formation. The acute pain, which lasts for several days, is aggravated by stretching the muscle, which occurs with knee flexion; therefore, patients tend to keep the knee in an extended position. Healing is primarily by scar formation rather than by regeneration of muscle fibers. As the scar contracts, it tends to shorten the muscle, so gentle quadriceps stretching exercises should begin as soon as

pain allows. Icing and nonsteroidal anti-inflammatory drugs (NSAIDs) for 24 to 48 h following injury reduce the pain and swelling. Prior to a return to full activities, more vigorous stretching and strengthening is needed to prevent reinjury. A common complication of a quadriceps contusion is *myositis ossificans,* in which bone forms in the injured soft tissues next to the bone. It appears on radiographs 3 to 4 weeks following injury (Fig. 13.34). Pain and restricted flexion of the knee are the primary clinical features. Treatment is largely symptomatic. Mild analgesics are used for discomfort, and continued gentle stretching is critical to regaining full motion. Vigorous passive stretching may cause additional injury and should be avoided. Usually, myositis ossificans is self-limiting, but the return to sports should be delayed until symptoms have subsided, which usually requires several months. Surgical excision is rarely needed and should never be performed during the acute, active phase of bone formation because of the high likelihood of recurrence.

Most *strains* occur when a muscle is suddenly stretched during an active contraction. They are especially common in the hamstring and adductor muscles. The tear generally occurs near the musculotendinous junction and causes immediate pain and diminished function of the involved muscle. Treatment includes rest, ice, compression, and elevation (RICE), with NSAIDs initially. As soon as pain subsides, gentle stretching is begun to minimize scar contracture within the muscle. Recovery often takes 4 to 6 weeks. A strengthening program should be instituted prior to return to full activities to prevent reinjury.

Knee

Fractures about the knee. These occur in the distal femur, the proximal tibia, or the patella.

Supracondylar and intercondylar fractures of the femur involve the distal femoral metaphysis and/or the medial and lateral femoral condyles. In young patients, they usually follow high-energy trauma, but in older, osteoporotic patients the trauma may be minimal. Most distal femoral fractures are displaced by the strong muscles that span the fracture, particularly the medial and lateral heads of the gastrocnemius. Although amenable to treatment in traction, most of these fractures benefit from open reduction and internal fixation, which minimizes immobilization, subsequent stiffness, and posttraumatic arthritis.

Fractures of the tibial plateau are common in older patients with osteoporotic bone and usually result from a valgus force against the knee. Treatment depends largely on the degree of displacement of the fracture fragments. Fractures displaced only 1 to 2 mm can be managed with a cast or brace. Displacement or

depression of 3 mm or more in the weight-bearing area requires operative reduction and fixation to minimize late deformity and osteoarthritis.

Patellar fractures disrupt continuity of the quadriceps extensor mechanism. The patella is surrounded by medial and lateral retinaculae, which act as strong checkreins. If a patellar fracture is nondisplaced, limited extensor power remains through the intact retinaculae. For a fracture to separate, the retinaculae must also be torn, which eliminates active extension of the knee (Fig. 13.35). Nondisplaced fractures can be treated by immobilization in full extension for 6 to 10 weeks. Displaced fractures require open reduction and internal fixation.

SOFT TISSUE INJURIES ABOUT THE KNEE Injuries to the soft tissues around the knee are common. Because of the flattened contour of its joint surfaces, the knee has little inherent stability and relies heavily on the spanning ligaments and muscles for this purpose. Four major ligaments are the prime stabilizers of the knee joint: the medial and lateral collateral ligaments, which are outside the joint and provide stability against valgus and varus forces; and the anterior and posterior cruciate ligaments, which are intraarticular and prevent excessive anterior and posterior translation of the tibia on the femur, although they also contribute to varus and valgus stability (Fig. 13.36).

Tears of the medial collateral ligament occur when an impact against the lateral aspect of the leg, as occurs in football or from the bumper of a moving car, produces enough valgus force to tear the medial collateral ligament anywhere between its origin on the femoral epicondyle and its insertion on the proximal tibia. The area of maximum tenderness mirrors

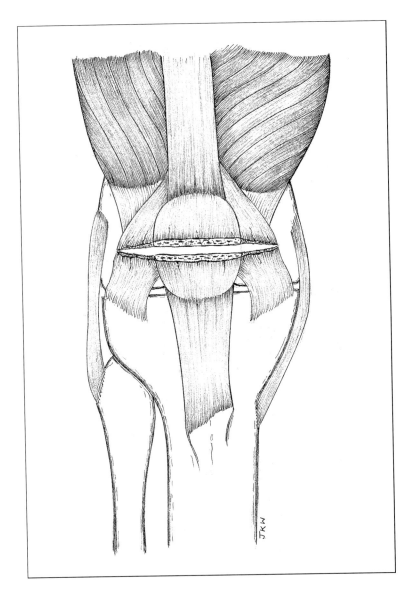

Figure 13.35 Displaced patellar fracture, with tears of the medial and lateral retinaculae.

the location of the tear. The degree of injury may be determined by testing the stability of the knee (see discussion under "Ligaments," above). Valgus stress testing should be done with the knee in slight flexion and compared to tests of the contralateral knee (Fig. 13.37).

Radiographs are recommended in adults to rule out an associated fracture of the tibial plateau, and stress radiographs are needed in children, since similar instability may result from a fracture through the growth plate rather than ligamentous injury.

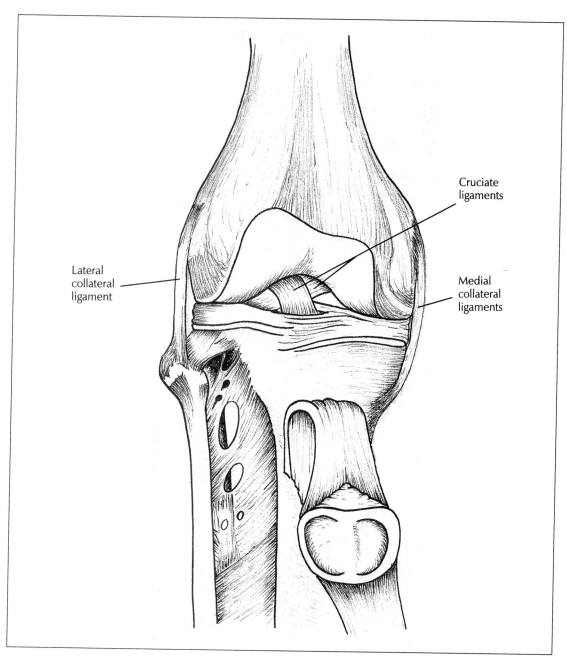

Cruciate
ligaments

Lateral
collateral
ligament

Medial
collateral
ligaments

Figure 13.36   Major ligaments in and around the knee. (Redrawn with
permission from Peterson L, Renström P: *Sports Injuries: Their Prevention
and Treatment.* Chicago, Year Book, 1983, p 285.)

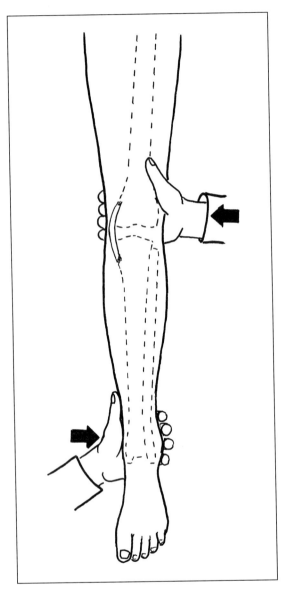

Figure 13.37 Application of valgus stress for integrity of the medial collateral ligament. The uninjured side is used for comparison.

Treatment of an isolated medial collateral ligament tear is generally nonoperative because of the excellent healing potential of this ligament. Grade I injuries can be treated by restriction of activities for 1 to 2 weeks and mild analgesics, with gradual return to full activities guided by pain. Grade II injuries may need as much as 4 weeks of restricted activity. For the first few days, crutches and a removable brace may be needed for control of pain. Full recovery can be expected in 4 to 8 weeks. Grade III tears can also be treated by early mobilization in a removable hinged brace if the cruciate ligaments are intact to serve as internal splints for the torn medial ligament.

Tears of the lateral collateral ligament, less common than those of the medial ligament, result from a varus force applied to the knee. The integrity of the lateral ligament can be determined by application of a varus force to the slightly flexed knee. Since the peroneal nerve is also susceptible to disruption by varus stress, its function should be carefully assessed. Treatment of isolated injuries of the lateral collateral ligament is similar to that for injuries of the medial collateral ligament.

Injuries of the anterior cruciate ligament, as opposed to tears of the collateral ligaments, have very limited healing potential. They are often associated with tears of the collateral ligaments and meniscal injuries. Unless the joint capsule is also torn, there is, within several hours, a tense hemarthrosis caused by bleeding from the torn ends of the ligament. The *Lachman test* is used to evaluate the anterior cruciate ligament (Fig. 13.38). The degree of instability and the presence or absence of a firm "endpoint," as described in the earlier section on ligaments, should be noted. The anterior cruciate ligament can also be assessed by the *pivot-shift test,* which is performed by apply-

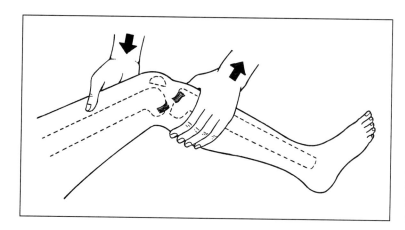

Figure 13.38 Lachman's test for integrity of the anterior cruciate ligament. If the ligament is torn, an anterior pull on the proximal tibia with the knee in 20° flexion displaces the tibia anteriorly.

ing valgus, internal rotation, and an axial load to the knee while bringing the knee from full extension into flexion. In the anterior cruciate–deficient knee, the tibia reduces (shifts) suddenly from its anteriorly subluxed position to its normal position at approximately 30° of flexion as a result of the pull of the iliotibial band (Fig. 13.39). The pivot shift test requires absolute relaxation of the hamstring muscles and may be difficult to perform in the acutely injured knee because of pain and swelling. Radiographs are usually obtained in patients with acute tears of the anterior cruciate ligament to rule out associated fractures, which can also cause an immediate hemarthrosis. Additional imaging studies, such as an MRI scan, are rarely needed if a careful examination is performed; however, an MRI scan may be useful if associated injuries, such as meniscal tears, are suspected. The early treatment of acute tears remains controversial. Since they have little or no healing potential, an unreconstructed tear leaves the knee with anteroposterior instability, which may cause giving way during vigorous activity and secondary damage to the menisci and articular cartilage. Many factors determine the degree to which

the anterior cruciate–deficient knee becomes symptomatic. Low-demand patients with only slight instability (3 to 5 mm excursion on a Lachman test) can probably be managed nonoperatively. After the initial swelling has subsided, a rehabilitation program is begun to strengthen the hamstring muscles, which compensate somewhat for the torn cruciate ligament. In an active patient with significant instability, neuromuscular compensation often fails to keep the tibia reduced during vigorous activity, leading to episodic giving way. Surgical reconstruction of the anterior cruciate ligament is usually accomplished by substituting a tendon autograft or allograft for the torn ligament.

Tears of the posterior cruciate ligament are much less common than those of the anterior cruciate ligament, and pain and swelling are usually less dramatic. Frequently, these injuries are unrecognized until the knee is examined later. Instability can be demonstrated by the *posterior drawer test* (Fig. 13.40). In many patients the instability does not cause giving way; however, the risk of late degenerative changes is increased, particularly in the patellofemoral and medial tibiofemoral joints.

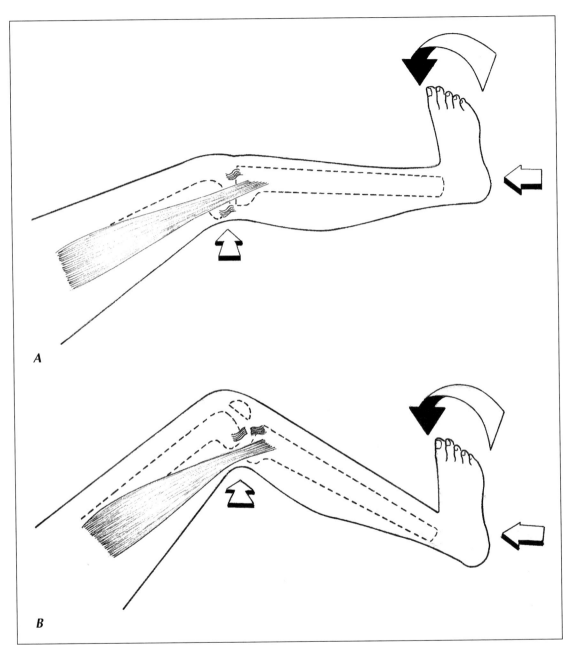

Figure 13.39   Pivot-shift test for integrity of the anterior cruciate ligament. Applying axial, internal rotation, and valgus forces in full extension subluxes the tibia anteriorly; as the knee is flexed, there is a sudden reduction of the tibia, which is felt as a "shift" if the ligament is torn.

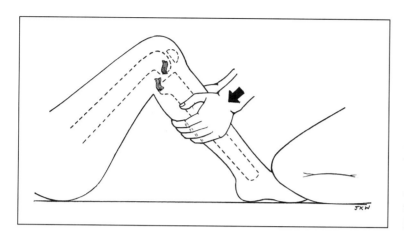

Figure 13.40 Posterior drawer test for integrity of the posterior cruciate ligament. A posteriorly directed force will displace the tibia posteriorly if the ligament is torn.

Treatment is usually nonsurgical, with emphasis on quadriceps strengthening to prevent posterior subluxation of the tibia.

MENISCAL INJURIES   Injuries to the knee joint often involve the menisci, which are load-dispersing structures that reduce contact stresses in the joint (Fig. 13.41). Twisting injuries sustained during axial compression may trap the meniscus between the femoral and tibial articular surfaces and produce a tear. In children, meniscal injuries are often associated with a *discoid meniscus,* in which the meniscus is a full disk, covering the condyle, instead of a C-shaped structure. Torn medial or lateral menisci cause pain and tenderness at a point along the joint line that corresponds to the location of the tear. Vertical tears involving the entire thickness of the meniscus often result in displacement of the inner "bucket-handle" fragment into the joint, which causes mechanical symptoms of catching, locking, and giving way. The instability of this meniscal fragment can be provoked by the *McMurray test,* in which the internally or externally rotated knee, when passively extended from a fully flexed position, produces a palpable, painful "pop" at the joint line (Fig. 13.42). Most meniscal tears,

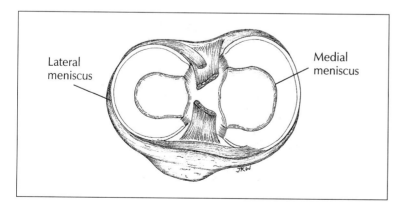

Lateral meniscus

Medial meniscus

Figure 13.41 Medial and lateral menisci in the knee joint.

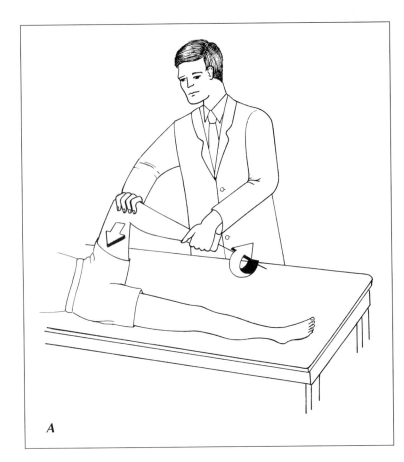

A

Figure 13.42 McMurray's test for a displaceable medial meniscal tear. Starting from full flexion, the knee is extended while the tibia is held in an externally rotated position. A painful pop is felt in the presence of a displaceable meniscal tear.

however, are small radial or horizontal tears, with only joint line tenderness. In patients without mechanical symptoms, an MRI scan may confirm the diagnosis. Such scans are noninvasive (as opposed to arthrography) and are highly sensitive and specific for meniscal tears.

Acute tears of the menisci may heal spontaneously if the tear is located at the vascularized periphery and the fragment is stable. Patients with suspected meniscal injuries without mechanical symptoms can therefore be treated by restricting activity for 4 to 6 weeks. If mechanical symptoms, such as locking or giving way, are present, arthroscopic treatment is generally advisable.

Degenerative meniscal tears occur in an older population than acute tears, presumably as a result of repetitive subacute trauma. Degenerative lesions are a common cause of chronic or recurrent pain, effusion, and mechanical symptoms, such as locking and catching. Arthroscopic debridement is not as effective for chronic as for acute tears since the

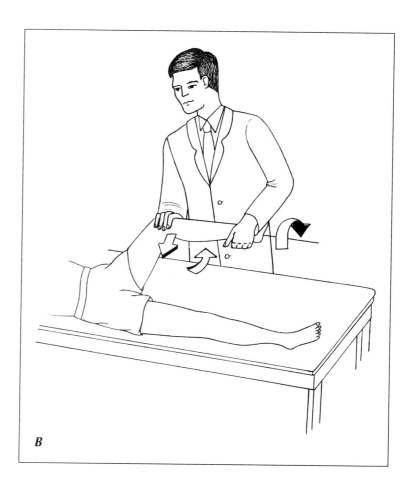

Figure 13.42 Continued

cleavage planes in chronic tears tend to extend horizontally in complex patterns. Early osteoarthritic changes are frequently associated findings.

SUBLUXATION AND DISLOCATION OF THE PATELLA   Valgus stress of the knee, particularly if combined with external rotation, can cause lateral patellar dislocation or subluxation, which tears the restraining fibers of the medial retinaculum (Fig. 13.43). If the dislo-

cation is unreduced, the diagnosis will be obvious. If not spontaneous, reduction usually follows passive extension of the knee. Occasionally medially-directed pressure on the patella is needed. If the patella reduced spontaneously, the only finding is tenderness over the medial retinaculum. Recurrent displacement of the patella is usually associated with a positive "apprehension sign," in which laterally directed pressure against the patella as the knee is flexed results in a sudden grimace by the

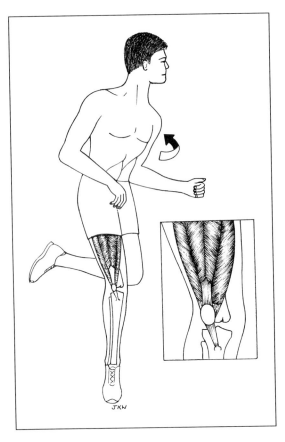

der, recurrence often requires operative stabilization.

RUPTURES OF TENDONS   Other acute injuries around the knee include ruptures of the quadriceps or patellar tendon, which usually follows violent contraction of the quadriceps and simultaneous passive flexion of the knee, such as a landing from a jump. The diagnosis can usually be made from the physical examination. A defect is palpable at the site of injury, and active extension of the knee is impossible if the rupture is complete; however, partial tendon ruptures may allow weak active extension. Radiographs are needed to rule out patellar fracture. A high-riding patella indicates rupture of the patellar tendon rather than the quadriceps tendon. Treatment of these ruptures is surgical.

Figure 13.43   Mechanism of injury for lateral patellar dislocation: valgus thrust at the knee and external rotation of the tibia.

SUBACUTE AND CHRONIC INJURIES ABOUT THE KNEE   One of the most frequent chronic knee problems is *retropatellar pain* (or *anterior knee pain*), which is exacerbated by activities that produce high patellofemoral contact forces, such as walking up and down stairs. While the specific etiology of this symptom complex is often unclear, it is often associated with patellar subluxation and chondromalacia.

Recurrent patellar subluxation is accompanied by acute pain and giving way as the patella slips laterally out of the trochlea of the femur. Spontaneous relocation is the rule. Predisposing anatomic variants are increased valgus, *patella alta* (high-riding patella), increased femoral anteversion, increased external tibial torsion, and generalized ligamentous laxity. The patellar apprehension test is

patient. Radiographs are needed to rule out an osteochondral fracture of the patella or femoral condyle. Flexion beyond 30 to 45° should be prevented for 4 to 6 weeks by use of a brace. Following this period of immobilization, intensive quadriceps strengthening, especially of the vastus medialis, reduces the likelihood of recurrence. As with dislocations of the shoul-

often positive in these patients. Standardized tangential radiographs (Laurin or Merchant views) often reveal tilting or lateral positioning of the patella in the trochlear groove (Fig. 13.44). Initial treatment entails strengthening of the vastus medialis obliquus portion of the quadriceps muscle, which increases the medial pull on the patella and thereby helps prevent lateral subluxation. A patellar brace can be used to augment this program. If recurrent subluxation continues, surgical realignment is advisable to prevent progressive degenerative changes.

Chondromalacia of the patella is often present in patients with patellar pain who have no evidence of malalignment. The name of this poorly defined syndrome suggests that the primary abnormality is in the articular cartilage of the patella, which is often "blistered," fibrillated, or absent, exposing underlying bone. The relationship between pathological findings and pain is unclear, since articular cartilage does not contain sensory nerve endings. No definitive treatment is available for this group of patients; however, increasing strength and flexibility of the knee and NSAIDs may improve the clinical picture. Arthroscopic shaving *(chondroplasty)* of the fibrillated cartilage may help temporarily but has not been shown to result in significant long-term improvement.

Leg

FRACTURES *Tibial and fibular shaft fractures* are common and more difficult to manage than to diagnose. The high energy force needed to fracture the adult tibia is frequently associated with extensive damage to the overlying skin and soft tissues. Indeed, the degree of injury to the soft tissues influences both treatment and prognosis. Open fractures have a higher incidence of infection, delayed union, and nonunion. Radiographs will define the amount of displacement and comminution. Closed fractures with displacement of less than 50 percent of the shaft's diameter can usually be managed by closed reduction and above-knee casting for 4 to 8 weeks. A below-knee cast is then used until healing occurs, usually another 8 to 20 weeks. When significant shortening or angulation cannot be corrected by manipulation, open reduction and internal fixation are indicated. Open fractures need emergent surgical debridement of contaminated and avascular tissues and stabilization by external or internal fixation.

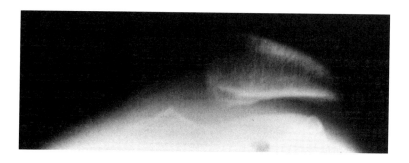

Figure 13.44 Merchant's view of the patella showing lateral patellar subluxation and secondary degenerative changes.

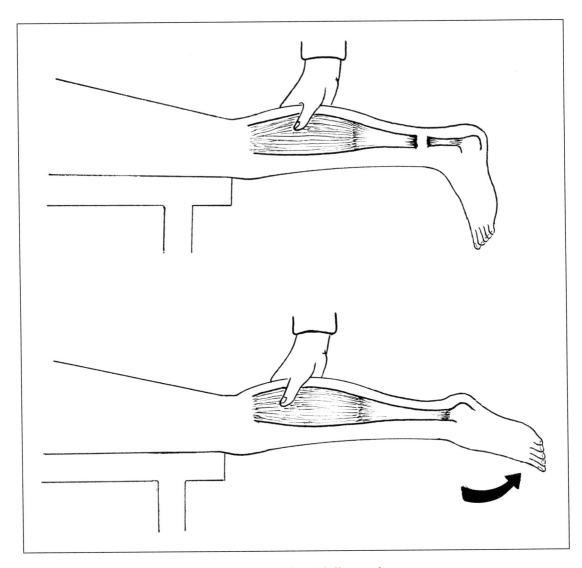

Figure 13.45   Thompson's test for integrity of the Achilles tendon.
Squeezing the calf causes plantar flexion of the ankle only if the tendon
is intact.

INJURIES OF MUSCLE AND TENDON   The muscles and tendons of the leg are especially susceptible to injuries during running and jumping activities. Most musculotendinous injuries occur in the calf.

Gastrocnemius strain or *"tennis leg"* usually involves the medial head, possibly because of the high content of fast twitch muscle fibers in that area. The patient usually experiences sudden pain and is unable to continue play or work. Local tenderness and swelling are present, but a defect is rarely palpable, since these are only partial tears of the muscle. The treatment is symptomatic, with ice and mild analgesics. Light stretching with progression to strengthening usually leads to resolution of symptoms in 4 to 6 weeks.

Rupture of the Achilles tendon is a more serious injury. Preexisting degenerative changes and a sudden contraction or stretch of the muscle are the usual etiologic factors. Active plantar flexion of the ankle is weakened but not absent. The diagnosis is confirmed by palpation of a defect in the tendon and the absence of plantar flexion of the ankle when the belly of the relaxed gastrocnemius muscle is squeezed (Fig. 13.45). The rupture can be treated by casting in equinus for 6 to 12 weeks followed by a heel lift or by surgical repair. The higher rerupture rate in casted patients must be balanced against the rate of infection following surgery.

Shin splints is a condition produced by prolonged running and jumping that results in small tears near the attachment of the muscles to the proximal tibia and fibula. Periostitis results from inflammation around the periosteal insertion of the muscles. Tenderness is localizable to the posteromedial aspect of the proximal tibia (Fig. 13.46). Shin splints are treated

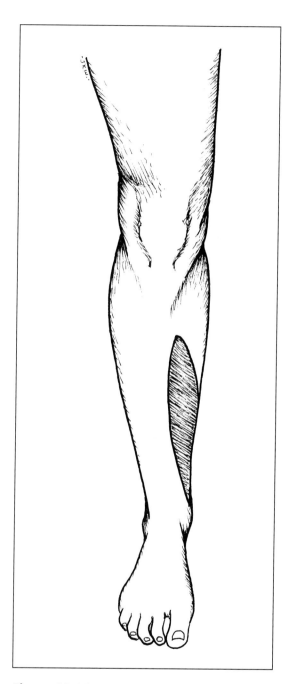

Figure 13.46   Area of pain in a patient with shin splints or traction periostitis.

by limiting running and jumping, especially on hard surfaces. The use of NSAIDs and supportive, shock-absorbing running shoes is helpful, and patients with flexible flat feet benefit from arch supports.

A *compartmental syndrome* occurs when the repetitive impact of running and jumping causes diffuse swelling of the leg muscles. Since the muscles of the leg are contained in well-defined fascial compartments with rigid boundaries, this swelling may create excessive pressure within the compartment, which slowly returns to normal after the exercise is stopped. Deep, activity-related muscle pain that disappears within minutes after the activity ceases is the usual complaint. In severe cases, transient pedal numbness may be noted. The diagnosis is made by measurement of compartmental pressure during or immediately after exercise. Symptoms are relieved by decreasing activity. Unremitting symptoms demand surgical release of the fascial walls of the compartment.

It is important to distinguish compartmental syndromes and shin splints from tibial or fibular *stress fractures.* The distinction is based on radiographic demonstration (usually not visible for 10 to 14 days) of the fracture or fracture callus; however, technetium bone scans are positive much sooner.

Ankle

FRACTURES OF THE ANKLE *Fractures of the lateral and/or medial malleolus* are suggested by the findings of malleolar tenderness and crepitus, with or without deformity of the ankle. Radiographs are used to assess the type of fracture and determine treatment, which depends upon the displacement and stability of the fracture. Isolated fractures of one malleo-

lus may be treated in a below-knee cast. Bimalleolar fractures are unstable injuries. Their requirements for precise reduction and rigid fixation to avoid talar shift are usually best met by open reduction and internal fixation, which minimizes the need for casting and permits earlier motion.

Fractures of the talus are much less common than malleolar fractures. Osteochondral fractures involving the lateral corner of the talar dome result from inversion injuries, although the distinction between this lesion and a localized area of avascular necrosis is not always clear (Fig. 13.47). Cast immobilization may lead to healing if the fragment is nondisplaced; however, if the osteochondral fragment becomes detached, causes pain, and/or causes locking, removal of the fragment and drilling of the talar defect are indicated. Other fractures of the talus are discussed under "Hindfoot," below.

INJURIES OF THE LIGAMENTS OF THE ANKLE Although an inversion injury can fracture the ankle, it more commonly results in tearing of the lateral ligaments. Injury of the anterior talofibular and calcaneofibular ligaments is common, while only a severe injury disrupts the posterior talofibular ligament. Physical findings include tenderness, swelling and ecchymosis directly over the injured ligament, and pain with inversion. The treatment is largely symptomatic: crutches, application of ice, compression with an elastic wrap, elevation, and NSAIDs. Casting is generally not needed, since the ankle joint is stable, and ligamentous healing is improved if gentle motion can be maintained. Healing often takes as long as 6 weeks. Bracing and taping allow an earlier return to sports. During recovery,

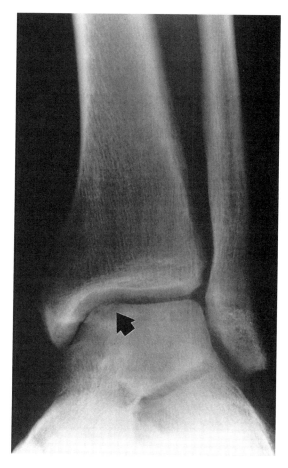

Figure 13.47 Osteochondritis dissecans of the talus *(arrow).*

strengthening exercises, especially of the peroneal muscles, may reduce the likelihood of recurrence.

SUBACUTE AND CHRONIC INJURIES OF THE ANKLE Recurrent sprains of the ankle lead to attrition of the lateral ligaments, which predisposes to further sprains. Stress radiographs usually show abnormal talar tilt when compared to the normal side. Management entails peroneal muscle strengthening and taping or bracing during activities. If this approach does not reduce the frequency of recurrent sprains, surgical reconstruction of the ligaments should be considered.

Inversion injuries can also disrupt the retinacular restraints of the peroneal tendons behind the lateral malleolus, allowing recurrent anterior displacement of the tendons, which often produces a sensation of giving way. *Subluxation of peroneal tendons* may be demonstrated by active dorsiflexion and eversion of the ankle. Treatment is surgical reconstruction of the peroneal retinaculum.

Hindfoot

FRACTURES OF THE HINDFOOT The hindfoot is especially vulnerable to injury in falls from a height.

Fractures of the calcaneus usually result from axial loading, without significant eversion or inversion. They are often extensively comminuted, with disruption of the talocalcaneal joint. A nonoperative approach is favored for injuries at the extremes of severity; nondisplaced and extensively comminuted fractures tend to fare better with compression, ice, elevation, and early motion. In certain displaced but less comminuted fractures, open reduction and internal fixation offer a better result. Both open and closed treatment are frequently followed by posttraumatic arthritis.

Fractures of the neck and body of the talus are less common. Fractures of the talar neck are frequently associated with tibiotalar or talocalcaneal dislocation, which may disrupt the blood supply to the body of the talus, causing avascular necrosis. Open reduction and internal fixation results in a stable anatomic reduction but has not been shown to reduce the incidence of avascular necrosis.

DISLOCATIONS OF THE HINDFOOT   Dislocation of the talocalcaneal joint *(subtalar dislocation)* is produced by forced eversion or inversion of the foot. Marked deformity of the hindfoot is obvious. Closed reduction is usually possible unless soft tissues are trapped in

the joint. Once reduced, the joint is relatively stable and requires only a short period of immobilization.

SUBACUTE AND CHRONIC HINDFOOT INJURIES   Tendinitis, which often follows partial rupture of deconditioned tendons, is common in the hindfoot (Fig. 13.48). Achilles tendinitis is characterized by pain with activity and upon arising. Tenderness is most pronounced 1 to 2 in. above the insertion of the tendon, and nod-

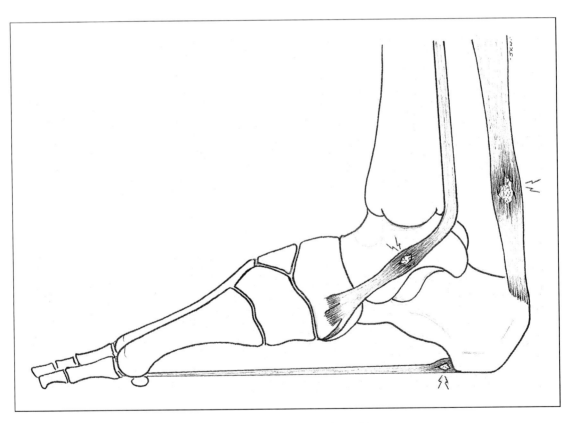

Figure 13.48   Tendons and plantar fascia commonly affected by overuse injuries.

ules, caused by thickening of the sheath surrounding the tendon, are often palpable. Treatment involves NSAIDs, calf stretching, and use of a heel pad in the shoe. The injection of steroids into the tendon increases the risk of tendon rupture and should be avoided. For resistant cases, surgical removal of the scarred tendon and/or tenosynovium is usually curative.

Peroneal and posterior tibial tendinitis are also characterized by localized pain and tenderness over the course of the involved tendon. Posterior tibial tendinitis occasionally progresses to complete rupture, with a resulting flatfoot deformity (Fig. 13.49). Reduced activity, NSAIDs, and arch supports provide symptomatic relief. Surgical repair may be successful if the injury is recognized early. Chronic symptoms, if disabling, may require triple arthrodesis (Fig. 10.14).

Forefoot

FRACTURES   *Fractures of the forefoot* result from direct impact or twisting injuries. Direct impact usually fractures the metatarsal shaft or phalanges, which, if minimally displaced, can

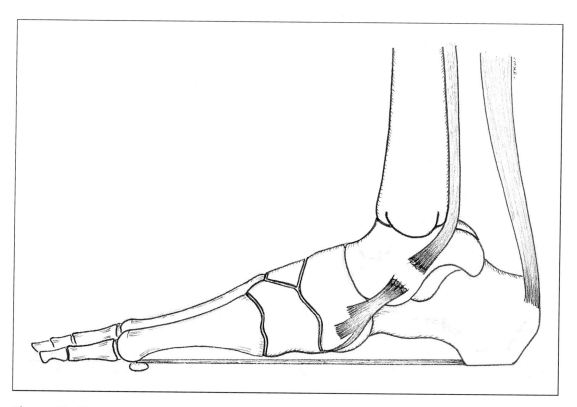

Figure 13.49   Flatfoot deformity caused by rupture of the posterior tibial tendon.

be treated in a below-knee cast or wooden-soled shoe. Twisting inversion injuries commonly produce an avulsion fracture at the base of the fifth metatarsal, which can be misdiagnosed as a sprained ankle if the point of maximum tenderness is not carefully determined (Fig. 13.50*A*). These fractures are most comfortably treated in a cast with a well-molded arch for 3 to 4 weeks but will also heal in a sturdy shoe.

Fractures of the proximal shaft of the fifth metatarsal (Jones fracture) have a poorer prognosis than avulsion fractures of the base of the metatarsal (Fig. 13.50*B*). These fractures require a non-weight-bearing cast for at least 6 to 8 weeks. Internal fixation reduces the rate of nonunion and the period of casting.

INJURIES TO THE JOINTS   A plantar flexion or twisting injury to the forefoot occasionally results in dislocation of some or all of the tarsometatarsal joints *(Lisfranc dislocation)*. These dislocations may be difficult to diagnose because of associated pain and swelling. Careful radiographic evaluation is needed to determine the presence and extent of injury. Fractures of the bases of the metatarsals are frequently associated. Open reduction and percutaneous pinning constitute optimal treatment, but late forefoot pain is common.

Dislocations of the metatarsophalangeal or interphalangeal joints are relatively infrequent because of protection from the shoe. Closed reduction and taping to the neighboring toe is usually successful.

SUBACUTE AND CHRONIC INJURIES   Tendinitis in the forefoot is less common than in the hindfoot. Chronic forefoot pain is more

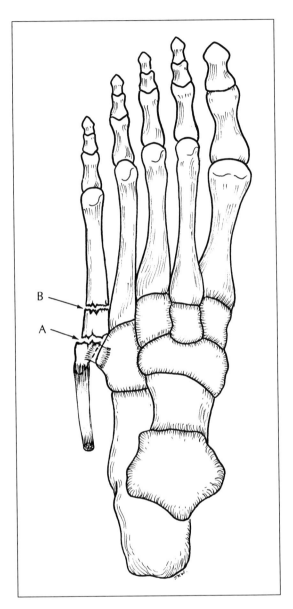

Figure 13.50   *A.* Avulsion fracture at the base of the fifth metatarsal. *B.* Fracture of the proximal shaft of the fifth metatarsal (Jones fracture).

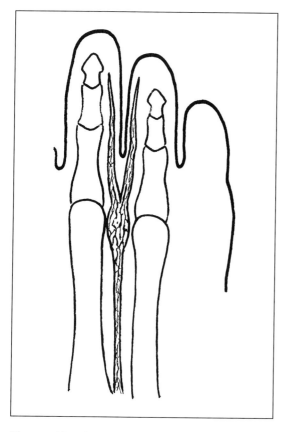

Figure 13.51   Morton neuroma.

likely to result from a *Morton neuroma,* in which repetitive trauma of the interdigital nerve causes perineural fibrosis and swelling of the nerve typically between the third and fourth toes (Fig. 13.51). These patients complain of forefoot pain accentuated by weight-bearing and accompanied by numbness in adjacent halves of the digits. Nonoperative treatment includes NSAIDs, a metatarsal pad, and corticosteroid injection. If unsuccessful, resection of the neuroma is simple and curative.

SUGGESTED READINGS

BROWNER BD, JUPITER JB, LEVINE AM, TRAFTON PG: *Skeletal Trauma.* Philadelphia, Saunders, 1992.

DeLEE JC, DREZ D: *Orthopaedic Sports Medicine: Principles and Practice.* Philadelphia, Saunders, 1994.

ROCKWOOD CA, GREEN DP, BUCHOLZ RW: *Fractures in Adults,* 3d ed. Philadelphia, Lippincott, 1991.

Chapter 14

Degenerative Diseases and Disorders

Frank C. Wilson

GENERAL ASPECTS

Aging is a complex process that may be defined as the sum of all the naturally occurring, degenerative changes that occur in humans with the passage of time.

Ageism is a term applied to traditional notions imprinted upon the elderly by society, which, like those of racism and sexism, are inappropriate in today's world.

The French philosopher Simone de Beauvoir observed that "the issues of age challenge the whole society and put the whole society to the test." Certainly the problems of aging are societal and political as well as personal and unique.

The Aging Population

By the year 2000, there will be some 36 million people in the United States—15 percent of the population—over the age of 65 years. In 1900, only 4 percent of the population were over 65. Compared to 1900, almost twice as many of those born now may expect to reach the age of 65. During the twentieth century, the average age at death has increased from 50 to 75 years—yet those who survive the longest live no longer today than they did 2000 years ago, The Book of Joshua states, "Moses was 120 when he died; his eye was not dim nor his natural force abated."

Change in the sex ratio of the population has been as dramatic as the change in life expectancy. In 1900, there were 102 older men for every 100 older women; today the ratio is 150 women to 100 men. However, this differential is seen only in countries that are highly developed socioeconomically, which suggests that the sex difference in survivorship may be accounted for in large part by diet and lifestyle,

both of which influence the onset and severity of atherosclerosis.

In the past, people tended to behave in a fashion that society considered appropriate for their age. The person who at age 50 decided to give up singles tennis was likely to be responding more to societal expectations than to changes in physical capability, thereby reinforcing the notion of functional impairment in the aged. Because of the broad range of individual variation, the best predictor of performance currently is a person's earlier performance rather than any normative studies based on age-related decline. Thus, an 80-year-old jogger may have better cardiovascular function than a 50-year-old librarian. Among the alterations in function modified by lifestyle are the maximum rate of oxygen consumption, muscular power, speed of recovery from physical stress, and performance on a standard glucose tolerance test.

Theories of Aging

In a biological sense, there is no survival value for a species with a life span beyond reproductive maturation; persons over the age of 45 or 50—when reproductive activity is complete and children have reached sexual maturity—are biologically superfluous.

The two major hypotheses of aging are the *theory of cellular degeneration,* caused by genetic instability and/or cellular damage, and the *immune theory,* in which active self-destruction is mediated by the immune system via genetic, environmental, and/or endocrine influences.

A hallmark of cellular aging is the intracellular accumulation of the chemically complex pigment *lipofuscin,* although the amount may differ even within a given tissue. In skeletal muscle, for example, more lipofuscin is deposited in the muscles of the limb than in the muscles of the trunk. Although lipofuscin has generally been regarded as inert, it may play a functional role through accumulation of inert intracellular material that progressively occupies cytoplasmic volume and thereby becomes a metabolic depressant of the cell (the "clinker" theory).

Important work by Hayflick and associates in 1979 with human fibroblasts in culture showed that these cells were capable on average of only 50 doublings before they stopped dividing and died. A finite proliferative capacity has now been demonstrated for a host of other normal cell types and is accepted as a general phenomenon; however, the probability that animals age because important cells lose their proliferative capacity is unlikely, since other functional losses produce physiologic decrements in cellular function long before these cells reach their maximum proliferative capacity.

Evidence for the role of the immune system in aging is more convincing for the *diseases* of old age than for normal aging; however, the theory of progressive immunodeficiency is attractive, since it may be more accessible to therapeutic manipulation.

Another theory of aging, proposed by Harmon in 1968, implicated free radicals as central to the changes seen with aging at the tissue, cellular, and subcellular levels. Free radicals are chemical intermediates containing an unpaired electron. These molecules, which may be formed from dietary or atmospheric materials, are highly reactive and usually have a brief half-life. The untoward effects of diffusable free radicals are expressed by impaired transfer of information in the cell, loss of membrane functions, and impaired enzymatic activity. There is limited evidence that reactions producing free radicals increase with age

and that protection against free radicals is enhanced by endurance exercises and dietary antioxidants, which has stimulated use of vitamins A, E, and C for their antioxidant properties. While the exact mechanism by which antioxidants act is unclear, possibilities include depression of appetite and reduction of food intake, suppression of tumor growth (a common cause of death in longevity studies), and slowing of the decline of immune processes.

Effects of Aging on Musculoskeletal Tissues

Involving as they do some 80 percent of the body, musculoskeletal problems are among the most common complaints in the elderly—affecting more the quality than the quantity of life and often leading to disabilities that are very costly to manage.

In *muscle,* the strength and speed of contraction of limb muscles is significantly decreased in the elderly, although overall muscle endurance is minimally affected; furthermore, athletic training can improve muscle strength in elderly patients, in part because muscle, as opposed to cartilage, has the ability to regenerate normally following injury.

Bone mass decreases steadily after about age 30, declining on average between 0.5 and 1 percent per year thereafter, with perhaps 2 to 5 percent lost per year in postmenopausal females. By age 80, however, gender differences in bone mass have almost disappeared.

Evaluation of the Elderly Patient

Unraveling the distinction between physiologic (successful) aging and pathologic (unsuccessful) aging is one of the more intriguing challenges of modern medicine. How does one distinguish normal aging from the sequelae of disease, especially given the breadth of the normal spectrum among persons and individual organ systems? Difficult as it may be, such distinction is critical, since disease-related disorders are often remediable. With age-related cognitive impairment a product more of disease states than senility and the ability to increase physical vigor in the elderly, we are obliged to reexamine traditional approaches and modes of thought in this segment of the population. Since the function of certain organs remains constant in some patients while declining in others, we must wonder too whether those who experience loss do so as the result of disease rather than normal aging. Certainly it is no longer appropriate to tell a patient that his hip hurts because he is 84 years old when his other, asymptomatic, hip is its contemporary.

Although gradual deterioration occurs with aging, the redundancy of most organ systems prevents this decrement from becoming functionally significant until the loss is moderately extensive. As a rough rule of thumb, organ systems lose about 1 percent of their function per year beginning about the age of 30, although recent data from longitudinal cohort studies have shown less pronounced and widely variable changes.

Just as with patients, the critical issue in organ systems is function, which depends upon the rate of deterioration, the level of function needed, and the extent to which the organ is overbuilt. The physician's role is to enhance the coping ability of the patient by identifying and treating remedial problems and by facilitating changes in the environment to maximize function in the face of problems that remain.

More than with other specialties, the com-prehensive medical evaluation of older patients entails awareness and sensitivity to their unique concerns, along with the patience, capability, and willingness to interact with a host of health professionals. Goals and progress must be measured on a different scale, since dramatic response to treatment and complete cure are less often possible.

Listening to the patient is just as important with the elderly as it is with the young, although—because of a reduction in the aged patient's response to stress, including that of disease—symptom intensity may be damp-ened by the "background noise" of aging. Since histories are longer and response times slower, greater patience is required to take the history of an elderly patient. Coexisting conditions are the rule and require considerable skill in prioritization of importance and order of treatment.

Interpretation of physical findings requires an awareness of age-related physical changes. Abnormalities in all physical systems should be carefully assessed, since identification and correction of incidental disabilities, such as those of hearing or seeing, may result in valuable functional gain in the patient's life.

Similarly, age-related changes in laboratory values may occur: for example, normal serum creatinine levels may be found despite significant reduction in renal function, because lean body mass and endogenous creatinine production decline with age. Formed blood elements, electrolytes, blood urea nitrogen, and liver function tests usually do not change, although changes in the sedimentation rate, chest radiographs, and electrocardiogram with aging are relatively frequent.

Functional status is especially critical with respect to the activities of daily living, which entail not only feeding, dressing, toileting, and bathing but also activities requiring instrumental manipulation, such as writing, cooking, using the telephone, and cleaning. Remediable conditions that impair these activities should be defined and corrected, which pleads the case for a multidisciplinary approach to geriatric patients. Environmental modification may be just as important as pharmacologic intervention, but the physician cannot reasonably be expected to provide comprehensive management of social and environmental needs along with the medical aspects of care.

From a skeletal standpoint, the major problem in the elderly is loss of bone mass *(osteopenia)*, which leads to the clinical syndrome of *osteoporosis* that affects 40 to 50 percent of women over the age of 50 with fractures of the vertebral bodies, hip, wrist, and shoulder. While there are many risk factors for osteopenia, including steroid usage, parathyroid and thyroid disorders, inanition, high caffeine and alcohol intake, and smoking, the major causative factor in postmenopausal women is the lowered estrogen levels that allow increased bone resorption (see Chap. 16).

The best "treatment" for osteopenia is prevention, which would greatly reduce the cost, morbidity, and mortality rates for fractures through bones weakened by this condition. There is agreement that regular exercise plays a significant role in protection against bone loss. Pharmacologic management is more controversial. Calcium (1200 to 1500 mg per day) and vitamin D (400 units per day), with estrogen replacement after menopause, has been shown to prevent bone loss. Calcium gluconate appears to be the most effective form of calcium replacement, although the antacid Tums, each tablet of which provides 200 mg of calcium, is a convenient and palatable alternative.

Cartilage loss, which produces *osteoarthritis,* is extremely common in the weight-bearing joints of the elderly, although these changes usually do not reach clinical significance. The prevention of osteoarthritis and the management of osteoarthritic joints are considered in subsequent sections of this chapter.

Preoperative Evaluation

It is of particular importance that elderly patients about to undergo operative procedures be assessed by an internist or geriatrician if significant problems exist in other organ systems. While no studies have shown convincingly that age alone increases surgical morbidity and mortality, these outcomes *are* affected by systemic illnesses such as cardiac or renal failure, obstructive pulmonary disease, and anemia. Medications must be scrutinized to determine what modifications, if any, are necessary before and after surgery. Prophylaxis for infection and thromboembolic disease should be strongly considered, especially if there is a history of these disorders. Only with a full understanding of the patient's general health can the appropriateness and risk-benefit ratio of proposed surgery be assessed accurately. Particular caution should be exercised in operating upon patients who have sustained a myocardial infarction within 6 months or who have pulmonary edema, unstable angina, or aortic stenosis; also, renal function must be known for patients in whom the use of nephrotoxic or renally excreted drugs is anticipated.

There is a common misconception that regional anesthesia is preferred for the elderly because of the increased risks from general anesthesia in this group; however, data do not support this contention, especially since many elderly patients require added intravenous sedation and/or analgesia. Also, since significant cardiovascular changes may occur during regional anesthesia, invasive monitoring may be required as well.

SPECIFIC DISEASES AND DISORDERS

Articular Diseases

Pathogenesis

Degenerative arthritis (osteoarthritis) is a disorder of movable joints resulting from cartilage degeneration. It is associated with a mild inflammatory reaction in the synovium and faulty bone and cartilage regeneration. Between one-third and one-half of the U.S. adult population has radiographic evidence of osteoarthritis, with a striking rise in prevalence that parallels advancing age. Although men and women are affected with nearly equal frequency, the findings are usually more advanced and more generalized in women.

While loss of articular cartilage follows both disuse or overuse, earlier and more marked changes result from any mechanical factor that increases surface loading and/or a genetic factor that increases the susceptibility of cartilage to degenerative changes.

In the early stages of the disease, cartilage loses its glistening appearance and develops a yellowish cast. With time, flaking and fissuring (fibrillation) of the cartilage occur. Sclerosis of the subchondral bone follows full-thickness loss of cartilage, leading to a polished and ivory-like (eburnated) appearance. Cysts may develop in the subchondral bone, occasionally communicating with fissures in the overlying

cartilage. Osteophytes form at the joint margins and enlarge slowly. Microscopically, faulty attempts at cartilage repair are seen in the deeper layers of cartilage. In the subchondral bone, thickened trabeculae and, occasionally, microfractures are found. The synovium is thickened and scarred, with low-grade inflammatory changes.

The inciting pathogenetic factor for primary degenerative arthritis is unknown. Cartilage and bone vie for the distinction of being the locus of the initial disturbance. The *cartilage theory* espouses damage to the chondrocyte as the primary lesion, which causes the release of enzymes that degrade matrix proteoglycans in spite of natural enzyme inhibitors and the synthesis of new proteoglycans. Changes in the proteoglycans permit the cartilage to imbibe excess water, which results in changes in its biomechanical properties that render it more vulnerable to mechanical stress. It is unknown, however, whether abnormalities of the matrix represent enzymatic degradation of existing components or the synthesis of altered constituents of the matrix.

According to the *bone theory*, repetitive mechanical stress produces microfractures in the subchondral bone. Healing of these fractures leads to more and harder bone, which, by reducing its shock-absorbing function, increases stress on the overlying cartilage.

The development of degenerative arthritis is hastened by acquired irregularities of the joint surfaces, which may result from fractures, meniscal injuries, loose bodies, or other arthritides. Extraarticular malalignment (e.g., bowleg or knock-knee), loss of ligamentous stability, and loss of "protective" sensory feedback also induce joint degeneration. The latter condition, which results in the generation of increased joint forces, may be encountered in diabetic neuropathy, tabes dorsalis, syringo-myelia, and following intraarticular steroid administration (see Chap. 10). Even remote causes, such as obesity and occupation, and iatrogenic conditions, such as prolonged immobilization and meniscectomy, may be responsible for more rapid joint wear.

Spine

Degenerative joint disease is even more common in the spine than in the limbs; in fact, over 75 percent of people who reach the age of 75 will have had one or more episodes of low back pain from disorders of the intervertebral disk, varying only in frequency and intensity.

THE AGING DISK   To understand the biochemical changes in the aging disk, it is important to realize that the disk has four main structural components: the nucleus pulposus, or central region, which is essentially a concentrated proteoglycan solution containing randomly distributed collagen fibers; and the annulus fibrosus and two cartilaginous end plates that surround the nucleus pulposus. In contrast to the nucleus, the annulus has a highly organized structure, with its collagen fibrils arranged into parallel bundles that form concentric lamellae around the nucleus. The outermost lamellae anchor directly into the vertebrae as Sharpey's fibers, whereas those of the inner annulus connect to the end plates.

The intervertebral disk allows spinal mobility while retaining axial stability. The disk is continually loaded in vivo, even in the supine position, as a result of compression by the surrounding muscles and ligaments. The hydrostatic pressure produced by these forces is balanced by the imbibition pressure produced by long proteoglycan chains in the nucleus that contain large negatively charged glycosami-noglycan molecules, which attract water into the extracellular matrix. An increase in the loading forces causes fluid to be expressed from the nucleus and, as fluid is lost, the concentration of the negatively charged glycosaminoglycans increases, which raises the imbibition pressure within the disk to balance the increased load. Unfortunately, the proteoglycan content of the human disk decreases with age, leading to lower imbibition pressure, reduced water content, and associated fibrous replacement of the nucleus pulposus. Accompanying these evolving changes in the nucleus, the fibers of the annulus show coarsening and hyalinization, with fissuring of the lamellae, especially in the lumbar and cervical regions, where motion and stress are maximal. This sequence of events often culminates in *extrusion of the nucleus pulposus* through the annulus fibrosus, usually posterolaterally, where the restraint of the posterior longitudinal ligament is least and where it may compress a spinal nerve root. As dehydration continues, the nucleus eventually contains insufficient fluid to be extruded through the increasingly fibrous annulus, so that the incidence of disk herniation decreases after the fifth decade.

Because of changes in the blood supply to the disk that occur with aging, repair cannot keep pace with degeneration. The disk receives its blood supply from two sources, the periphery of the annulus and the vertebral bodies. The nucleus and inner annulus are almost entirely dependent on blood supply from the vertebral bodies, while the outer annulus is nourished by adjacent peripheral vessels. Because the arteries that feed the inner zones of the disk are subject to degeneration, the blood supply to the nucleus decreases with age. Nutrition of the nucleus is further impaired by increasing calcification of the cartilaginous end plates, which creates an impermeable barrier to transport of solutes.

Degenerated disks have the following characteristics: decreased disk height, increased lateral bulging, reduced imbibition pressure, and increased mobility. Decreased disk height leads to abnormal loading of the facet joints: lateral bulging can produce nerve root compression; reduced internal pressure causes an increase in end-plate loading; and increased mobility produces greater stresses on adjacent soft structures. Thus, degenerative disk disease is a syndrome initiated by degenerative changes in the disk, which secondarily involves other spinal elements that contribute to the symptom complex; therefore, it is often impossible to isolate a single cause of low back pain. The capsule of the facet joint is richly supplied with nerve endings, so that overloading of the facets, which stretches the capsule, provokes a painful response. Increased ligamentous stress, which results from loss of disk height and overloading of the facets, causes stimulation of mechanical pain receptors in ligamentous tissue. With progressive hypertrophy of the facet and bulging of the annulus, compression of adjacent nerve roots is common, producing radicular pain or *sciatica*. Another frequent source of pain is adjacent spinal musculature. The trunk muscles maintain stability of the vertebral column and control intervertebral movement. When spinal instability occurs, greater demands are placed upon these muscles to maintain spinal alignment and prevent painful motion. This overuse leads to painful muscle spasm and limited movement.

In the early stages of disk degeneration, the annulus fibrosus fibrillates and develops central cracks that extend toward the periphery. A specific traumatic event, which often involves bending and twisting, may lead to herniation of the nucleus. Disks can be *protruded* (annulus intact), *extruded* (through the annulus but contained under the posterior longitudinal ligament), or *sequestrated* (free in the spinal canal) (Fig. 14.1). Again, continued dessication and fibrosis make herniation less frequent in the elderly.

Degenerative disk disease is uncommon in youth, although premature aging of the disks does occur as a familial trait.

IMAGING   The pathoanatomic features of degenerative disk disease are manifest on routine anteroposterior (AP), lateral, and oblique radiographs as narrowing of the disk spaces, reduction in lordosis, sclerosis and narrowing of the facet joints, and osteophyte formation. If significant osteopenia is also present, concavity of the vertebral end plates may be seen, producing the so-called *codfish vertebrae* (Fig. 14.2). Pathologic examination of these vertebrae shows small intravertebral disk herniations through the end plate *(Schmorl nodes)*. Degenerative spondylolisthesis may also be seen.

Both computed tomography with multiplanar reformation (CT/MPR) and magnetic resonance imaging (MRI) provide excellent delineation of the morphologic changes of disk degeneration. The major difference between the two lies in the ability of MRI to delineate the chemical changes in degenerating disks prior to the development of morphologic abnormalities. Magnetic resonance imaging also allows determination of whether the disk material is contained by the annulus and posterior longitudinal ligament or whether it has become a sequestrated fragment. Computed tomography, because of its excellent delineation of osseous structures and superior spatial resolution, is more accurate than MRI in determining

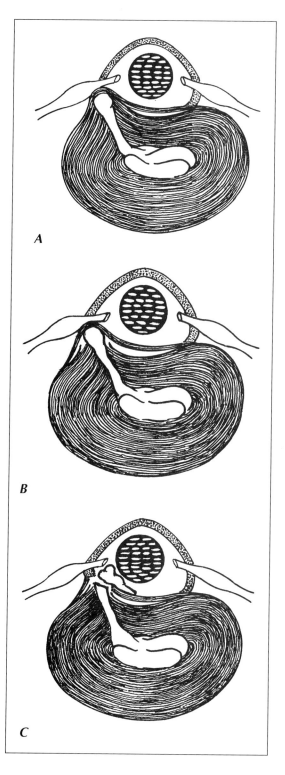

Figure 14.1 Types of lumbar disk herniation: *(A)* protruded disk, *(B)* extruded disk, *(C)* sequestrated disk.

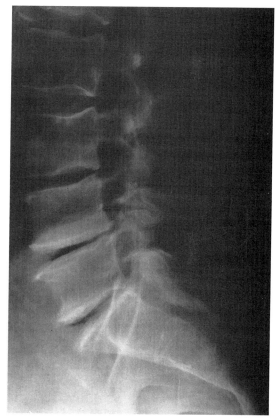

Figure 14.2 Degenerative disk disease in the lumbar spine. Note the narrowing of the disk spaces, osteophytes on L5, and end-plate concavities.

the location and size of end-plate spurs, which are hard to distinguish from herniated disk material by MRI. Because of the excellent sensitivity, specificity, and accuracy of MRI and CT in the diagnosis of disk disease, invasive studies such as myelography are less often necessary. It should be pointed out, however, that positive imaging studies are not always of clinical significance.

CERVICAL DISK DISEASE   The cervical spine, being subject to greater motion stress, and the lumbar spine, subject to greater weight-bearing stress, are the spinal segments most prone to degeneration. Pain is the predominant symptom in both areas. Degenerative disk disease in the cervical spine, often termed *cervical spondylosis,* while involving the same sequence of biochemical and anatomic changes seen in the lumbar spine, carries the additional risk of compression of the nearby spinal cord. The clinical expression of cervical spondylosis may thus take one of three forms: cervical pain, cervical radiculopathy, and cervical myelopathy.

Cervical pain results from stimulation of sinovertebral nerve fibers to the annulus, facet joint capsules, and spinal ligaments or from nerves innervating the paravertebral soft tissues. This pain is more diffuse and less well localized than radicular pain. However, without neurologic involvement, the distinction between a herniated disk, cervical spondylosis, and neck strain is clinically irrelevant, since these patients are treated in the same manner: immobilization with a well-fitted soft felt collar that is worn day and night, nonsteroidal anti-inflammatory drugs (NSAIDs), and injection of tender trigger points with a local anesthetic and corticosteroid preparation.

Patients with *cervical radiculopathy* report aching or burning pain that follows a radicular distribution. Herniations are usually intraforaminal or posterolateral, the latter often producing a preponderance of motor signs (Fig. 14.3). Most often, the C5-6 or C6-7 interspaces are involved, with compromise of the sixth and seventh cervical roots, respectively. Although location of the pain is similar for both (neck, shoulder, medial border of scapula, lateral arm, and dorsal forearm), compromise of C6 produces sensory changes in the thumb and index finger (versus the index and middle fingers for C7 lesions), and motor and reflex changes involving the biceps (versus the triceps for C7). The majority of these patients respond to the same nonoperative program outlined for cervical pain. If no improvement has occurred within 10 days, cervical traction (5 to 10 lb pulling in slight flexion) may be added with a home traction device. If muscle spasm is a predominant feature, a muscle relaxant, such as methocarbanol or carisoprodol, is commonly utilized. With subsidence of acute symptoms, a six-part program of isometric strengthening exercises should be begun and continued as prophylaxis against further episodes: using the hand for resistance, muscles controlling flexion-extension, rotation, and lateral bend should be strengthened. With failure to respond to these measures, especially in the presence of motor weakness, operative management is indicated. Manipulation of the cervical spine should be approached with extreme care if at all.

Patients with premorbid narrowing of the spinal canal and a midline protrusion are more likely to develop *cervical myelopathy* and at a younger age (Fig. 14.4). The anteroposterior diameter of the cervical spine is further reduced by flexion and extension, which stretches the cord over vertebral osteophytes

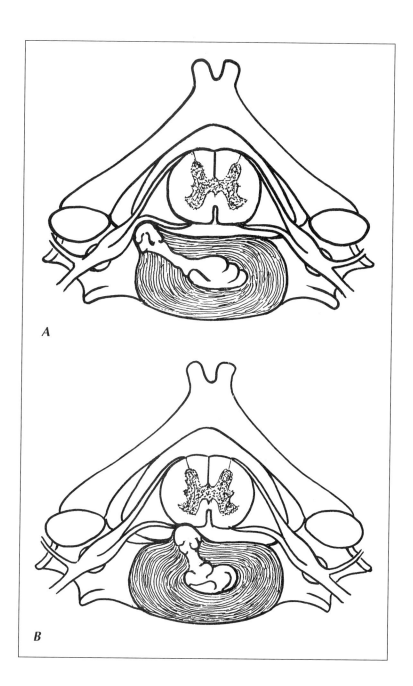

Figure 14.3 Common directions of cervical disk herniations: *(A)* intraforaminal; *(B)* posterolateral.

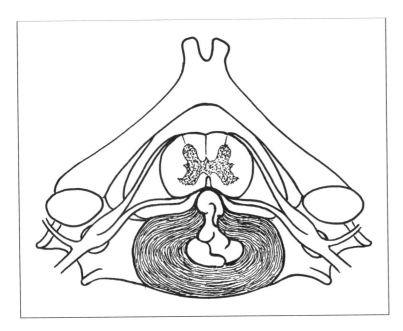

Figure 14.4 Midline cervical disk protrusion, which may cause cervical myelopathy.

and causes buckling of the ligamentum flavum, respectively. Older males are more commonly involved, typically with sensory findings paramount in the upper limbs and weakness and spasticity in the lower. Clumsiness may be manifest in the handling of objects and in disturbances of gait. Abnormalities of urination, which occur in about one-third of the cases, suggest more severe involvement of the cord. Posterior column deficits (loss of vibration and position sense) are more common in the feet than in the hands. Coexistence of a radiculopathy may confound the diagnosis. Because of the severity of the disability resulting from progressive myelopathy, diagnosis is tantamount to surgical decompression, which yields satisfactory results in 70 to 85 percent of cases.

For patients in whom the predominant symptom is arm pain *(brachialgia),* it is critical to rule out localized compression of vascular structures or peripheral nerves in the limb, which may cause similar findings. Peripheral entrapment syndromes can usually be distinguished by a pattern of motor and sensory loss that corresponds to the distribution of a peripheral nerve rather than a specific nerve root and by electrodiagnostic testing. Nerve conduction studies are particularly valuable to corroborate the diagnosis of peripheral compression syndromes, whereas electromyography is more useful when cervical radiculopathy or myopathy is suspected, especially if symptoms have been present for a month or more.

LUMBAR DISK DISEASE   In lumbar disk disease, the history typically involves a young or middle-aged male with episodic low back pain, followed at some point by radiation into the lower limb below the knee. Pain that radiates only into the buttock and thigh is more likely to be referred from adjacent spinal joints or muscles rather than the nerve root. Compression or stretching of the nerve root leads to inflammatory, ischemic, and eventually fibrotic changes, which may be permanent. Characteristically, the pain is relieved by recumbency and aggravated by movement. Sitting, because it produces greater pressure on lumbar disks than other postures, also accen-

tuates the pain of an acute protrusion, as does coughing or sneezing, which increase intrathecal pressure. Asymmetrical lumbar muscle spasm can cause *sciatic scoliosis*. Spinal movement is restricted by pain and muscle spasm, and localized tenderness is found in the affected interspinous space. With the patient supine, passive straight leg–raising reproduces the offending back and/or leg pain, which then disappears if the knee is flexed (*Lasègue's sign*) (Fig. 14.5). This back and leg pain must be distinguished from the discom-

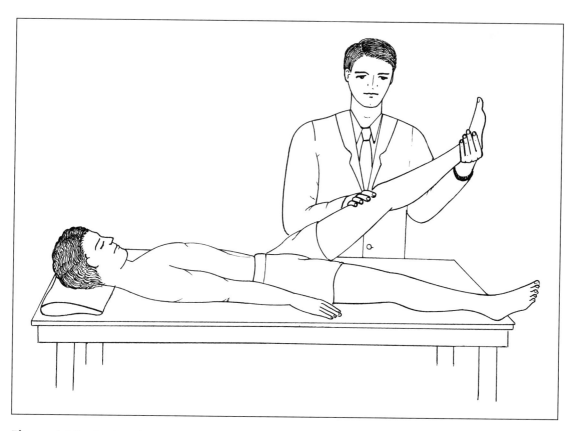

Figure 14.5 Lasègue's test: passive straight leg raising reproduces the back and/or leg pain of lower lumbar disk herniation.

fort in the posterior thigh that results from stretching tight hamstring muscles, which is usually present on the uninvolved side as well. The pain in a positive Lasègue's test is produced by increased tension in the nerve root as it is pulled distally over the protruded disk by elevation of the leg. If pain on the affected side is reproduced by a straight leg–raising maneuver of the opposite leg, the finding is even more reliable, since this maneuver produces less movement and tension on the compromised nerve root. Neurologic changes, if present, are related to the level and location of the protrusion. Midline protrusions are rare in the lumbar spine because of the thickness of the posterior longitudinal ligament in that area. Some 90 percent of symptomatic lumbar protrusions occur posterolaterally at the L4-5 or L5/S1 interspaces. Because the lumbar nerves exit the spine through the superior aspect of the intervertebral foramina, the nerve root most likely to be affected corresponds to the lower vertebral level of the herniation (Fig. 14.6). Thus, the fifth nerve root is more likely to be compromised by a protrusion from the L4-5 disk space, while a lesion at the L5-S1 level usually compresses the S1 nerve root. Involvement of the L5 nerve root produces a sensory deficit on the lateral calf and dorsum of the foot and big toe, with weakness in the posterior tibial, extensor digitorum longus, and extensor hallucis longus muscles. Occasionally, the posterior tibial reflex will be diminished. Compromise of the first sacral root produces sensory loss in the posterior calf and plantar aspect of the foot and little toe, associated with weakness in the gastrocnemius-soleus and flexor hallucis longus muscles. The ankle jerk is characteristically diminished. Disk herniation at higher lumbar levels in-

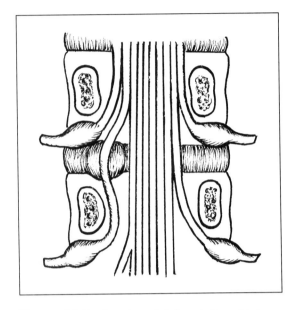

Figure 14.6   Lumbar disk herniation. Note compression of the nerve root corresponding to the lower vertebral level. (Redrawn with permission from Mercier LR: *Practical Orthopaedics,* 2d ed. Chicago, Year Book, 1987, p 107.)

volves roots of the femoral nerve, producing sensory loss in the anterior thigh (L2-L3) or medial calf (L4), with motor weakness in the hip flexors (L1-L3), quadriceps, and/or tibialis anterior (L4). The knee jerk is most likely to be diminished with compression of the fourth lumbar root.

Central prolapse of a lumbar disk, although rare, may precipitate the *cauda equina syndrome,* a surgical emergency associated with back pain, bowel or bladder dysfunction (usually urinary retention), saddle anesthesia, and loss of strength in the lower limb.

Low back pain resulting from acute or degenerative disk disease must be distinguished from other causes of lumbar pain, such as genitourinary lesions, vascular disorders, spinal or paraspinal infections, neoplasia (primary and secondary), osteoporosis (microfractures), and soft tissue disorders such as neuropathies, myofascial lesions, or muscle strains. These conditions should be ruled out by a careful history and physical examination, abetted by appropriate laboratory studies and radiographs.

The treatment of lumbar disk disease must be tailored to the individual patient. Rest, weight reduction, exercise, braces, drugs, heat, and modification of activities constitute the front line of therapy; if employed judiciously, these measures result in subsidence of symptoms in over 95 percent of patients.

While subacute and chronic symptoms often subside with limitation of pain-producing activities, acute symptoms, especially when accompanied by radiculopathy, will abate more quickly and surely with a short period (3 to 7 days) of rest on a firm bed with the knees well supported. Gentle stretching of the lumbar paraspinal muscles, performed by pulling the knees to the chest, will relieve symptoms due to muscle spasm. Usually, NSAIDs will provide sufficient analgesia, although opiates may be needed initially. When ambulation can be tolerated without accentuating discomfort, bed rest should be alternated with increasing periods of ambulation, avoiding sitting as much as possible. This program is followed by a comprehensive back rehabilitation and fitness program that involves stretching (especially of the hamstring muscles), strengthening (especially of the abdominal muscles), aerobic conditioning, and instruction in proper posture and techniques for sitting, lifting, and standing (Fig. 14.7). If lumbosacral support is used as

ambulation is being resumed, it should be gradually discontinued as symptoms subside and the exercise program becomes well established.

Surgical intervention should be considered for unremitting pain in spite of adequate nonoperative treatment, a picture that suggests a sequestrated fragment. A second indication is found in patients with frequent and disabling episodes of back pain. Emergent intervention should be considered in the patient with myelopathy or who develops a nerve root deficit while complying with a nonoperative treatment program. *Microdiskectomy* and *percutaneous diskectomy,* which restrict visualization of herniated disk fragments and lateral root stenosis, have limited indications. Enzyme therapy *(chemonucleolysis),* which has approximately the same indications as surgery, has fallen out of favor because of the seriousness of its complications (anaphylaxis and transverse myelitis) and lack of efficacy for certain types of disk herniations, e.g., sequestrated fragments. Spinal manipulation may be useful for locked facets resulting from segmental instability.

Two other syndromes that represent end-stage degenerative disk disease are segmental instability and spinal stenosis. With thinning and damage, the disk becomes less able to resist shear forces. Associated ligamentous laxity may then allow rotatory instability, classically manifest as a sudden painful snapping or "catch" of the spinal facets with extension. Segmental instability may also be manifest by forward slippage of one vertebra on another, known as *spondylolisthesis.* Degenerative spondylolisthesis, which is especially common at the L4-L5 disk space, is predisposed to by degeneration of cartilage in the facet joints

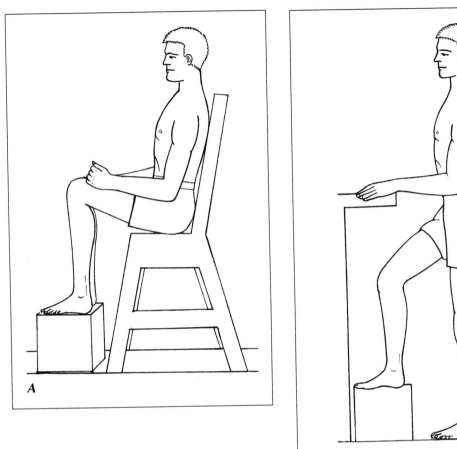
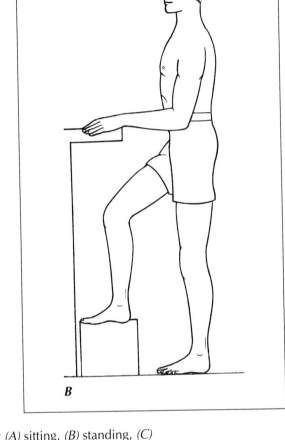

Figure 14.7   Proper lumbar spinal posture for *(A)* sitting, *(B)* standing, *(C)* lifting.

(Fig. 14.8). It is not associated with defects in the pars interarticularis, as is the case with spondylolisthesis of childhood.

Spinal stenosis, or narrowing of the spinal canal and/or neural foramina, is often associated with spondylolisthesis and is manifest clinically as neurogenic claudication (Fig. 14.9). Because spinal extension causes posterior bulging of the annulus with compromise

of the spinal canal and further displacement of the facets into the neural foramina, patients are usually more comfortable sitting (with the spine flexed) than standing or walking—a reversal of the picture seen with *acute* disk herniation. The pain and paresthesias that radiate into *both* buttocks and legs do not subside when walking stops, which differs from the pain of *vascular* claudication that subsides

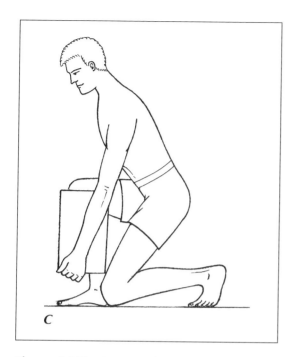

Figure 14.7   Continued

when movement ceases. Also, pain from neurogenic claudication proceeds from proximal to distal, whereas vascular claudication produces its initial discomfort distally and spreads proximally. Treatment of spinal stenosis is usually surgical.

Upper Limb

The joints of the upper limb, which are used more for activities that do not include superimposed body weight, are less affected by degenerative changes than those in the spine and lower limb; however, several joints in the upper limb commonly except this rule.

ACROMIOCLAVICULAR JOINT   Degenerative arthritis in the acromioclavicular joint may result from repetitive stress (e.g., occupational overuse), but it is more often a late sequela of

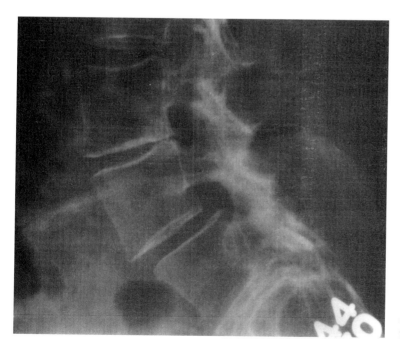

Figure 14.8   Degenerative spondylolisthesis of L4 on L5, which is caused by loss of cartilage in the facet joints posteriorly. This type of spondylolisthesis is not associated with a defect in the pars interarticularis.

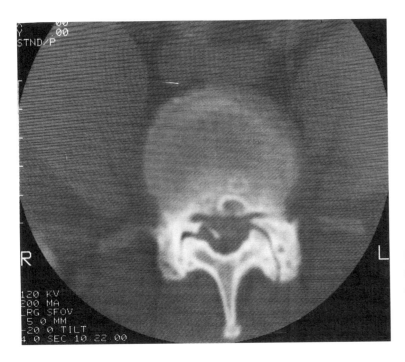

Figure 14.9 Spinal stenosis. Note narrowing and deformity of facet joints and protrusion of osteophytes into the vertebral canal on this CT scan.

joint damage from a fall or blow on the shoulder that damages the cartilage or results in joint incongruity (Fig. 14.10). Intermittent aching and tenderness in the joint are characteristic, especially after overuse and during bad weather. Lipping of the articular margins may make the joint more prominent, and compression of the joint by adducting the arm across the body often accentuates symptoms. The diagnosis is confirmed by pain relief following instillation of a local anesthetic and acromioclavicular radiographs that show either joint narrowing, osteophytes, or both. Rest, NSAIDs, and steroid injections usually suffice for mild, episodic discomfort; however, if symptoms are disabling and/or prolonged, excision of the outer clavicle provides definitive relief with little morbidity or loss of function.

GLENOHUMERAL JOINT   Although they may also occur without known cause, recurrent subluxations or dislocations, common in the glenohumeral joint, are most often responsible for degenerative changes in this articulation. Absent this history, other causes for these changes should be sought (e.g., avascular necrosis or metabolic forms of arthritis), since significant degenerative changes in nonweight-bearing joints are unusual. Because this joint is more critical to shoulder function than the acromioclavicular joint, pain and limited motion are more likely to cause significant disability. If nonsteroidals and rest do not restore adequate comfort and functional levels, surgical intervention in the form of joint replacement may be indicated. While rehabilitation is more prolonged than with most joint replacements, pain relief is equally striking, and motion is usually improved.

ELBOW AND WRIST JOINTS   Degenerative changes in the elbow and wrist joints are also

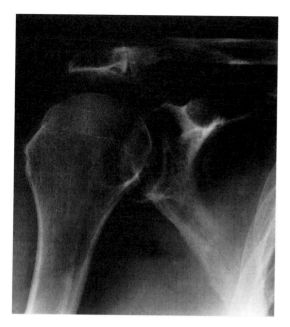

Figure 14.10   Degenerative arthritis of the acromioclavicular joint. Note the narrowing, sclerosis, and osteophyte formation.

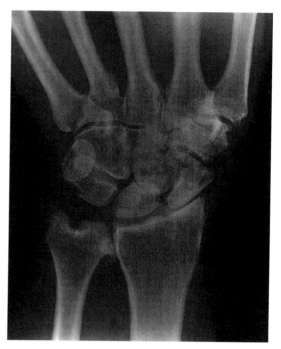

Figure 14.11   Radiocarpal arthritis. Note the narrowing and sclerosis between the distal radius and navicular. Degenerative changes are also present at the radioulnar and first carpometacarpal joint.

uncommon without prior injury. Fractures of either end of the radius, through cartilage damage or residual joint incongruity, may hasten wear-and-tear changes in the elbow or wrist joints (Fig. 14.11). The proximal end of the radius may be excised for severe symptoms; however, disabling arthritis of the wrist, whether from radial or carpal injury, often entails more complex surgical treatment, such as arthrodesis or arthroplasty.

CARPOMETACARPAL JOINT   Degenerative changes in the carpometacarpal joint of the thumb, a frequent result of occupational overuse, cause activity-related pain at the base of the thumb (Fig. 14.12). This condition is more common in the dominant limb and in women, perhaps because that digit is used extensively

in such activities as sewing, knitting, and typing. Rest in a splint and nonsteroidals constitute the first line of treatment. If these measures are unsuccessful, injection of steroids and a change of occupation should be considered, with arthroplasty or fusion of the joint as a final resort. Degenerative changes in the other carpometacarpal joints are rare.

INTERPHALANGEAL JOINT   Osteoarthritis of the interphalangeal joints usually accompanies generalized osteoarthritis. Proliferative changes at the joint margins of the distal joints produce *Heberden nodes;* similar proliferations in the proximal interphalangeal joints are

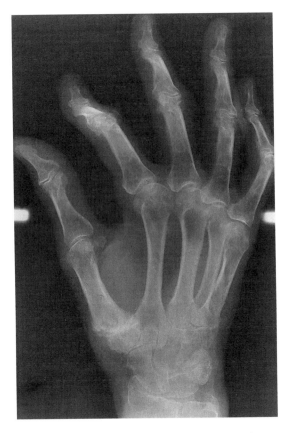

Figure 14.12 Degenerative changes in the carpometacarpal joint of the thumb, which may follow occupational overuse.

termed *Bouchard nodes* (Fig. 14.13). Although these changes, along with frequently associated radial deviation, are disfiguring, they rarely require specific treatment. Intractable pain is effectively relieved with arthrodesis.

Lower Limb

While primary degenerative arthritis of the upper limb is relatively rare and usually related to occupational overuse, weight-bearing forces increase the frequency and severity of this condition in the lower limb.

HIP JOINT   Primary osteoarthritis isolated to the hip often results from a preexisting disorder, such as congenital displacement, coxa plana, slipped epiphysis, or avascular necrosis. Although frequently difficult to incriminate in retrospect, it is likely that congenital displacement or dysplasia of the hip, which is more common in females, accounts in large measure for the greater prevalence of osteoarthritis of the hip in women.

Since both the clinical and radiographic pictures are striking and typical, the diagnosis is rarely difficult. Minor stiffness or pain aggravated by activity and relieved by rest is common, as is starting discomfort after prolonged sitting or lying. Stiffness upon arising is characteristic of both rheumatoid and osteoarthritis; however, osteoarthritic symptoms dissipate more quickly with activity. As symptoms progress, activity is subconsciously restricted, weight gain occurs, symptoms worsen, and activity is further reduced. As pain increases, muscle spasm is induced, which increases pain and further restricts motion, especially abduction and extension. Eventually, the pain radiates down the anterior and medial aspects of the thigh, following the course of the femoral and/or obturator nerves. Gradually, the hip becomes more fixed in flexion, adduction, and external rotation. The rate of progression is extremely variable; some patients become disabled within a year of the onset of symptoms; others experience little progression over many years. With progressive loss of cartilage and bone, the leg becomes shortened, which compounds the disability.

Characteristic findings on routine radiographs include joint narrowing, subchondral sclerosis, and osteophytes. Since these changes occur to some degree in asymptomatic individuals and symptoms of hip disease may be mimicked by other conditions, e.g., lumbar

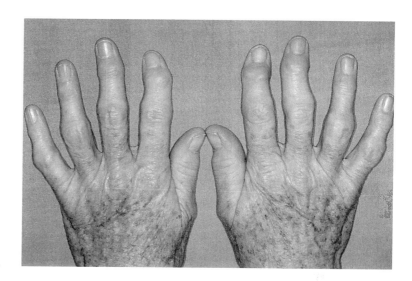

Figure 14.13 Heberden nodes (DIP joints), and Bouchard nodes (PIP joints).

disk disease, it is important to confirm the hip as the primary source of symptoms before undertaking treatment. Extension of pain below the knee and/or a neurologic deficit should, for example, suggest the spine rather than the hip as the source of symptoms.

The treatment of osteoarthritis of the hip should be tailored to the disability it is producing. Mild symptoms require only reassurance, observance of mechanisms for joint protection, and occasional analgesics. When a more aggressive approach is warranted, specific nonoperative measures should be considered: reduction or elimination of factors causing excessive joint loading (including obesity), physical therapy, drug therapy, and occasionally psychological counseling.

Among factors causing excessive joint loading, the most important is weight-bearing. Since each pound of additional weight results in the transmission of roughly $3\frac{1}{2}$ more pounds across the hip joint with each step, reduction of body weight, especially in the obese, is paramount. Modification of the workplace to permit sitting instead of standing and

obviate kneeling or squatting often reduces work-related disability significantly, as do frequent short rest periods during the day. Lifting and jogging should be avoided as exercises. Swimming is an excellent alternative. Use of higher chairs or stools for sitting and the avoidance of stairs should also be encouraged. While seen as an unacceptable admission of disability by many, use of a cane in the opposite hand may reduce weight-bearing forces across the hip by more than 50 percent.

Physical therapy includes the use of heat or cold and an appropriate exercise program. Since heat loosens tight periarticular tissues, exercise should be preceded by the application of heat, preferably moist. Ultrasound or diathermy are sometimes useful for such deep-seated joints as the hip. Exercises are designed to preserve motion, stretch contracted tissues, and strengthen muscles spanning the joint. Frequent short periods of exercise are preferable to single long periods. As a rule of thumb, any discomfort caused by the exercise should subside completely before the next set of exercises is undertaken.

It is important for both patient and physician to realize that drug therapy does not cure osteoarthritis, although it plays a critical role in symptomatic relief. The pain in osteoarthritis is multifactorial, with contributions from inflamed synovium, subchondral microfractures, and abnormal tension on scarred capsular and ligamentous structures. Cartilage, being aneural, is not a source of pain. In general, four levels of drug therapy are employed, depending upon severity of the clinical picture: analgesics, NSAIDs, phenylbutazone, and intraarticular steroids. Frequently employed analgesics include acetaminophen and mild narcotics such as propoxyphene (Darvon). If these agents do not effectively relieve pain, NSAIDs should be considered (Table 15.2). In general, they are likely to be more effective where synovial inflammation (warmth, erythema, and effusion) are present. Although producing less gastric irritation than salicylates, all NSAIDs inhibit prostaglandin synthesis and are thus to some extent contraindicated in patients with gastrointestinal complaints. It should also be remembered that NSAIDs, again through inhibition of prostaglandin synthesis, may diminish renal blood flow and function, leading to a rise in blood urea nitrogen (BUN) and creatinine (see Chap. 15). This complication is more common among the elderly, many of whom have nephrosclerosis. Indomethacin, for reasons yet unclear, has been reported to be particularly effective for osteoarthritis of the hip. Symptomatic improvement following intraarticular steroid injection is usual, although temporary, with shorter periods of relief after subsequent injections. Since animal experiments have shown a loss of proteoglycans in articular cartilage following intraarticular injections of steroids and potential harmful effects may result from overuse if symptoms are masked, repeated injections are not recommended.

Surgery should be reserved for patients with disabling symptoms in spite of the above measures. Joint replacement is usually the favored procedure, although osteotomy or arthrodesis should be considered for the young laborer with single-joint disease.

KNEE JOINT   Many of the same principles apply to osteoarthritis of the knee. Certain mechanical features of the knee, however, make it uniquely susceptible to wear-and-tear changes:

1. It has relatively little bony stability or protection.
2. It rests at the end of the two longest lever arms in the body and is therefore subject to great angular stresses.
3. Unlike the hip, where motions in all planes are permitted, certain knee motions must be restrained, which increases stresses on the joint surfaces.
4. Irregularities of the joint surfaces are common, most often from meniscal injuries.
5. Ligamentous injury is frequent, which allows abnormal motion and stress concentrations in the knee.

As with the hip, muscle forces acting across the joint amplify weight-bearing forces acting across the knee by approximately threefold.

Degenerative changes in the knee often begin in the patellofemoral joint, which is predisposed to abnormal wear by tibiofemoral malalignment or by an idiopathic condition known as chondromalacia patella, in which the patellar articular cartilage undergoes softening and degeneration (see Chap. 13).

As with degenerative changes in other arthritic joints, pain occurs after immobilization, subsides quickly with activity, and recurs with fatigue. Night pain is more characteristic of patellofemoral arthritis, as is pain with stair ascent or squatting. Discomfort is also increased by a drop in the barometric pressure, which allows distention of scarred joint capsules and stretching of pain fibers located there. Giving way or locking usually indicates a specific internal derangement, such as a loose body or a torn meniscus rather than degenerative arthritis—although the two often coexist.

The most characteristic physical finding is joint-line tenderness, especially if synovitis exists. Crepitus, resulting from joint irregularities, may be present during movement of the joint. If the crepitus is patellofemoral, it will be increased by patellar compression against the femoral condyle as the knee is actively flexed and extended. Effusion and warmth indicate more active synovitis. Progressive loss of cartilage may allow subluxation of joint surfaces with increased deformity, often manifest during weight-bearing as a sudden lateral (or medial) movement or "thrust."

The management of degenerative changes in the knee begins with an analysis of the roles played by contributing factors. Skeletal malalignments, such as bowlegs or knock knees—or even foot deformities—may contribute to the development of degenerative changes. In the latter cases, an appropriate shoe wedge may be surprisingly effective in relieving symptoms in the knee. Because excessive weight increases the disability of osteoarthritis, weight reduction is important for obese patients. It must be emphasized to the patient at the outset that this is not a condition that can be cured by a pill, an operation, or by any means, and that his or her cooperation and effort will be necessary for symptomatic and functional improvement.

Physical therapy is useful to maintain motion, prevent muscle atrophy, and relieve muscle spasm. Strengthening the muscles that cross a joint reduces stresses on the joint surface. Short arc or isometric exercises are less painful, and, since joint movement appears to retard cartilage degeneration, non-weight-bearing, range-of-motion exercises should also be performed regularly. Preliminary heat, preferably moist, enhances the effectiveness of an exercise program. Since they involve less weight-bearing, swimming and bicycling are preferable to jogging. Stoics must be cautioned against excessive exercise, which may aggravate symptoms. As a general rule, exercise-related discomfort should subside within several hours; if not, the program should be reduced. Use of a cane will significantly increase walking distance. In varus knees, the cane should be used in the ipsilateral hand, contrary to its customary use on the contralateral side.

Anti-inflammatory medications are used in the same manner as for the treatment of degenerative arthritis in other joints.

Those patients who have knee pain with each step (not just morning pain upon arising, which will not change with surgery) and who have anatomical alterations such as deformity, excessive cartilage or bone loss, or instability, should be considered for surgery. The surgical alternatives for osteoarthritis of the tibiofemoral joint are: debridement, osteotomy, arthroplasty, and arthrodesis.

The first two categories may be considered "therapeutic" surgery and the last two "salvage" surgery. Arthroscopic debridement is used for less severely damaged knees with torn

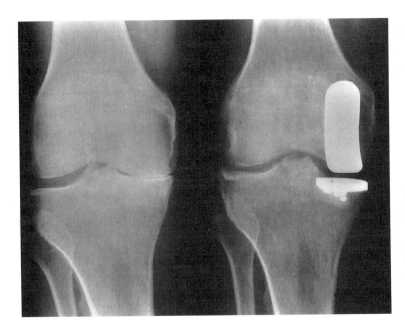

Figure 14.14
Degenerative arthritis involving the medial compartment of the knee treated by replacement of the medial compartment (*hemiarthroplasty* or *unicondylar arthroplasty*).

menisci or loose bodies but without deformity or instability.

Treatment of patients with unicompartmental arthritis of the knee by osteotomy of the proximal tibia or distal femur to shift weight-bearing forces from a damaged to the more normal compartment may be preferable for the patient under 65; however, such problems in the more elderly, because of the shorter rehabilitation period, are preferentially dealt with by partial or complete knee replacement (Fig. 14.14).

The need for complete replacement of the knee joint is suggested by the presence of degenerative changes in all compartments. Contraindications to replacement include local or systemic sepsis or claudication. When circulation is impaired, the increased activity afforded by surgery leads to increased ischemia.

The primary indication now for arthrodesis of the knee is failure of joint replacement, al-though fusion should also be considered for infection and in the young, heavy, male laborer whose occupation does not require significant knee flexion.

ANKLE JOINT   Primary degenerative arthritis in the ankle joint is rare. When present, it usually follows trauma to the ankle, such as repeated sprains or fractures involving the articular surface. Even when present, symptoms are rarely severe enough to justify arthrodesis, which is the cornerstone of surgical treatment. Replacement arthroplasty of the ankle joint is not sufficiently reliable to be recommended, especially for younger, more active patients. Ankle braces, such as the Aircast, and NSAIDs often provide gratifying symptomatic relief.

SUBTALAR AND MIDTARSAL JOINTS   Degenerative arthritis of the subtalar or midtarsal joints is also uncommon without antecedent trauma involving the articular surfaces. If a rigid, molded arch support and a supportive shoe do not provide sufficient relief, arthrodesis will, with little functional loss.

METATARSOPHALANGEAL JOINT   Degenerative arthritis in the first metatarsophalangeal joint is relatively common, usually in association with long-standing hallux valgus. When plantar- and dorsiflexion of the metatarsophalangeal joint are limited by limited osteophytes, the condition is referred to as *hallux rigidus.* If shoes with a wide toe box and rigid soles do not provide needed symptomatic relief, arthrodesis, arthroplasty, or resection of the proximal portion of the proximal phalanx (Keller procedure) relieves symptoms with little morbidity or late disability.

Nonarticular Disorders

Upper Limb

CALCIFIC TENDINITIS   Calcific tendinitis is a degenerative condition involving the tendons of the rotator cuff, commonly the supraspinatus, culminating in a localized deposit of calcium, which frequently causes inflammation of the overlying bursa (bursitis). It is one of the most frequent nontraumatic causes of shoulder pain, occurring in 2 to 3 percent of the adult population, although many deposits are asymptomatic. Middle-aged males are predilected, as is the dominant shoulder, which suggests a connection to use and activity. Over 25 percent of patients have bilateral involvement.

The shoulder is anatomically unique in having its intrinsic musculature located between the "pestle" of the humeral head and the "mortar" of the coracoacromial arch. With overhead use, the cuff is compressed by these two structures, which leads to increased wear. Since the lateral portion of the supraspinatus tendon is relatively avascular, repair cannot keep pace with breakdown.

Calcific tendinitis begins with cloudy swelling and culminates in tissue necrosis. The more alkaline local environment produced by necrotic debris favors, in a faulty attempt at repair, the precipitation of amorphous calcium hydroxyapatite crystals. The crystal is similar to bone crystal although slightly larger, but the calcium is laid down randomly on the collagen fibrils rather than with the 640 Å periodicity that occurs in bone collagen. Since circulation for the area is limited, there is little or no inflammatory response, which accounts for many patients being asymptomatic. If, however, the tendon fibers overlying the deposit rupture, bringing it into contact with the bursal floor, a painful inflammation is produced in the bursa.

The chronic form, without bursitis, is often clinically silent. In the acute form, the amount of pain is related to the extent of bursal inflammation. There is point tenderness over the greater tuberosity, and active abduction, especially from 60 to 90°, is often extremely painful. Accompanying spasm in the deltoid muscle may produce pain at its insertion. Intermittent aching or a "catch" sometimes precedes the acute picture by many years.

The diagnosis is confirmed by routine anteroposterior radiographs, with the shoulder in internal, neutral, and external rotation to visualize the entire rotator cuff. Chronic calcium deposits have hazy, irregular, ill-defined margins; whereas acute deposits are more sharply circumscribed, with distinct margins (Fig. 14.15).

Usually, calcium deposits resolve spontaneously, with subsidence of symptoms in 7 to

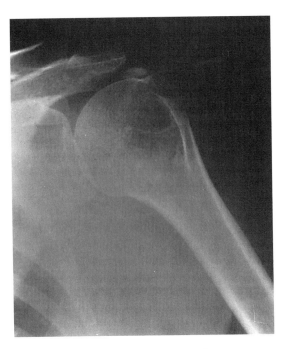

Figure 14.15 Acute calcific tendinitis involving the rotator cuff, probably the supraspinatus. Note circumscribed, distinct margins of the calcium deposit, suggesting an acute process.

10 days. The rate of absorption depends upon the intensity of the inflammatory response. More intense pain, indicating a greater inflammatory response, usually results in earlier rupture of the deposit into the bursa, with more rapid resolution. Large deposits may persist, with the periodic aching that discourages use of the shoulder and often leads to a frozen shoulder.

Acutely painful deposits are best treated by injection of a local anesthetic, with aspiration of as much of the deposit as possible and rupture of the remainder into the overlying subdeltoid bursa. The instillation of cortisone, although reducing the inflammatory response and pain, inhibits the fibrogenesis necessary for repair, so repeated instillation should be avoided. Adjunctive treatment includes ice, analgesics, and the temporary use of a sling. A small number of patients with recurrent or persistently symptomatic deposits require surgical excision, accompanied by division of the coracoacromial ligament and partial acromionectomy.

The most frequent complication of calcific tendinitis is a frozen shoulder, which follows limited use. Infection may follow injection or excision.

FROZEN SHOULDER   The term *frozen shoulder* or *adhesive capsulitis* refers to an acquired limitation of active and passive glenohumeral motion as a result of capsular contracture. This condition affects approximately 2 percent of the adult population, favoring females in a ratio of 3:2. Probably because of the correlation between the frozen shoulder and inactivity, the nondominant shoulder of older patients is predilected.

Restricted use of the shoulder invariably precedes the development of a frozen shoulder. Local or remote pathology, such as calcific tendinitis or a Colles' fracture, predisposes the shoulder to limited movement. Inactivity leads to venous and lymphatic stasis in dependent capsular tissues, followed by serofibrinous exudation and the deposition of fibrin, which forms adhesions between redundant inferior capsular folds.

Grossly, adhesions are present between the synovium and capsule, between the layers of synovial membrane that surround the biceps tendon, and between the walls of the subdeltoid bursa. Microscopically, the picture is one of dense connective tissue containing many fibroblasts. Fibrosis and fibroplasia cause retraction of the capsule, cuff, and even the adductor muscles. Disuse and a commonly associated vasomotor dystrophy may lead to marked osteopenia.

Although restriction of glenohumeral motion occurs slowly and to a degree that varies among patients, the loss is frequently unnoticed until normal activities become limited by stiffness and discomfort. Tenderness is common over the proximal portion of the biceps tendon. Especially in tense, highly strung patients, pain may lead to muscle spasm and chronic sympathetic overstimulation, with edema, sweating, and neurologic symptoms (hypesthesia and hyperreflexia) often extending distally to the hand, a condition known as the *shoulder-hand syndrome.*

The pathology may be demonstrated by an arthrogram, which shows capsular contracture. Whereas the normal glenohumeral joint has a capacity of about 15 mL, in frozen shoulders it is often reduced to 5 or 6 mL. Osteoporosis is the rule, and a calcium deposit in the rotator cuff is seen in 10 to 20 percent of patients.

For reasons that are unclear, this condition is usually self-limited. The time to recovery is proportional to the original degree of stiffness, but is usually less than 18 months.

There are three general types of treatment. The first is exercise, which should be gentle and frequent. The emphasis is on simple exercises that can be performed by the patient. Passive is followed by active-assisted and then by active-unassisted exercises only to the point of discomfort. The regimen begins with pendulum exercises and progresses to include abduction, forward flexion, external rotation, and internal rotation (Fig. 14.16). Ice may reduce discomfort after exercise.

Manipulation under general anesthesia may be useful in the tight or resistant shoulder that has less than 90° of abduction after 6 months of treatment. Exercises must be started promptly to maintain the motion obtained by manipulation. Continuous passive motion devices, which allow the patient to be ambulatory, reduce the cost and discomfort of hospital rehabilitation.

Operative division of tight anterior structures, including the capsule, subscapularis, and biceps tendon, is necessary only for extremely resistant cases.

Fundamental to the treatment of all frozen shoulders is the recognition and elimination of underlying or remote conditions that led to limited shoulder movement.

TEARS OF THE ROTATOR CUFF   These lesions are defined by a disruption of the tendinous portion of the rotator cuff, usually the supraspinatus, and commonly beginning at its insertion. Complete ruptures of the rotator cuff have been found in 5 to 33 percent of autopsy specimens on persons over the age of 60. There is no predilection of sex or side.

As with calcific deposits, the attritional changes in the cuff that result from its impingement between the coracoacromial arch and the humeral head lead to degenerative changes that, because of poor regional circulation, have little potential for repair. Thinning and weakening of the cuff by these changes predispose the tendons to rupture, often as the result of surprisingly little trauma. Tears of the cuff are rarely seen in young patients without massive trauma.

Tears of the rotator cuff may be complete or incomplete. Complete tears usually begin as avulsions of the supraspinatus tendon just medial to its insertion on the greater tuberosity. Thereafter, divergent pull by the cuff tendons produces a vertical component extending me-

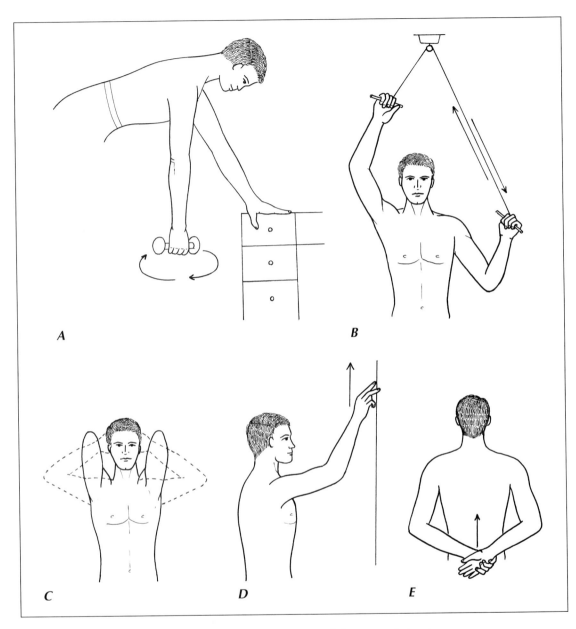

Figure 14.16 Exercises for a frozen shoulder: *(A)* pendulum, *(B)* abduction, *(C)* external rotation, *(D)* forward flexion, *(E)* internal rotation.

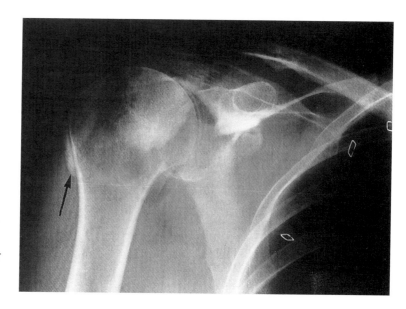

Figure 14.17 Arthrogram of the shoulder showing a tear of the rotator cuff. Extension of the dye distally beyond the attachment of the rotator cuff to the greater tuberosity indicates a torn cuff.

dially from one end of the transverse tear. From this L-shaped configuration, continued retraction enlarges the tear, which typically evolves from a triangular to an oval defect. In contrast to the degenerative tears in older patients, tears in young patients occur typically through healthy tendons, usually as the result of major trauma. A tear of the cuff should be suspected when a minor shoulder injury in an older patient is followed by persistent aching in the shoulder, especially at night and with overhead use. Long-standing cuff tears are often associated with selective myopathy: spinati atrophy and deltoid hypertrophy. In thin patients, it may be possible to palpate the defect or soft tissue crepitus. Passive motion is usually full, although large lesions (greater than 3 cm) usually preclude full active motion. With either active or passive movement, pain typically occurs between 70 and 120° of abduction, especially if the shoulder is not allowed to rotate externally as it is abducted. Large tears are usually associated with weak-

ness in abduction; with attempted abduction, superior migration of the head produces asymmetrical abduction. When the underlying biceps tendon is exposed by the cuff tear, as is often the case, it becomes subject to similar impingement and secondary bicipital tendinitis.

The diagnosis may be established by arthrography of the glenohumeral joint, although ultrasonography and MRI are increasingly reliable and are noninvasive (Fig. 14.17).

Cuff tears do not invariably require operative repair. Nonoperative management is accomplished by a sling and passive range-of-motion exercises performed three to four times a day. If symptoms do not abate within a month, surgery should be considered; otherwise progressive enlargement of the tear makes repair more difficult and compromises surgical results.

Incomplete tears *(rim rents)* may occur in the superficial, deep, or middle fibers of the tendon. These lesions, while painful, produce less typical clinical and radiograph findings and thus defy diagnosis. Definitive diagnosis and treatment may require surgery.

Large, long-standing tears frequently allow proximal migration of the humeral head with secondary degenerative changes in the joint, a condition termed *cuff-tear arthropathy.* In the advanced stage of this disorder, a bumpy, deformed humeral head may erode the overlying acromioclavicular arch.

IMPINGEMENT SYNDROME   *Impingement syndrome* is the term for a condition in which the interval between the humeral head and the overlying coracoclavicular arch is, for any reason, narrowed, subjecting the rotator cuff to abnormal compressive forces and accelerated degenerative changes. It often precedes a cuff tear or a frozen shoulder. The condition is especially common in persons between the ages of 25 and 55. No predilection for sex or side has been noted.

A common predisposing factor is an abnormality of the acromion that results in narrowing of the humeroacromial interval. Such abnormalities may be congenital or acquired. The acquired variety is more common and results from spur formation on the anteroinferior aspect of the acromion, which may be related to excessive overhead use of the limb, as occurs in certain occupations and sports. Weakness of the muscles that depress the humeral head (biceps and rotators) has also been incriminated.

Neer has described the pathology of rotator cuff impingement in three stages: I, edema and hemorrhage; II, tendinitis and fibrosis; and III, tendon ruptures and bone changes. If compression is unrelieved, stage I, which is reversible, often progresses to stage III, which is irreversible.

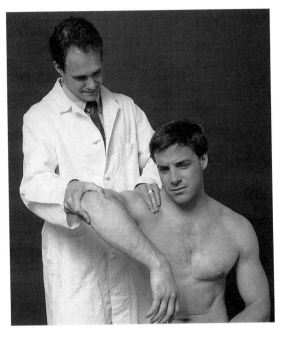

Figure 14.18   Positive impingement sign. Abduction of the internally rotated shoulder produces pain just distal to the anterior acromion.

Patients commonly complain early of chronic aching in the shoulder that is more noticeable at night and with active abduction of the shoulder, especially in the arc between 60 and 120°. Accentuation of the pain occurs if the shoulder is passively elevated in the internally rotated position and slightly forward of the coronal plane of the body (positive *impingement sign*) (Fig. 14.18). Tenderness is present just below the anterolateral acromion and over the bicipital groove. With disuse or tendon rupture, weakness and atrophy follow.

Another useful diagnostic finding is relief of pain following injection of a local anesthetic into the acromiohumeral interval (positive *impingement test*).

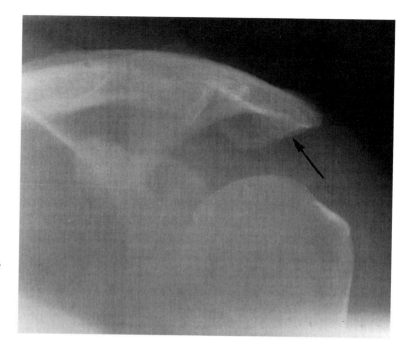

Figure 14.19   Spur projecting inferiorly from the anterior acromion *(arrow).* This spur was large enough to be seen on a routine anteroposterior radiograph.

Special radiographs are also helpful. Acromial sclerosis or spurring can be identified by a supraspinatus outlet view that profiles the anteroinferior aspect of the acromion (Fig. 14.19). An axillary view aids in the identification of a bipartite acromion and in recognition of degenerative changes in the acromioclavicular joint. Arthrography is specific for the diagnosis of a cuff tear.

Avoidance of pain-producing activities forms the cornerstone of treatment for stages I and II, which are often reversible by gentle, daily stretching and strengthening exercises to restore flexibility (especially in adduction and internal rotation) and strength (especially of the rotator muscles). If symptoms persist for over 6 months despite these measures, anterior acromioplasty, with excision of the coraco-acromial ligament and bursectomy, should be considered. In stage III, the surgical proce-

dures are extended to include repair of the rotator cuff (and biceps tendon if ruptured) and excision of the outer clavicle if there are degenerative changes in the acromioclavicular joint.

A frozen shoulder may result from disuse of the shoulder during any stage of impingement. Complications occurring in stage III are bicipital tendinitis and rupture and cuff tear arthropathy.

TENNIS ELBOW   Tennis elbow is an overuse syndrome involving rupture of aponeurotic extensor fibers at their origin from the lateral epicondyle or, less often, of the flexor aponeurosis from the medial epicondyle. This condition favors the dominant elbow of male patients over the age of 30, especially those with occupations that entail repetitive motions of the elbow while grasping an implement. It results from repetitive loading of the extensor or flexor musculature, as occurs in activities requiring grasping or lifting with repeated flexion and extension of the elbow, especially when pronation and supination are added.

Partial rupture of the aponeurotic origin, which may be evident only microscopically, leads to an inflammatory reaction followed by the formation and maturation of a collagenous scar, which "heals" the rupture.

Epicondylar pain in the predominant clinical finding, ranging from mild and nonincapacitating to acute and disabling. It is exacerbated by activities producing tension in the finger or wrist extensors or flexors. There is tenderness over the epicondyle and often around the radial neck (annular ligament). Symptoms diminish with subsidence of the inflammatory reaction, which may induce a false sense of recovery, since several additional months must pass before the scar is sufficiently mature to withstand vigorous use.

With few exceptions, patients who have not had multiple cortisone injections can be successfully treated without surgery. Rest, ice, analgesics, and gentle, passive stretching exercises are the essentials of treatment. The use of a sling may be temporarily necessary for severe symptoms; however, casts are contraindicated. As acute symptoms subside, strengthening exercises should be added, since the strength of a muscle's tendinous attachment parallels the strength in that muscle. Injection of a local anesthetic will relieve acute symptoms, and scarifying the epicondyle with the needle fosters healing. Infiltration with cortisone relieves pain because of its anti-inflammatory effect, although repeated injections prevent formation of the scar tissue necessary for healing. Surgery is indicated for persistent

symptoms and usually entails stripping of the lateral epicondyle, with transfer of the origin of the extensor aponeurosis distal to the elbow.

OLECRANON BURSITIS   Although many bursae have been described about the elbow, only one, the *olecranon bursa,* has clinical significance. This bursa, situated between the tip of the olecranon and the skin, is subject to repetitive friction and compression by activities or occupations that entail leaning on the elbow, although it may be produced by a single injury.

The diagnosis is made from a history of trauma to the area, followed by the appearance of a fluctuant, nontender swelling. Redness and tenderness, especially if associated with an open injury and fever, should alert the physician to the possibility of *septic* bursitis. Radiographs contribute little to the diagnosis, although an olecranon spur is frequently present.

Treatment depends largely upon the chronicity of the lesion. For acute bursitis, aspiration, compression, and avoidance of the offending trauma usually suffice. If infection is suspected, the aspirated fluid should be stained and cultured, and, if organisms are found, open surgical drainage carried out. In chronic cases, the bursal sac is thickened and usually contains fibrinous loose *"rice" bodies.* For such patients, excision of the bursa may be necessary to eliminate the swelling.

GANGLION   A ganglion is a benign cystic structure with fibrous walls that contains clear, mucinous fluid and is associated with degenerative changes in a nearby joint capsule or tendon sheath. It occurs usually between the ages of 15 and 35, with no gender predilection. It is most commonly found on the radial and dorsal aspects of the wrist.

Clinically, ganglia present nontender, localized swellings that sometimes induce mild discomfort from compression of adjacent structures (Fig. 14.20). Gradual enlargement is common. The lesion is firm and somewhat mobile, depending upon the length of its pedicle. Unlike the dorsal tenosynovitis of rheumatoid arthritis, with which a dorsoradial ganglion may be confused, extension of the fingers does not cause tucking-in of the most distal portion of the swelling (negative *tuck sign*).

Treatment is indicated for discomfort, neural compression, or cosmesis. Aspiration, even with a large-bore needle, is usually ineffective. Surgical excision is the treatment of choice, although it must not be undertaken casually, since recurrence is common after incomplete excision.

TRIGGER FINGER OR THUMB   This term refers to a localized stenosis of the digital flexor tendon sheath, with secondary nodule formation in the tendons, which often limits active (and occasionally passive) motion and produces a snapping sensation during flexion and extension of the affected digit. The condition occurs often in adults with rheumatoid arthritis; the idiopathic variety favors middle-aged females. In children, the condition is congenital, with the digit (usually the thumb) fixed in the flexed position.

In patients with rheumatoid arthritis, synovial inflammation and scarring lead to thickening and stenosis of the tendon sheath and eventually to invasion and localized thickening and nodule formation in the tendon itself.

In the idiopathic variety, *stenosing tenosynovitis,* which causes thickening and scarring of the tendon sheath, is the primary pathologic process. The lining layer of synovial cells is thickened by extensive fibrosis, which occasionally evolves to fibrocartilaginous metaplasia. Secondarily, nodules develop in the tendon; with passage in and out of the proximal end of the sheath, these cause snapping during flexion and extension.

Patients with trigger fingers experience difficulty during flexion and extension of the digit, especially the proximal interphalangeal joint, often with a sensation of snapping. There may be a small, tender, palpable nodule that moves with the sheath of the flexor tendon. If the disproportion between the thickened tendon and the contracted opening in the tendon sheath becomes sufficiently great, the tendon can no longer glide into the tendon sheath and the joint becomes trapped, usually in flexion. In the adult, nodules are less frequent in thumb than in finger tendons, so that locking is less common in the thumb.

Persistence of the condition in spite of splinting and one injection of hydrocortisone suggests the need for operative release of the tendon sheath and excision of nodules in the tendon.

DEQUERVAIN DISEASE   DeQuervain disease is a localized stenosis of the common sheath of the abductor pollicis longus and the extensor pollicis brevis tendons at the wrist. Middle-aged females are predilected. Occasionally, there is an enlarged or deformed radial styloid process; however, the usual predisposing factor is repetitive use of the thumb, as in cutting or sewing.

The pathologic changes are the same as those encountered in trigger thumb, although

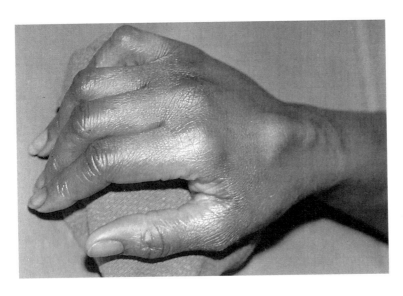

Figure 14.20   Ganglion. These cystic degenerative lesions are commonly located on the dorsoradial aspect of the wrist.

nodules do not form in the tendon and locking of the digit does not occur.

This condition is usually more painful than a trigger thumb. The pain is reproduced by ulnar deviation of the wrist with the thumb flexed (positive *Finkelstein's test*) (Fig. 14.21). Because there are no nodules or locking, there is no snapping with movement of the thumb.

If NSAIDs, rest of the digit by splinting, and steroid injection do not eliminate triggering,

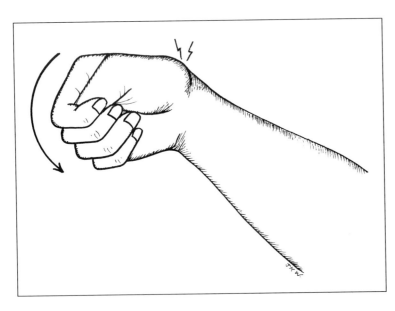

Figure 14.21   Finkelstein's test. Ulnar deviation of the wrist with the thumb flexed in the palm produces pain over the radial styloid process in de Quervain disease.

surgical release of the constriction in the tendon sheath is indicated.

Lower Limb

BURSITIS   Bursae are sacs lined with synovial tissue that exist normally between tendon and bone or tendon and skin to protect the tendons from compression and/or friction at their insertional sites. When pressure or excessive friction is applied to these bursae, the synovial lining becomes inflamed, which increases the production of synovial fluid to further "cushion" the tendon. At unexpected sites of friction caused by bony prominences, metal implants, or constricting shoes, adventitious bursae may form from pluripotential connective tissue cells in the region.

Three major bursae existing normally about the *hip* may be of clinical significance: the iliopectineal or iliopsoas bursa, the ischiogluteal bursa, and the trochanteric bursae.

The *iliopectineal* bursa is located between the iliopsoas muscle and pelvis above, and the anterior hip joint capsule below (Fig. 14.22A). It frequently communicates with the hip joint. Inflammation in this bursa is felt as pain in the groin, often radiating into the anterior thigh. Increasing pain with ambulation and tenderness over the anterior aspect of the hip muddy the distinction between this condition and arthritis of the hip. A subtle difference lies in the fact that the pain of iliopectineal bursitis is increased by isometric flexion of the hip against resistance, which is an uncommon finding in the arthritic hip. There are no definitive laboratory tests, and radiographs are useful only to rule out arthritis. Treatment consists of rest, NSAIDs, and application of ice (if early and acute) or heat (if late and chronic) until reso-

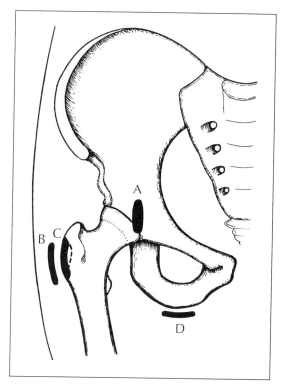

Figure 14.22   Bursae about the hip: A, iliopectineal; B, superficial trochanteric; C, deep trochanteric; D, ischiogluteal.

lution occurs, which may be expected in a matter of weeks.

There are two *trochanteric* bursae: a deep bursa that lies above the tendinous portion of the gluteus maximus muscle behind the trochanter and a superficial bursa that rests between the lateral aspect of the trochanter and the skin and subcutaneous tissue (Fig. 14.22B and C). Either may become inflamed, producing pain and tenderness in the trochanteric area. Swelling and redness are more apparent when the superficial bursa is involved, and pain is reproduced by marked adduction of the

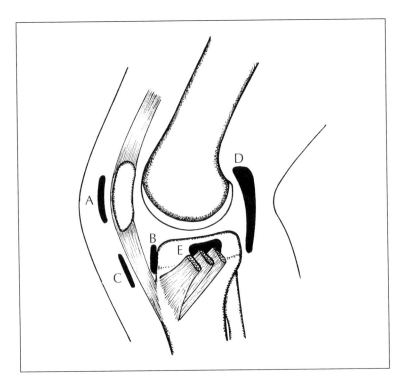

Figure 14.23 Bursae about the knee: A, prepatellar; B, deep infrapatellar; C, superficial pretibial; D, popliteal; E, anserine.

hip. With inflammation of the deep bursa, the hollow behind the greater trochanter is obliterated and the leg tends to be held in abduction and external rotation. Pain emanating from the deep bursa is reproduced by passive internal rotation and adduction or active external rotation and abduction.

After ruling out infection of the femur and/or hip joint, trochanteric bursitis may be treated by rest, NSAIDs, and avoidance of pain-producing positions or movements. Although usually unnecessary, cortisone instillation may hasten recovery. Care must be taken to avoid placing cortisone into the tendon, and the injection should not be repeated.

The *ischiogluteal* bursa is located superficial to the tuberosity of the ischium and is sub-

ject to irritation in persons whose occupations involve prolonged sitting, especially on hard surfaces, such as tailors or weavers *("weaver's bottom")*, truck drivers, and boatmen (Fig. 14.22D). Buttock pain is reproduced by direct pressure over the ischium and straight leg raising. The sciatic nerve, which lies nearby, may be irritated by the inflamed bursa, producing a picture of sciatica that is difficult to distinguish from that of lumbar disk disease. Avoidance of pressure and NSAIDs usually effect cure.

While there are some 18 bursal sacs about the *knee*, those of clinical importance are the prepatellar, deep infrapatellar, superficial pretibial, popliteal, and anserine bursae (Fig. 14.23A through *E*).

The *prepatellar* bursa, which lies anterior

to the lower patella and upper patellar ligament, becomes inflamed after repeated or prolonged kneeling, leading to its designation as
"housemaid's knee." Since splinters and needles may be encountered in this position, the
superficial swelling, redness, and tenderness
resulting from simple friction must be distinguished from that of an infected bursa by aspiration and culture of bursal fluid. Avoidance
of repeated irritation as well as the use of
NSAIDs and heat will usually effect a cure.
Infected bursae are treated by drainage and antibiotics.

The *deep infrapatellar* bursa is situated between the lower portion of the patellar tendon
and the upper tibia. Swelling here obliterates
the depressions that normally occupy either
side of the patellar tendon. Pain is reproduced
by passive flexion and active extension of the
knee, both of which compress the tendon
against the inflamed bursa.

Inflammation of the *superficial pretibial*
bursa, which overlies the insertion of the patellar tendon, follows acute or repetitive
trauma and is distinguishable from prepatellar
bursitis primarily by its location. Treatment is
similar to that for prepatellar bursitis.

Inflammation of the bursa at the insertion of
the *anserine* tendons is more difficult to diagnose, especially if it is not considered. The
condition occurs typically in individuals car-
rying out strenuous weight-bearing exercises.
Pain and tenderness localized to the antero-
medial face of the upper tibia are constant but
must be distinguished from that caused by
sprains of the medial collateral ligament, medial meniscal injury, and arthritis in the medial
compartment of the knee. Significant injury
usually precedes ligamentous or meniscal pathology, and radiographs will define the status
of the joint. Rest, heat, and NSAIDs form the
keystones of treatment, although recovery
from particularly acute or recalcitrant episodes
may be hastened by an injection of cortisone.

Of the many *popliteal* bursae, inflammation
in the one that exists between the medial head
of the gastrocnemius and the semimembrano-
sus *"Baker's cyst"* (or *popliteal cyst*) is the
most common. Since this bursa usually communicates with the synovial cavity of the knee,
intraarticular pathology that causes an effusion
in the joint produces distention of the bursa,
resulting in a painless, nontender, mass in the
popliteal area. Unless it ruptures, patients are
usually unaware of small enlargements of this
bursa, simulating a muscle tear or thrombophlebitis. Confirmation of the diagnosis is by
arthrography, and treatment entails correction
of the underlying intraarticular pathology. Except for extremely large cysts, seen most commonly in patients with rheumatoid arthritis,
surgical removal of the cyst itself is rarely necessary.

Two bursae exist to protect the insertion of
the Achilles' tendon: superficial and deep (Fig.
14.24*A* and *B*). The *superficial calcaneal
bursa* intervenes between the insertion of the
Achilles' tendon and the skin to protect the
tendon from the pressure of a tight shoe. A
second, larger, bursa, the *deep calcaneal
bursa,* pads the tendon just proximal to its insertion into the calcaneus. Bursitis in this location is more likely to result from abnormal
prominence of the posterosuperior angle of the
calcaneus. Localized redness and swelling are
less prominent with deep calcaneal bursitis,
and symptoms are increased by passive dorsiflexion of the ankle. The frequent occurrence
of calcaneal bursitis in women who wear
close-fitting high-heeled shoes has led to their

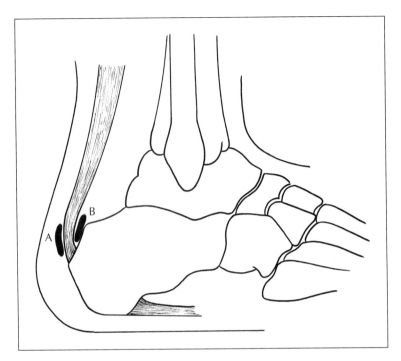

Figure 14.24   Calcaneal bursae: A, superficial; B, deep.

descriptive designation as *"pump bumps"* (Fig. 14.25).

Successful treatment of inflammation in either bursa requires that the offending pressure be relieved, which usually entails a change or modification of footwear. A 1/2-in heel lift (bilaterally) and NSAIDs are useful adjunctive treatment. If lateral radiographs of the foot reveal posterosuperior prominence of the calcaneus in the face of recalcitrant symptoms, ostectomy of this portion of the bone may be indicated.

Mechanical irritation of the *metatarsal bursae* that lie beneath the metatarsal heads is one of the causes of *metatarsalgia.* Obesity, prolonged standing, and thin-soled, high-heeled shoes predispose to this condition. In addition to metatarsal pain, the condition is manifest clinically by tenderness and swelling beneath the metatarsal heads. Often, the bursal effusion is palpable. This condition responds readily to correction of the predisposing factors mentioned above, with the addition of metatarsal bars to the shoes, which is the most effective means of relieving weight-bearing pressure on the metatarsal heads.

TENDINITIS Tendinitis is perhaps the most common manifestation of overuse, which occurs when the load placed on the musculotendinous unit exceeds its ability to meet this demand. The condition occurs frequently in deconditioned persons who attempt to compensate for a sedentary work week by prolonged weekend physicality. Additional predisposing factors are weight gain, which increases stress on the tendon, and aging, which reduces the elasticity of the musculo-

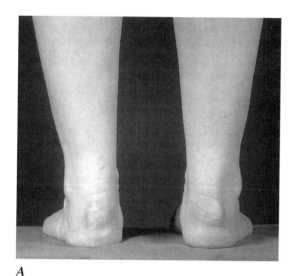

A

Figure 14.25 Bilateral calcaneal bursitis ("pump bumps"). *A.* Clinical appearance. *B.* Note the prominent posterosuperior angle of the calcaneus.

tendinous unit. Because tendons are less vascular than muscles, repair does not keep pace with attritional breakdown, which further predisposes the tendon to injury. Since healing is slow and problematic, prevention by regular stretching and strengthening of muscle groups used in sport or recreational activity is of particular value.

In the lower limb, tendinitis is most common in those tendons associated with extension of the knee and plantarflexion of the ankle, i.e., the quadriceps and Achilles' tendons. *Quadriceps tendinitis* may occur in the supra- or infrapatellar portions of the tendon at the junction of the tendon with the patella. Because jumping is associated with the delivery of explosive acceleration and deceleration stresses to the tendon, this condition is often referred to as *"jumper's knee,"* although it is also frequent in runners. Tenderness at the pa-

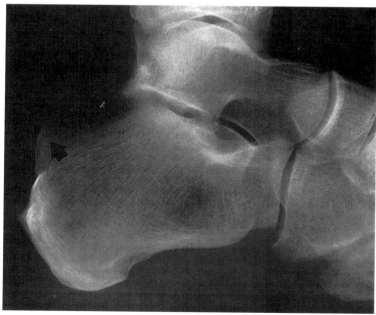

B

tellotendinous junction is common, and pain is reproduced by resisted extension and prolonged sitting or sleeping with the knees acutely flexed. Avoidance of pain-producing activity and posture is critical to resolution of this condition. Symptoms are minimized by icing immediately after exercise, but steroid injections are contraindicated because they further weaken the tendon. Since it is impractical to eliminate activities involving weight-bearing flexion and extension of the knee, it is difficult to achieve the rest needed for full recovery. If symptoms persist for longer than 6 months in patients who have been compliant with rest, stretching, and NSAIDs, surgical exploration with excision of scar and necrotic debris should be considered.

The occurrence of tenderness at the attachment of the tendon to the inferior pole of the patella seen in adolescent males and known as *Sinding-Larsen-Johansson syndrome* is a traction injury similar to that seen at the junction of the other end of the infrapatellar tendon to the tibial tubercle called *Osgood-Schlatter disease* (see Chap. 9).

Tendinitis also occurs in the distal portion of the iliotibial tract. This condensation of fibers of the fascia lata runs over the lateral condyle of the femur to insert at Gerdy's tubercle on the proximal tibia. Repeated passage of this tract over the underlying structures, most often a result of running, produces inflammation, especially in persons whose iliotibial tract is exceptionally tight. Tenderness over the distal course of the tendon is increased by its compression against the underlying structures as the knee is moved through its range of motion. This condition occurs often in association with *popliteal tendinitis,* which is also common in runners, especially cross-country runners who do a lot of downhill running. Rest, stretching

of the iliotibial tract, and NSAIDs form the basis of treatment.

Both tendinitis and stress fractures (another manifestation of overuse) in the lower limbs may be related to underlying metabolic bone disease (especially common in aging women) and in patients with pronated feet and increased external tibial torsion. Shoe inserts in the form of arch supports and outer sole wedges may be helpful for the latter conditions.

PLANTAR FASCIITIS   Plantar fasciitis is perhaps the commonest cause of heel pain. It favors overweight, middle-aged females whose activities entail prolonged standing. Gradual settling of the arch as a result of these factors increases stress on the plantar fascia, which runs between the medial tubercle of the calcaneus and the metatarsal heads. Continuation of this stress leads to tearing of the fascial origin from the calcaneus, followed by an inflammatory reaction. The plantar heel pain is typically reproduced by dorsiflexion of the metatarsophalangeal joints, and tenderness is confined to the medial tuberosity of the calcaneus. Classically, symptoms are worse immediately after periods of non-weight-bearing, as when arising from bed in the morning or from a seated position. Since rheumatoid arthritis, gout, and Reiter syndrome also cause heel pain in this location, a sedimentation rate, rheumatoid factor, and serum uric acid may be needed to exclude other etiologies. Lateral radiographs of the foot often disclose a small spur on the calcaneus at the origin of the plantar fascia, which makes excision tempting; however, such spurs are at least as common in asymptomatic patients, and excision is as likely to increase as to relieve symptoms; therefore, management of this condition is routinely nonoperative, consisting of well-molded, firm arch supports, weight reduction, shorter periods of standing, and NSAIDs. Heel cups are more effective for those patients with heel pain resulting from breakdown of the fat pad beneath the calcaneus. In such patients, tenderness is more diffuse and is not accentuated by stretching of the plantar fascia.

SUGGESTED READINGS

ANDERSON F, WILLIAMS B: *Practical Management of the Elderly,* 5th ed. Oxford, Blackwell, 1989.

BODEN SM, WIESEL SW, LAWS ER JR, ROTHMAN RH: *The Aging Spine.* Philadelphia, Saunders, 1991.

BRASHEAR HR JR, RANEY RB SR: *Handbook of Orthopaedic Surgery,* 10th ed. St Louis, Mosby, 1986.

CARSTENSEN LL, EDELSTEIN BA: *Handbook of Clinical Gerontology.* New York, Pergamon, 1987.

FERRARO KF: *Gerontology: Perspectives and Issues.* New York, Springer, 1990.

FRYMOYER JW, GORDON SL: *New Perspectives on Low Back Pain.* Park Ridge, IL, American Academy of Orthopaedic Surgeons, 1989.

HARMAN D: Free radical theory of aging: Effect of free radical inhibitors on the mortality rate of LAF1 mice. *Gerontology* 23:476, 1968.

HAYFLICK L: The cell biology of aging. *Clin Geriatr Med* 1:15-27, 1985.

KANE RL, OUSLANDER JG, ABRASS IB: *Essentials of Clinical Geriatrics,* 2d ed. New York, McGraw-Hill, 1989.

KENNEY RA: *Physiology of Aging: A Synopsis,* 2d ed. Chicago, Year Book, 1989.

MILLER MD: *Review of Orthopaedics.* Philadelphia, Saunders, 1992.

NEER CS: *Shoulder Reconstruction.* New York, Saunders, 1990.

SALTER RB: *Textbook of Disorders and Injuries of the Musculoskeletal System,* 2d ed. Baltimore, Williams & Wilkins, 1983.

Chapter 15

Rheumatic Diseases

Mary Anne Dooley and Frank C. Wilson

GENERAL ASPECTS

The rheumatic diseases include over a hundred disorders ranging in severity from localized tendinitis to life-threatening vasculitis. The diagnosis and differentiation of one disorder from another may be difficult, since findings are rarely specific or pathognomonic for any one disease. Moreover, the physician must exclude other conditions, such as infection, allergic drug reactions, or neoplasms in which arthritis is the presenting complaint.

Despite continued advances in radiographic and laboratory technology, a careful history and physical examination remain the keystones of evaluation. Most rheumatic diseases are systemic illnesses, with both general and local findings. Often the diagnosis requires repeated examinations or simply the lapse of time for nonspecific findings to develop into a clinically recognizable pattern. Indeed, during the development of rheumatic disease, patients are often seen for multiple, seemingly unrelated complaints that in time fuse into the pattern of a single diagnostic entity.

The medical history should include a detailed search for possible initiating events, such as viral or bacterial illness, medications, inoculations, recent pregnancy, environmental exposure (e.g., sunlight), or trauma. A history of previous episodes, responses to therapies, and family history are also important elements. Inflammatory disease is suggested by morning stiffness lasting longer than 1 h and *gel phenomena* (stiffness with inactivity) during the day. Joint swelling, discoloration, fatigue, or fever are also important features. The distribution of joints affected is significant in that monarticular disease is more characteristic of infection, trauma, or crystal-induced arthritis, while polyarticular involvement is more sug-

gestive of rheumatic disease. In addition, the distribution of polyarticular arthritis may provide helpful diagnostic clues.

The physical examination should pay attention to the skin, scalp, nails, and genital areas, as well as the musculoskeletal system. The emphasis given to various parts of the examination depends upon the patient's symptoms and the practitioner's diagnostic suspicions; thus, oral and nasal ulcers may be asymptomatic but important for the diagnosis of Reiter syndrome or lupus. A psoriatic patch in the scalp or pitting of the nails provides diagnostic clues for the patient with asymmetrical polyarthritis and sacroiliitis.

When a systemic disorder is suspected, each joint should be assessed for warmth, erythema, synovial thickening, deformity, range of motion, pain with movement, tenderness, and stability. Intraarticular disease produces diffuse pain with movement rather than pain localized to bony prominences, tendons, or ligaments.

Immunology

Most rheumatic diseases are characterized by inflammation, which may damage joints and/or other organs. While the specific etiology may be impossible to pinpoint, it is theorized that an abnormal immune response to an exogenous challenge often initiates the pathologic processes. Genetic influences determine to a large extent how the immune system reacts to antigens.

Immune Mechanisms

The cells of the immune system arise from pluripotent stem cells, which diverge into lymphoid and myeloid lineages. Specificity of the immune response is provided by lymphocytes. The two major lymphocyte populations include *T cells,* which generate cellular immune responses, and *B cells,* which produce antibody and generate humoral immune responses. After activation by an antigen, T cells can proliferate and become helper cells for antibody production, or they can become cytotoxic T cells. With few exceptions, T cells recognize antigens only when they are attached to molecules of the *major histocompatibility complex* (MHC) on the surface of the cells. There are two classes of cell-surface MHC molecules: class I molecules, which are present on the surface of all cells; and class II molecules, which are restricted to certain cells, such as macrophages, B cells, and activated T cell populations. In contrast to T cells, B cells are able to recognize free antigen in solution through their immunoglobulin receptors. B cells differentiate into plasma cells, which produce antibodies. *Cytokines* are hormonelike substances produced by cells, particularly activated T cells and macrophages. These proteins have a host of regulatory functions that influence cells involved in the processes of inflammation and repair.

Autoimmunity

Many rheumatic diseases have been considered autoimmune in origin because of characteristic antibody formation to self proteins *(autoantibodies).* Autoantibodies target a highly diverse set of antigens, including extracellular matrix, cell surface proteins, and molecules of the cellular nucleus (see below). The presence of autoantibodies alone does not explain fully the pathogenesis of rheumatic disorders, since relatives of patients with rheumatic disease may manifest autoantibodies without clinical disease. Furthermore, individuals with rheumatic disease usually have abnormalities of T cells and other components of

cellular immunity in addition to abnormal antibody production *(humoral immunity).*

Diagnostic Studies

Acute-Phase Reactants

Acute-phase reactants are a diverse group of hepatically synthesized proteins that are rapidly induced in the setting of inflammation or tissue necrosis. Well recognized examples include (1) the coagulation proteins fibrinogen and prothrombin; (2) transport proteins, such as haptoglobin, transferrin, and ceruloplasmin; (3) complement components, such as C3 and C4; and (4) proteins such as albumin, fibronectin, *C-reactive protein* (CRP), and serum amyloid-A–related protein.

In clinical practice, the tests most commonly used to detect inflammation are the *erythrocyte sedimentation rate* (ESR) and the CRP. The CRP is a more sensitive measure of inflammation than the ESR, since CRP levels respond to changes in inflammatory activity more rapidly; however, CRP is assayed by radioimmunodiffusion, which requires more sophisticated equipment and time to perform. Both the ESR and CRP are nonspecific tests, and both may be elevated in the absence of disease. The ESR is higher in women and rises with pregnancy, age, anemia, renal failure or trauma. It is important to note that elevation of the ESR is a specific diagnostic criterion of *giant-cell arteritis* (GCA) and *polymyalgia rheumatica* (PMR); its level is useful in monitoring the activity of these diseases. The ESR is also a helpful marker of disease activity in patients with rheumatoid arthritis (RA); it is less valuable in patients with systemic lupus erythematosus (SLE) and the spondyloarthropathies.

Autoantibodies

Autoantibodies are immunoglobins directed against self-antigens located in the intracellular, cell surface, or extracellular milieu. Detection of these proteins is problematic. Individual laboratories employ different techniques of measurement, which can vary substantially; and there is no widely accepted standardization of either methods or expression of results. Moreover, the titer of some antibodies fluctuate, and positive serologic tests may become negative with repeated testing. It is also important to understand that autoantibodies may be present in low titers in normal patients and in disease states other than rheumatic disorders, including infection, malignancy, and chronic liver disease. The use of certain medications is also associated with the presence of autoantibodies. For these reasons, one cannot base the diagnosis of rheumatologic disease solely on the presence of autoantibodies.

Antinuclear Antibodies

Testing for antinuclear antibodies (ANA) is most useful when the rheumatologic disease suspected is SLE, since the test is highly sensitive in this disease. In SLE, the ANA test is positive in at least 95 percent of patients, making the disease unlikely in a patient with a negative result; however, the usefulness of the ANA test is limited by its lack of specificity. A positive ANA test may be associated with other rheumatic diseases, such as systemic sclerosis, Sjögren syndrome, and rheumatoid arthritis. Older patients, patients with infectious disease, or patients taking certain medications (e.g., procainamide, hydralazine, phenytoin) can also have a positive test for ANA. A small number of patients on medication develop drug-induced lupus.

Rheumatoid Factor

Rheumatoid factors (RF) are primarily IgM antibodies directed against the Fc portion of immunoglobulin G (IgG). Rheumatoid factor is detected by agglutination of IgG-sensitized sheep red blood cells or latex particles coated with human IgG. Among patients with rheumatoid arthritis, high levels of RF are associated with severe disease, rheumatoid nodules, and extraarticular manifestations. Rheumatoid factors are not specific for rheumatoid arthritis and are also found in patients with sustained hypergammaglobulinemia, as occurs with chronic infections (e.g., subacute bacterial endocarditis) or chronic inflammation (e.g., *Wegener's granulomatosis,* a systemic vasculitis).

Complement

More than 20 biologically active proteins and inhibitors produced in the liver contribute to the complement cascade. Patients with hereditary deficiencies of certain complement components are at increased risk of autoimmune disease or recurrent pyogenic infections. The *classic pathway* of complement activation is responsible for the lysis of abnormal cells, such as virally infected cells, which are coated with antibodies. In contrast, complement activation by the *alternative pathway* does not require surface-bound antibodies. Complement may be assayed by techniques measuring either the presence of one of its components or its overall function. The best screening test for a complement abnormality is the CH50, which is a functional assay of the entire classic pathway. A low level suggests either complement consumption or complement component deficiency.

The activation of complement can be triggered by exposure to a foreign protein, especially one bound to a host antibody (immune complex). Examples of conditions characterized by the formation of immune complexes and subsequent hypocomplementemia include SLE (especially with nephritis), idiopathic membranoproliferative glomerulonephritis (GN), and serum sickness. Hypocomplementemia also occurs without demonstrable immune complex formation in hemolytic-uremic syndrome, septic shock, liver failure, severe malnutrition, pancreatitis, severe burns, malaria, and porphyria.

HLA Typing

The association of the HLA-B27 allele with the spondyloarthropathies makes this marker potentially useful in the evaluation of patients with musculoskeletal symptoms. In caucasian populations, the diagnostic sensitivity of this test is 95 percent in ankylosing spondylitis, 80 percent in Reiter syndrome, 50 percent in symptomatic spondylitis associated with inflammatory bowel disease, and 70 percent in patients with spondylitis and psoriasis. The prevalence of HLA-B27 positivity with spondyloarthropathy in other ethnic groups may be less than 50 percent. The utility of the test is also limited by the background prevalence of this genetic marker (6 to 10 percent in Caucasian populations) and the fact that only a small minority of HLA-B27–positive individuals ever develop a spondyloarthropathy.

Interpretation of Diagnostic Tests

The importance of proper interpretation of laboratory tests is underscored by the rheumatic diseases, which often cannot be diagnosed by single parameters. The utility of a laboratory test is measured by its sensitivity and specificity. *Sensitivity* refers to a test's ability to identify correctly those patients with a particular disease. *Specificity* refers to the test's ability to identify those patients who do not have the disease.

Two other measures of test performance are important: *positive predictive value* and *negative predictive value*. *Positive predictive value* refers to the probability that a patient with a positive result has a given disease. The term *negative predictive value* refers to the probability that a patient with a negative value on the test does not have the disease. The positive and negative predictive values are dependent on the sensitivity and specificity of the test as well as the prevalence of disease in the population tested. The higher the likelihood of a disease, the more likely that a positive test result is a true positive result, and that a negative test result is a true negative result. The relationship is such that a test is most helpful clinically when the pretest probability that the patient has a specific disease is meaningfully elevated.

For example, the clinical utility of RF testing is limited for the general population, despite being positive in 75 to 90 percent of patients with RA. The RF performs poorly as a screening test because of the prevalence of false-positive results (2 to 25 percent in persons over 75 years of age).

SPECIFIC DISEASES

Rheumatoid Arthritis

Rheumatoid arthritis (RA) is a systemic, autoimmune disorder of unknown etiology characterized by a destructive synovitis. The arthritis is typically symmetrical and favors the small joints of the hands, wrists, feet, and an-

Table 15.1 The American Rheumatism Association 1987 Revised Criteria[a] for the Classification of Rheumatoid Arthritis

Criterion	*Definition*
1. Morning stiffness	Morning stiffness in and around the joints, lasting at least 1 hour before maximal improvement
2. Arthritis of three or more joint areas	At least three joint areas simultaneously have had soft tissue swelling or fluid (not bony overgrowth alone) observed by a physician
	The 14 possible areas are right or left PIP, MCP, wrist, elbow, knee, ankle, and MTP joints
3. Arthritis of hand joints	At least one area swollen (as defined above) in a wrist, MCP, or PIP joint
4. Symmetrical arthritis	Simultaneous involvement of the same joint areas (as defined in item 2 above) on both sides of the body (bilateral involvement of PIPs, MCPs, or MTPs is acceptable without absolute symmetry)
5. Rheumatoid nodules	Subcutaneous nodules, over bony prominences, or extensor surfaces, or in juxtaarticular regions, observed by a physician
6. Serum rheumatoid factor	Demonstration of abnormal amounts of serum rheumatoid factor by any method for which the result has been positive in $<5\%$ of normal control subjects
7. Radiographic changes	Radiographic changes typical of rheumatoid arthritis on posteroanterior hand and wrist radiographs, which must include erosions or unequivocal bony decalcification localized in or most marked adjacent to the involved joints (osteoarthritis changes alone do not qualify)

[a] For classification purposes, a patient is said to have rheumatoid arthritis if he or she has satisfied at least four of these seven criteria. Criteria 1 through 4 must have been present for at least 6 weeks. Patients with two clinical diagnoses are not excluded. Designation as classic, definite, or probable rheumatoid arthritis is *not* to be made.

kles. Criteria established by the American Rheumatism Association (ARA) in 1955 and revised in 1987 highlight the importance of clinical findings to the diagnosis (Table 15.1). The existence of at least four of the seven criteria for at least 6 weeks establishes the diagnosis of RA. Laboratory tests, in contrast, are not essential or specific for the diagnosis. For example, approximately 20 percent of patients are negative for rheumatoid factor.

The initial pathologic event in RA is unknown, but it likely reflects activation or damage of endothelial cells in synovial tissue by one or more as yet unidentified agents. In addition to proliferation of synovial cells, an immune reaction develops in periarticular soft tissues. Polymorphonuclear cells accumulate in the synovium and in synovial fluid. Mononuclear cells—including T cells, B cells, fibroblasts, and plasma cells—gather and multiply around the small blood vessels deeper in the synovial tissue. Together, the leukocytes and synovial cells produce the *pannus,* a proliferative and invasive granulation tissue that often contains rheumatoid factors. As the disease progresses, periarticular bone and cartilage are eroded and destroyed, and the joint capsule is distended or ruptured, allowing subluxation or dislocation to occur. Loss of subchondral bone results in bony collapse and skeletal deformities, such as valgus deformities of the knees. Limited and painful movement from incongruous joint surfaces compounds disability.

Epidemiology

The prevalence of RA is 1 to 2 percent in most populations and increases with age in both sexes. Women are affected more often than men in a ratio of 2.5 : 1. The influence of sex hormones on the incidence of RA is suggested by the increased risk of disease in nulliparous women, decreased incidence in oral contraceptive users, and remissions with pregnancy. Exacerbations of RA are frequent in the postpartum period, and onset of symptoms at menopause is also common.

The role of genetic factors in the development of RA is suggested by familial aggregation of the disease, increased prevalence of the class II HLA-DR4 antigen in patients with RA, and a higher concordance rate of RA in monozygotic than dizygotic twins.

Clinical Features

The peak onset of RA is in the fourth and fifth decades of life. The presentation is typically gradual, with development of symptoms over a period of several weeks; however, an explosive, acute, polyarticular onset is occasionally seen. Early in its course, RA may lack the symmetry of joint involvement that characterizes the chronic state, but the appearance of RA as an acute, disabling, monarticular arthritis is rare and suggests infection as a more likely diagnosis.

Palindromic rheumatism is a clinical syndrome of isolated and less severe attacks of monarticular synovitis, usually lasting 3 to 5 days, with periods of complete remission. Approximately one-third of these patients will develop RA.

Rheumatoid arthritis is a systemic disease, and most individuals experience extraarticular manifestations that include morning stiffness, generalized malaise, or fatigue. In patients who are positive for rheumatoid factor, synovitis often affects areas of the musculoskeletal system other than joints, most notably the tenosynovium of the hands and feet, which may lead to ruptures of tendons, producing significant disability and deformity (Fig. 15.1).

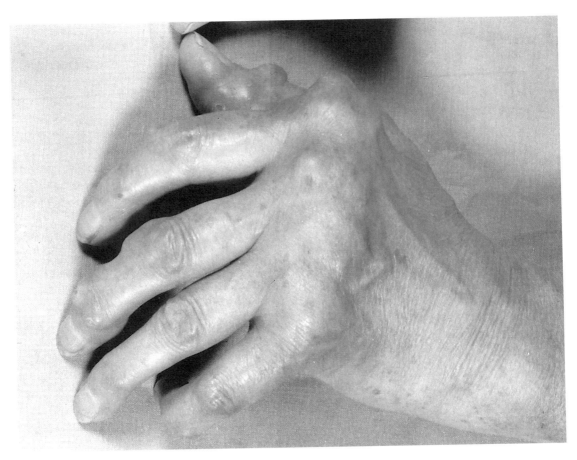

Figure 15.1   Rheumatoid arthritis (RA) of the hand. Note the rheumatoid nodules, ulnar drift, and metacarpophalangeal subluxation.

These complications may be prevented by tenosynovectomy. The presence of rheumatoid nodules or severe erosive disease is also associated with increased risk of extraarticular manifestations. Rheumatoid nodules are present in up to 50 percent of patients. They typically form over pressure points, such as the olecranon or Achilles' tendon, and can involute or disappear over time, although they commonly recur after excision.

Vasculitic lesions are frequent in RA; small vessels may be affected by a leukocytoclastic vasculitis, manifest by palpable purpura or small nail-fold infarcts. The presence of such lesions does not necessarily imply a coexistent systemic vasculitis.

Ophthalmologic involvement includes keratoconjunctivitis sicca and secondary *Sjögren syndrome*. Episodes of episcleritis are common. Scleritis occurs with more serious involvement and is termed *scleromalacia perforans,* which may result in loss of vision.

Pulmonary involvement in RA is common, but pulmonary symptoms are relatively infrequent because of lower levels of physical exertion. Solitary or multiple pulmonary nodules *(Caplan syndrome)* seen on radiographs of the chest are more frequent in the setting of exposure to environmental agents. Pleural effusions occur commonly and have characteristically low levels of glucose. Inflammatory pericarditis is found in close to 50 percent of patients with rheumatoid arthritis. Pain or altered cardiovascular function is uncommon, but chronic constrictive pericarditis may develop with time. Other cardiac derangements include inflammatory lesions similar to rheumatoid nodules that may involve both the myocardium and the valves, leading to valvular dysfunction and embolic phenomena, conduction defects, or cardiomyopathy. Aortitis may lead to dilation of the aortic root, with aortic insufficiency.

Involvement of the cervical spine is common and must be recognized. Clinical manifestations include cervical pain and stiffness, which may progress to devastating neurologic consequences. As with peripheral joint involvement, rheumatoid synovitis of the cervical spine damages ligaments and causes loss of articular cartilage and bone, which often leads to atlantoaxial instability and subluxation, with progressive neurologic changes and even death. Basilar invagination of the odontoid is a worrisome radiographic sign and constitutes an indication for surgical fusion (Fig. 15.2).

Radiographic hallmarks of RA in peripheral joints are osteopenia (versus the osteosclerosis of osteoarthritis), uniform narrowing of the joint (cartilage) space, and subchondral erosions (Figs. 15.3 and 15.4).

Treatment

Management of patients with RA is demanding and requires a comprehensive approach, including education, exercise, orthotics, medication, and surgery. Education is important for enhancing patients' psychological well-being as well as their ability to participate in self-care. Therapy includes range-of-motion exercises, strengthening, and cardiovascular exercises. Orthotics encompass walking aids, shoe modifications, and special devices for the hand. Physical and occupational therapy help maximize function.

Drugs are a particularly important aspect of the management of patients with RA; the major classes used are nonsteroidal anti-inflammatory drugs (NSAIDs), slow-acting antirheumatic drugs (e.g., gold), corticosteroids, and cytotoxic agents (e.g., methotrexate). Clinical improvement with drug therapy is variable. Complete control of synovial inflammation is uncommon, and relapses of synovitis may occur despite therapy.

The NSAIDs exhibit analgesic, antipyretic, and anti-inflammatory effects. Suppression of prostaglandin synthesis is the principal anti-inflammatory action of NSAIDs, which impairs the production of a host of mediators of inflammation including bradykinin, leukotrienes, and oxygen radicals. The NSAIDs have not been shown to affect the basic underlying disease processes.

Although NSAIDs are widely used for musculoskeletal complaints and are generally safe, serious side effects occasionally occur. Upper gastrointestinal bleeding may develop as a result of increased acid production and decreased mucosal proliferation. Thus, NSAIDs should be avoided in patients with peptic ulcer disease. Renal ischemia, caused by the loss of vasodilatory effects of renal prostaglandins, may lead to decreased creatinine clearance. Reversible hepatotoxicity, with elevated transaminases, is seen in up to 15 percent of patients receiving NSAIDs. Rare hypersensitivity responses include anaphylaxis or the syndrome of rhinitis, nasal polyposis, and exacerbation of asthma. All NSAIDs alter platelet function and increase bleeding time. Patients should be followed closely during the introduction of NSAID therapy, and periodic monitoring of blood counts, renal and hepatic function, and stool guaiac is advised for patients on long-term therapy.

In choosing an NSAID for an individual patient, dosing schedule and previous responses to therapy are important factors. The optimal dose of an NSAID varies considerably, even among patients with the same condition. Low doses may provide analgesia without significant anti-inflammatory effect. Patients with inflammatory arthritis generally require the maximum recommended or tolerated dose to achieve benefit. There is no clear advantage to combination NSAID therapy, and toxicity is increased. Patients often exhibit striking variation in response to different NSAIDs, and benefits may decline with prolonged use. A

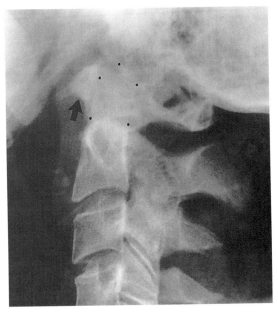

A

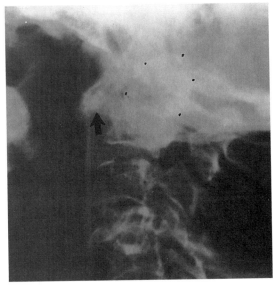

B

Figure 15.2   Involvement of the cervical spine in RA. The odontoid is outlined by dots. The arrow indicates C1. *A*. Normal for comparision. *B*. Instability of C1-C2 with displacement of the odontoid upward into the base of the skull. Note also the increased atlanto-dens interval.

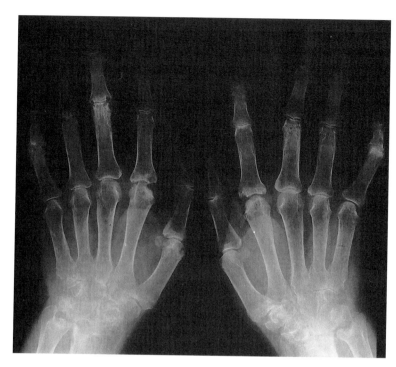

Figure 15.3 Rheumatoid arthritis of hands. Note the subchondral erosions of multiple small joints.

general recommendation is to select from another class of drugs when altering NSAID therapy (Table 15.2).

Many patients with rheumatoid arthritis require medications such as gold, steroids, or methotrexate in addition to NSAIDs. These drugs are associated with greater toxicities and more serious side effects than NSAIDs. Gold compounds are among the most effective agents for arresting florid synovitis or rapidly progressive disease. Toxic reactions develop in 15 percent of patients, most commonly affecting skin and mucosal membranes, which may preclude prolonged use. Corticosteroids are effective agents for symptomatic relief but do not stop progression of the disease. Side effects are well known, including adrenal insufficiency from rapid withdrawal, hyperten-

sion, hyperglycemia, obesity, osteopenia, peptic ulcers, susceptibility to infection, and osseous avascular necrosis. Immunosuppressants, such as methotrexate and azathioprine, have been used in low doses for patients with severe, refractory RA. Methotrexate is rarely associated with hepatic fibrosis and hypersensitivity pneumonitis, and, like azathioprine, can cause bone marrow suppression.

In the past, medications for rheumatoid arthritis were given sequentially, starting at the bottom of the "pyramid" with the least toxic drugs. When the diagnosis is certain, the use of more toxic agents may be warranted in an effort to stop or slow the progression of disease before permanent articular damage occurs.

Assessing the results of nonoperative management of RA is difficult. The effects of treat-

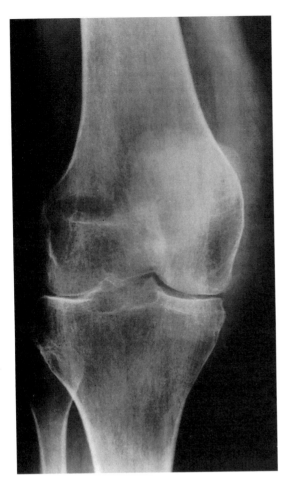

Figure 15.4   Rheumatoid arthritis of knee. Note the osteopenia, uniform narrowing of the joint and lack of osteophytes.

tures of tendons. Persistent, disabling arthralgia and radiographic evidence of joint destruction are indications for joint replacement, which markedly reduces pain and improves function in over 90 percent of patients. Joint replacements are most successful in the hip and knee, but replacement of other joints such as the shoulder, elbow, and metacarpophalangeal joints also reduces pain and restores function to severely compromised joints. Fusion or arthrodesis is also effective in relieving pain, but this approach must be used judiciously in selected areas, since stiffness is especially debilitating for patients with RA.

Felty syndrome is a triad of RA, leukopenia, and splenomegaly found in 1 percent of patients with RA. It occurs typically in patients with advanced erosive disease, systemic features, and a frequent history of infections. Some patients with Felty syndrome have increased numbers of large, granular lymphocytes, which may produce an apparently normal white blood cell count, but the lymphocytes do not function normally, and these patients have increased susceptibility to infections. Peripheral smears should be examined for these lymphocytes. Treatment of symptomatic patients includes corticosteroids or immunosuppressive therapy. Splenectomy has not been helpful.

ment may be monitored by the sedimentation rate, number of inflamed joints, and functional parameters. Plain radiographs do not capture early or subtle joint damage.

Surgical intervention is necessary when the disease progresses despite optimal medical management. Tenosynovectomy in the wrist and hand for uncontrolled synovitis may prevent the loss of function that results from rup-

Juvenile Chronic Arthritis (Juvenile Rheumatoid Arthritis)

Juvenile chronic arthritis (JCA), previously known in the United States as juvenile rheumatoid arthritis, is characterized by chronic synovial inflammation of unknown cause that affects children under age 16. Approximately 200,000 children in the United States are affected. The new terminology acknowledges

Table 15.2   NSAIDs by Chemical Class

Class	Generic Name	Brand Name	Tablet Size, mg	Dosage
Carboxylic acids	Acetylsalicylic acid	Aspirin	325, 500	325–500 mg q4–6h
	Choline magnesium salicylate	Trilisate	500, 750, 1000	1000–1500 mg bid
	Salsalate	Disalcid	500, 750	1000–1500 mg bid
	Diflunisal	Dolobid	250, 500	250–500 mg bid
Acetic acids	Phenylacetic acids Diclofenac	Voltaren,	25, 50, 75	50–75 mg bid
		Cataflam	50	50 mg tid
	Carbo- and heterocyclic acids			
	Indomethacin	Indocin	25, 50, 75SR	25–50 mg tid, 75SR mg qd
	Etodolac	Lodine	200, 300	200–300 mg tid/qid
	Sulindac	Clinoril	150, 200	150–200 mg bid
	Tolmetin	Tolectin	200, 400, 600	200–600 mg tid
	Ketorolac	Toradol	10	30 mg IM/IV q6h
Propionic acids	Ibuprofen	Advil, Nuprin	200	200–800 mg tid/qid
	Naproxen	Motrin	200, 400, 600, 800	
	Flurbiprofen	Naprosyn, Aleve	250, 375, 500	250–500 mg bid/tid
	Ketoprofen	Ansaid	50, 100	100–150 mg bid
	Fenoprofen	Orudis	50, 75	50–75 mg tid
	Oxaprozin	Oruvail	100, 150, 200	100–200 mg qd
		Nalfon	300, 600	300–600 mg qid
		Daypro	600	600–1800 mg qd
Fenamic acids	Mefenamic acid	Meclomen	50, 100	50–100 mg qid
Enolic acids	Phenylbutazone	Butazolidin	100	100–200 mg qd to tid
	Piroxicam	Feldene	10, 20	10–20 mg qd
Nonacidic compounds	Nabumetone	Relafen	500, 750	1000–2000 mg qd

fundamental differences between adult and pediatric arthritis.

There are three subtypes of JCA: pauciarticular, polyarticular, and systemic. No laboratory test is diagnostic for JCA; but the presence of rheumatoid factor or antinuclear antibodies may assist in classifying patients. Radiographs of joints are useful to establish a baseline and assess articular growth, but radiographic changes are not diagnostic, particularly in younger children with less ossified bone. There is no clear evidence of a genetic predisposition for JCA with the possible exceptions of familial spondyloarthropathy, which may be associated with HLA-B27, and pauciarticular disease in older children.

Pauciarticular Onset

Approximately 40 percent of children with JCA have a pauciarticular onset, defined as four or fewer joints affected within the first 6 months of disease. One subgroup of pauciarticular JCA is characterized by early age of onset (usually below age 6), female predominance, positive antinuclear antibody testing, and lack of systemic features. The knees, ankles, wrists, and elbows are the most frequently affected joints. Another subgroup is defined by older patients, predominantly males, about 50 percent of whom are HLA-B27–positive. The family history may be positive for spondyloarthropathy, and the arthritis is typically asymmetrical, affecting predominantly joints of the lower limb. Sacroiliitis may be present at the outset, either silently or symptomatically.

Eye involvement (iridocyclitis) develops in 10 to 50 percent of patients with pauciarticular JCA and usually begins with or precedes joint complaints, but it may develop as long as 10 years after the onset of arthritis. Chronic eye involvement is common and may lead to impaired vision. Children are usually asymptomatic, and only regular examinations by an ophthalmologist can detect early changes.

Polyarticular Onset

Approximately 40 percent of patients have a polyarticular onset of arthritis. This form of JCA may begin at any point in childhood, with girls twice as likely to be affected as boys. Findings include low-grade fever, malaise, growth retardation, weight loss, adenopathy, and anemia. Antinuclear antibodies are found in 25 to 40 percent of patients. Rheumatoid factor is present in approximately 15 percent, typically in children over 8 years of age at the onset of disease. The presence of rheumatoid factor heralds a more severe course of arthritis, with destructive and disabling joint disease occurring in approximately 50 percent, versus 10 to 15 percent in rheumatoid factor–negative patients. Impaired growth of the mandible may result from temporomandibular joint arthritis, leading to characteristic micrognathia (Fig. 15.5). Generalized retardation of growth can be seen with systemic and polyarticular JCA, and local overgrowth from the epiphyseal stimulation of synovial hyperemia may lead to significant limb-length discrepancies. Cervical spine involvement, characteristically at the C2-C3 apophyseal joints, occurs frequently.

Systemic Onset

A systemic onset (Still disease) occurs in about 20 percent of children with JCA. The ratio of males to females is approximately equal. Clinical manifestations include quotidian fevers, an evanescent, salmon-pink rash, generalized lymphadenopathy, hepatosplenomegaly, and pericardial or pleural effusions. Constitutional symptoms, including fatigue, muscle atrophy, and weight loss, may be severe. Antinuclear antibodies and rheumatoid factor are typically negative. About 25 percent of patients will subsequently develop severe, chronic arthritis that continues after systemic manifestations have resolved (Fig. 15.6). Approximately 50 percent of affected children have more than one systemic attack, ranging in duration from

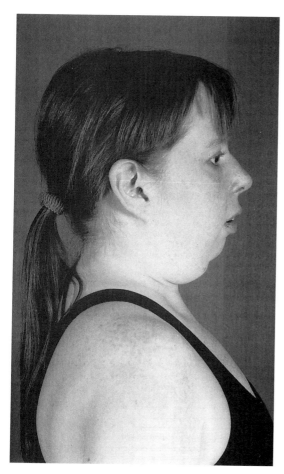

Figure 15.5   Juvenile chronic arthritis, polyarticular onset. Note the micrognathia.

days to months, even after intervals of several years.

Systemic Lupus Erythematosus

Systemic lupus erythematosus (SLE) is a systemic, autoimmune disease characterized by the production of numerous autoantibodies directed primarily against various components of the cellular nucleus. Females predominate in a proportion of at least 9 to 1, with higher ratios in the childbearing years. This condition is more common in certain racial groups, including African Americans, Chinese, and other Asian populations, and it has a familial prevalence.

Criteria for the classification of SLE were revised in 1982 (Table 15.3). Musculoskeletal complaints, including arthralgias and arthritis, are among the most common presenting features of lupus. The arthritis in lupus is characteristically symmetrical but nonerosive, affecting predominately small joints of the hand, the wrists, and the knees. Deformities of joints resulting from ligamentous laxity define *Jaccoud syndrome.* As rheumatoid factors may be found in the sera of up to 40 percent of lupus patients, an initial diagnosis of RA is not uncommon. Osteonecrosis is seen with increased frequency in lupus, even in patients not exposed to corticosteroids, and spontaneous tendon rupture is well documented.

The manifestations of lupus are protean, potentially affecting every bodily system. The best-recognized dermal manifestation of lupus is the "butterfly" or malar rash, which often follows exposure to the sun (Fig. 15.7). Discoid lesions are chronic, scarring cutaneous lesions that may produce atrophy and hypopigmentation. Approximately 25 percent of patients with discoid lupus progress to systemic lupus. A screening urinalysis in patients supected to have lupus is essential, as about 70 percent develop renal involvement and symptoms of renal involvement occur only with advanced disease. Abnormal urinary sediment, proteinuria, and rising creatinine levels are indications for detailed renal assessment including renal biopsy. Severe renal involvement

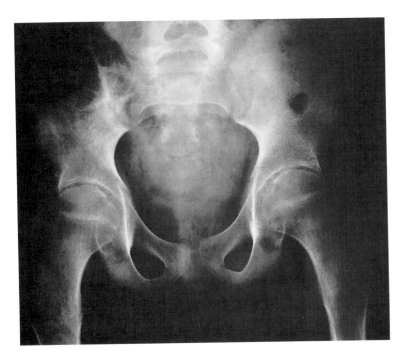

Figure 15.6 Juvenile chronic arthritis of the hips, systemic onset. Note the marked arthritis, osteopenia, and open physes.

may require high-dose corticosteroids and antimetabolite therapy. Serositis, presenting as pleuritis, pericarditis or peritonitis, is common in lupus. Neuropsychiatric manifestations are also frequent.

The correlation of disease activity with complement or anti-double-stranded DNA levels varies among patients with SLE, but serial measurements may be useful markers of disease activity for individual patients.

Seronegative Spondyloarthropathies

The seronegative spondyloarthropathies are a group of disorders associated with HLA-B27 that have similar clinical and radiographic features. Included in this group of diseases are ankylosing spondylitis, Reiter syndrome, psoriatic arthritis, reactive arthritis, arthritis asso-

ciated with inflammatory bowel disease, and Behet syndrome. Common clinical features include onset prior to the fourth decade, familial clustering, male predominance, prominent involvement of the spine and sacroiliac joints, *enthesitis* (inflammation at sites of tendon insertion into bone), and extraarticular features including eye, skin, and gastrointestinal manifestations.

Ankylosing Spondylitis

In the past, anklyosing spondylitis (AS) was considered to affect predominantly men; however, recent studies note a more even sex distribution, with milder disease in women. Women tend to have more peripheral joint and cervical spine involvement and are less likely to have progressive spinal disease. Ankylosing spondylitis predilects the sacroiliac joints, var-

Table 15.3   The American Rheumatism Association 1982 Revised Criteria[a] for the Classification of Systemic Lupus Erythematosus

Criterion	Definition
1. Malar rash	Fixed erythema, flat or raised, over the malar eminences, tending to spare the nasolabial folds
2. Discoid rash	Erythematous raised patches with adherent keratotic scaling and follicular plugging; atrophic scarring may occur in older lesions
3. Photosensitivity	Skin rash as a result of unusual reaction to sunlight, by patient history or physician observation
4. Oral ulcers	Oral or nasopharyngeal ulceration, usually painless, observed by a physician
5. Arthritis	Nonerosive arthritis involving two or more peripheral joints, characterized by tenderness, swelling, or effusion
6. Serositis	a. Pleuritis—convincing history of pleuritic pain or rub heard by a physician or evidence of pleural effusion OR b. Pericarditis—documented by ECG or rub or evidence of pericardial effusion
7. Renal disorder	a. Persistent proteinuria greater than 0.5 g/day or greater than 3+ if quantitation not performed OR b. Cellular casts—may be red cell, hemoglobin, granular, tubular, or mixed
8. Neurologic disorder	a. Seizures—in the absence of offending drugs or known metabolic derangements, e.g., uremia, ketoacidosis, or electrolyte imbalance OR b. Psychosis—in the absence of offending drugs or known metabolic derangements, e.g., uremia, ketoacidosis, or electrolyte imbalance
9. Hematologic disorder	a. Hemolytic anemia—with reticulocytosis OR b. Leukopenia—less than 4000/mm³ total on two or more occasions OR

Table 15.3   The American Rheumatism Association 1982 Revised Criteria[a] for the Classification of Systemic Lupus Erythematosus *(Continued)*

Criterion	Definition
	c. Lymphopenia—less than 1500/mm^3 on two or more occasions OR d. Thrombocytopenia—less than 100,000/mm^3 in the absence of offending drugs
10. Immunologic disorder	a. Positive LE cell preparation OR b. Anti-DNA: antibody to native DNA in abnormal titer OR c. Anti-Sm: presence of antibody to Sm nuclear antigen OR d. False-positive serologic test for syphilis known to be positive for at least 6 months and confirmed by *Treponema pallidum* immobilization or fluorescent treponemal antibody absorption test
11. Antinuclear antibody	An abnormal titer of antinuclear antibody by immunofluorescence or an equivalent assay at any point in time and in the absence of drugs known to be associated with "drug-induced lupus" syndrome

[a] For the purpose of identifying patients in clinical studies, a person is said to have systemic lupus erythematosus if any four or more of the eleven criteria are present, serially or simultaneously, during any interval of observation.

SOURCE: Tan EM, Cohen AS, Fries JF, et al: The 1982 revised criteria for the classification of systemic lupus erythematosus (SLE). *Arthritis Rheum* 25:1271–1277, 1982. With permission.

iably affects the rest of the spine, and affects the peripheral joints to a much lesser extent. Extraarticular manifestations—such as uveitis, carditis, or enthesitis—may occur. The association of HLA-B27 positivity with AS is strongest in Caucasian patients, with over 95 percent being HLA-B27–positive, compared to 6 to 10 percent of normal individuals. The sedimentation rate is frequently elevated, but there are no pathognomonic tests for AS.

Physical findings in AS include paraspinal muscle spasm and loss of normal lordosis. The degree of restriction of forward flexion can be documented by the *Schober test*, which measures the distraction of two points with flexion. The lower point is marked at the lumbosacral

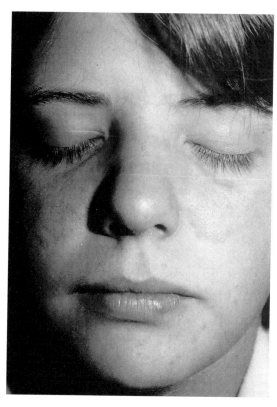

Figure 15.7 Systemic lupus erythematosus. Note the characteristic "butterfly" or malar rash.

junction and the upper point 10 cm above this level. Forward flexion in a normal individual produces distraction of 5 to 10 cm, versus zero to 7 or 8 cm in a patient with AS. Peripheral articular involvement with synovitis, particularly in the lower limbs, occurs in 20 to 30 percent of patients with AS. The frequency of peripheral joint involvement increases with the severity of the disease. Disease of the hip and shoulder may produce progressive contractures. A lower age at onset is also associated with more pronounced peripheral joint disease

and a greater likelihood of progression to joint replacement. Manifestations of enthesitis include plantar fasciitis, costochondritis, and Achilles tendinitis. Neurologic symptoms may result from cord compression by vertebral fractures or the cauda equina syndrome. Acute neck or back pain, especially following trauma, should raise diagnostic suspicion of a fracture through an ankylosed, osteoporotic spine. Fractures are most common in the cervical spine and may be difficult to identify on plain radiographs. A bone scan should be employed if diagnostic suspicion is high.

Early radiographic findings in AS include squaring of the superior and anterior margins of the vetebral bodies, which is produced by inflammatory disease at the insertion of the outer fibers of the annulus fibrosus. Later manifestations include bridging *syndesmophytes* (Fig. 15.8). Similar radiographic features, albeit less symmetrical, may be seen in seronegative spondyloarthropathy associated with inflammatory bowel disease, Reiter syndrome, psoriatic arthropathy, or Behet syndrome. Ankylosis of the spine in AS should also be distinguished from the bridging osteophytes of *diffuse idiopathic skeletal hyperostosis* (DISH), which is an advanced degenerative condition of the spine that occurs in the elderly. Patients with DISH have flowing hyperostosis at three or more vertebral levels, reflecting long-standing spondylosis (Fig. 15.9).

Nonmusculoskeletal features include fatigue, weight loss, and low-grade fever. Uveitis develops in up to 25 percent of patients with AS, occasionally with progressive visual impairment. The episodes are usually self-limiting but may require local corticosteroid therapy for control. The best-recognized cardiac feature of AS is isolated aortic insufficiency,

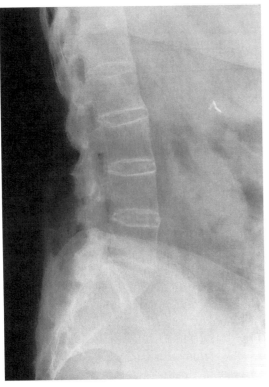

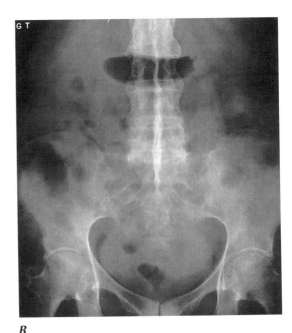

B

A

Figure 15.8   Ankylosing spondylitis. Note the bridging syndesmophytes.

although conduction defects, with varying degrees of heart block, also occur. Inflammation and fibrosis at the base of the aortic valve extending into the interventricular septum may lead to coexistent aortic insufficiency and heart block, for which valvular replacement and a pacemaker may be required.

Reiter Syndrome

Reiter syndrome, as described by H. Reiter in 1916, consisted of the triad of arthritis, urethritis, and conjunctivitis. In the past, patients with the triad were described as having the complete syndrome and patients with two features alone as having an incomplete syndrome. The current definition of Reiter syndrome is a seronegative arthritis that follows urethritis, cervicitis, or dysentery. Possible associated features include inflammatory eye disease and lesions of the skin and mucous membranes.

The prevalence of Reiter syndrome has not been well documented. Previously, the syndrome was described as overwhelmingly predilecting males. Recognizing that the initiating episode may include silent cystitis or cervicitis, the male to female ratio is declining and may now approach 4 or 5 to 1.

Clinical features of Reiter syndrome include

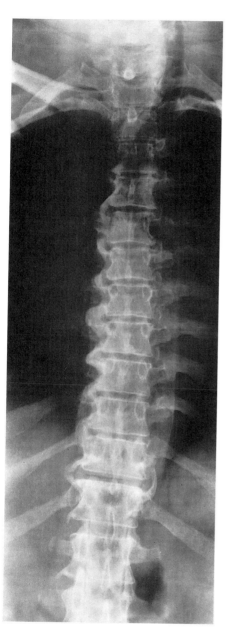

Figure 15.9   Diffuse idiopathic skeletal hyperostosis (DISH). Note the flowing osteophytes at more than three levels.

arthritis that typically develops 2 to 6 weeks following the onset of infection. The arthritis is acute in onset and commonly consists of an asymmetrical poly- or oligoarthritis affecting mostly large joints in the lower limbs. Three typical musculoskeletal manifestations include *"sausage digit,"* a diffuse swelling of an entire finger or toe; Achilles' tendinitis, with swelling at the insertion of the Achilles' tendon; and low back pain, consistent with sacroiliitis. Conjunctivitis, which may be unilateral or bilateral, is typically culture-negative, occurs in about 40 percent of patients, may be mild and transient, and appears early in the disease. Iritis occurs in about 5 percent, and permanently impaired vision has been reported in as many as 3 percent of patients. Uveitis, episcleritis, and corneal ulceration have also been described. Cutaneous lesions include *balanitis circinata,* which are typically small, shallow, painless ulcers on the glans penis and urethral meatus that occur in 25 to 50 percent of patients. *Keratoderma blenorrhagicum* is a hyperkeratotic skin lesion indistinguishable from pustular psoriasis, which occurs in approximately 10 percent of patients. It occurs predominantly on the soles of the feet but is also found on the palms, scrotum, and elsewhere. Painless, superficial oral ulcers may also be present. Cardiac involvement occurs in less than 10 percent of patients, with conduction abnormalities in early disease and aortic insufficiency late, often requiring valvular replacement.

Laboratory findings include synovial fluid cell counts in the 5000-to-50,000 range, predominantly PMNs. While 80 percent of Caucasian patients may be HLA-B27–positive, this marker is seen in less than 50 percent of African American patients. A small number of patients have one self-limiting episode of ar-

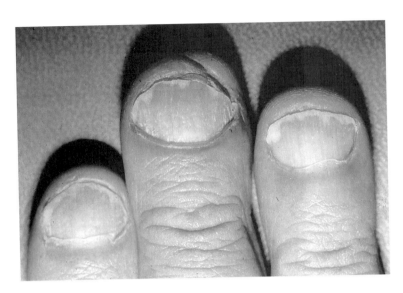

Figure 15.10   Psoriatic arthritis. Note the pitting, onycholysis, and irregularity of the nails.

thritis; an even smaller group suffer a continuous, unremitting course, and the majority of patients experience chronic, recurrent episodes of arthritis, often associated with infection. The severity of inflammation at the onset of arthritis does not appear to be a prognostic factor.

Enteropathic Arthritis

Two patterns of rheumatic involvement may be seen with inflammatory bowel diseases such as ulcerative colitis or Crohn disease. *Spondyloarthritis* (spinal arthritis) occurs in up to 8 percent of patients with inflammatory bowel disease; 50 to 75 percent of these patients have the HLA-B27 molecule, and there is a male predominance. The spectrum of disease is varied, ranging from sacroiliitis to ankylosing spondylitis. There is no relation of spondyloarthritis to the activity of the bowel disease; in fact, spondyloarthritis may precede inflammatory bowel disease by many years.

Peripheral arthritis occurs in as many as 20 percent of patients with inflammatory bowel disease, more commonly in those with Crohn disease than in those with ulcerative colitis, and with a slight female predominance. The arthritis is usually asymmetrical and most often involves the knee and ankle. The synovitis usually responds to treatment of the underlying bowel disease, and articular damage is rare. Here, the course of the peripheral polyarthritis does parallel inflammation in the bowel.

Psoriatic Arthritis

Inflammatory arthritis associated with psoriasis is relatively uncommon, affecting only 7 to 10 percent of patients with psoriasis. Sexual distribution is equal. The usual age of onset is in the thirties and forties, often with skin disease preceding joint disease by months to years. The pattern of joint involvement is variable. Involvement of nails is a clue to the diagnosis of psoriatic arthritis. Eighty percent of patients with psoriatic arthritis have nail abnormalities, including pitting, transverse or longitudinal ridging, or onycholysis (Fig. 15.10). Systemic involvement, with inflammation of the eye, occurs in approximately 30 percent of patients. Abnormal laboratory findings include elevation of the sedimentation rate and normocytic, normochromic anemia. Hyperuricemia occurs, particularly in patients with severe skin involvement.

Therapy

There is currently no cure for the seronegative spondyloarthropathies. Regular exercise is important, particularly in AS, to preserve function and minimize deformities. Spinal extension exercises help prevent ankylosis in a dysfunctional, flexed position. Patients are advised to sleep on firm mattresses, preferably without pillows. Deep-breathing exercises help maintain chest excursion.

Pharmacologic therapy includes NSAIDs, of which indomethacin may be the most efficacious. Phenylbutazone, now rarely used because of the risk of aplastic anemia or hepatitis, remains effective therapy for severely affected patients. *Sulfasalazine* has been shown to benefit AS, especially in patients with peripheral arthritis and short duration of disease. Sulfasalazine has been used in Reiter syndrome, but its superiority to NSAID therapy has not been shown. Oral corticosteroids are not indicated for the long-term management of these disorders because of the potential for serious side effects and lack of impact on the progression of the disease. Uveitis may require local corticosteroid drops. In psoriatic arthritis, corticosteroid tapers may be associated with flares of skin disease. In the therapy of psoriasis, methotrexate is often used to treat both skin and joint disease, but careful monitoring for potential hepatic damage or bone marrow suppression is essential. While no controlled study of methotrexate therapy for Reiter syndrome has been reported, clinical

experience shows that methotrexate is effective in treating reactive arthritis. Caution must be exercised, as Reiter syndrome may be associated with human immunodeficiency virus (HIV) and methotrexate use increases the risk of conversion of HIV positivity to acquired immunodeficiency syndrome (AIDS). Early and prolonged treatment with tetracycline may shorten the duration of reactive arthritis triggered by infection with chlamydia.

Surgery is often indicated for painful, end-stage arthropathy. Joint replacement is effective for hips, knees, and shoulders. Although spinal osteotomy is an option for patients with AS and ankylosis of the spine in marked flexion, patients should be aware of the considerable risks involved.

Crystal Arthritis

Features of crystal arthritis often include the sudden, unexplained onset of erythema, warmth, swelling, and pain in a single joint. Infection and trauma must be excluded. The formation of crystals within a joint induces an inflammatory reaction, which in time can result in destruction of the joint.

Analysis of Synovial Fluid

Synovial fluid should be analyzed for crystals while the specimen is fresh; otherwise, crystals may decay and escape detection. The calcium pyrophosphate dihydrate (CPPD) crystals of pseudogout, for example, decline markedly within a day and are completely undetectable within 2 to 8 weeks. Monosodium urate (MSU) crystals in gout are more stable and may remain detectable for weeks to months but become less strongly birefringent over time. Reducing the storage temperature of synovial fluid from 44° to 22°C will retard the disappearance of MSU crystals and also reduce the appearance of artifactual crystals.

Gout

The term *gout* encompasses a group of disorders caused by tissue deposition of uric acid crystals from supersaturated extracellular fluids. These negatively birefringent crystals stimulate the release of inflammatory mediators (C5a, bradykinin, kallikrein) from phagocytes and synovial lining cells. Clinical manifestations of gout include (1) recurrent attacks of acute gouty arthritis; (2) tophi; (3) gouty nephropathy (caused by precipitation of uric acid in renal tubules); and (4) renal stones. Hyperuricemia is the common pathogenetic factor giving rise to the clinical manifestations of gout; asymptomatic hyperuricemia is not a disease state.

The prevalence of gout in the United States is estimated to be 0.3 percent. The risk of developing gout increases with age and increasing concentrations of serum uric acid.

Acute arthritis is the most frequent manifestation of gout; however, in perhaps 10 percent of patients, the first joint symptoms are preceded by nephrolithiasis. The acute arthritis of gout most commonly affects the metatarsophalangeal (MTP) joint of the great toe *(podagra),* but the ankle, tarsus, and knee are also frequent sites of involvement. Some 75 percent of patients will have podagra at some time in their course.

Thomas Sydenham was the first to describe, in 1683, an attack of acute gouty arthritis, which typically begins abruptly in a single joint during the night, producing dramatic and unexplained joint pain, swelling, and erythema. The intense periarticular erythema that often accompanies attacks can be confused with cellulitis, thrombophlebitis, or a septic joint. Systemic effects include fever, chills, and desquamation of the skin overlying the affected joint as the inflammation subsides. Early attacks tend to subside spontaneously over 3 to 10 days, even without specific therapy. Patients may then be symptom-free until the next episode, which may not occur for months or years. Over time, attacks occur more frequently, involve more joints, and persist for longer periods of time. Chronic gouty arthritis can mimic rheumatoid arthritis, although the pattern of joint involvement is usually less symmetrical.

The intervals between attacks constitute the *intercritical stage* of gout. Initially, patients are symptom-free during the intercritical periods; however, even during asymptomatic periods, MSU crystals can be aspirated from previously involved joints and even joints that have not been overtly affected. Thus, a definitive diagnosis can be made during an asymptomatic interval by aspiration.

Tophi are noted an average of 10 years following the first episode of acute gout. They occur most frequently in synovium, subchondral bone, olecranon bursae, infrapatellar and Achilles' tendons, and subcutaneous tissue on the extensor surfaces of the forearms or overlying joints (Fig. 15.11). Tophi have also been described in aortic walls, heart valves, nasal cartilage, and carpal tunnels but curiously do not involve the central nervous system. They may also form on tendon sheaths in the hand and wrist, causing trigger finger or carpal tunnel syndrome. Tophi may be confused with rheumatoid nodules unless examined under polarizing microscopy.

Radiographs early in the disease show soft tissue swelling surrounding affected joints. Tophi produce irregular, asymmetrical soft tissue swellings and are sometimes calcified.

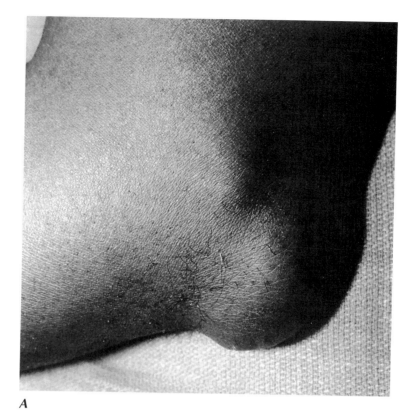

A

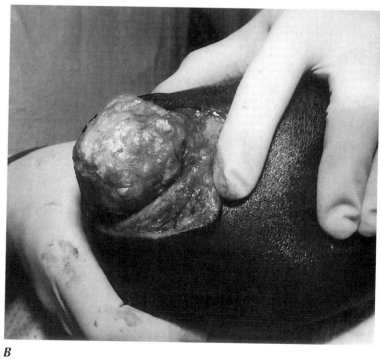

Figure 15.11 Gout. The large, symptomatic tophus over the olecranon was excised.

B

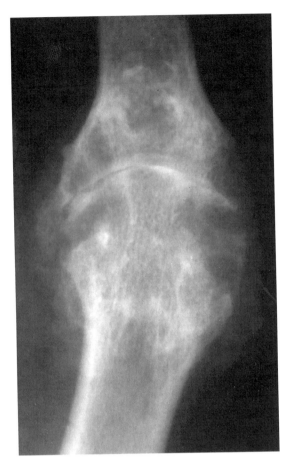

Figure 15.12   Gout of the first MTP joint. Note the subchondral erosions with a characteristic "overhanging lip" of bone at the joint margin and an adjacent calcified soft tissue tophus.

Bony erosions in chronic disease are characteristically round or oval in shape, with a sclerotic margin. Often a thin, overhanging edge of bone may be seen, but joint spaces are relatively well preserved until late in the course of the disease (Fig. 15.12).

Demonstration of intracellular, negatively birefringent MSU crystals is the "gold standard" for establishing the diagnosis of gout. The crystals occur intra- or extracellularly, are typically rod- or needle-shaped and 3 to 20 mm in length; they may be visible with a light microscope. Synovial fluid leukocyte counts in acute gouty arthritis range from 2 to 100,000 cells per cubic millimeter, predominantly neutrophils. Effusions are often cloudy because of the high cell count and concentration of crystals. Masses of crystals may produce thick, pasty, white joint fluid. Although uncommon, infection can coexist with uric acid crystals, and joint fluid should be cultured if this possibility is considered.

Serum uric acid levels during an acute attack may be spuriously low and thus of less value than normal intercurrent uric acid levels. Overproduction of uric acid may be determined if more than 750 mg are excreted in the urine during a 24-h period on a regular diet.

The treatment of acute gout is determined by the clinical manifestations of the individual patient. The goals of therapy are to bring acute attacks to a quick end with minimal drug-related side effects, prevent recurrences, minimize or prevent complications of the disease resulting from deposits of MSU crystals, and prevent the formation of renal stones.

The mainstay of drug therapy for acute gout is colchicine, which interferes with leukocyte migration and function by binding to microtubules. Colchicine may be given in doses of 0.6 mg every 1 to 2 h until significant improvement in inflammation occurs or gastrointestinal side effects become prominent. The agent is most effective if administered promptly following the onset of an acute attack. The total dose needed to achieve a loading effect is typically 4 to 6 mg, varying by body size and hepatic and renal function. The maximum oral dose should not exceed 6 to 8 mg in 24 h. Since the drug is excreted slowly, no further colchicine should be given for seven days after a loading dose. Patients who suffer from recurrent acute attacks may benefit from low-dose, daily therapy for prophylaxis, but these patients should not receive full loading doses for acute gouty flares because of the likelihood of toxic reactions, including bone marrow suppression. Gastrointestinal side effects are common, and approximately 80 percent of patients treated for acute gout experience cramping, diarrhea, and/or nausea and vomiting. Intravenous colchicine greatly reduces gastrointestinal side effects; however, serious potential complications, including local chemical thrombophlebitis and fatal overdosing preclude its use except when alternate routes of administration are not possible.

In addition to colchicine, nonsteroidal antiinflammatory drugs have been shown to be effective, even when therapy is delayed following the onset of an acute attack. Traditionally, indomethacin has been used to treat acute gout, but other NSAIDs, such as ibuprofen, in adequately high doses are also effective. Therapy during intercritical stages employs allopurinol or uricosuric agents for appropriate patients. Allopurinol, a xanthine oxidase inhibitor, reduces the synthesis of uric acid and is beneficial for patients who produce excessive amounts of uric acid. Potentially serious side effects limit routine use of the drug to appropriate patients. Uricosuric agents (e.g., probenecid and sulfinpyrazone) are used in patients who excrete insufficient amounts of uric acid, provided renal function is adequate. In long-standing cases of gout with joint destruction, arthrodesis or joint replacement may be necessary to relieve pain and disability.

Calcium Pyrophosphate Dihydrate Crystal Deposition Disease

The relationship between calcium pyrophosphate dihydrate crystal deposition disease (CPPD) crystals and arthritis remains unclear despite much investigative attention. The recognition of weakly positive, birefringent CPPD crystals in a diversity of clinical settings has challenged the recognition of CPPD deposition as a discrete clinical entity. However, demonstration that CPPD crystals are potent inflammatory agents and the production of synovitis by injection of CPPD crystals into normal joints have led to general acceptance of CPPD crystal deposition as a causal agent of arthropathy. The manifestations of CPPD deposition disease are protean and may mimic gout (pseudogout), rheumatoid arthritis, osteoarthritis, or neuropathic joint disease. Three common presentations of CPPD deposition disease include chondrocalcinosis, pseudogout, and chronic pyrophosphate arthropathy.

CHONDROCALCINOSIS   Chondrocalcinosis (radiographically apparent calcification of articular fibro- or hyaline cartilage) is a common but usually asymptomatic finding (Fig. 15.13). Chondrocalcinosis has a female predominance, affecting 2 to 7 times as many women as men. Prevalence climbs steadily with age, being rare under age 50 and soaring to 30 to 60 percent in those over age 85. No racial, genetic, or geographic predispositions are noted, although familial forms have been identified. Familial occurrence may be associated with a

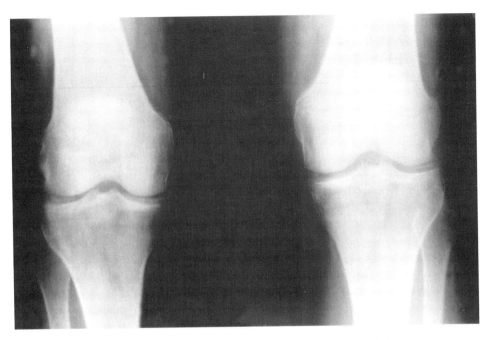

Figure 15.13 Chondrocalcinosis of the knee. Note the faint calcifications outlining both menisci.

younger age at presentation and polyarticular involvement.

PSEUDOGOUT   The typical attack of pseudogout clinically mimics gout, with rapid onset of severe joint pain, swelling, and erythema. Fever and leukocytosis are common. Elderly patients appear systemically ill and confused. Acute attacks are self-limited, subsiding in 1 to 4 weeks. Although episodes may develop spontaneously, several provocative factors are recognized: trauma, intercurrent illness, surgery (especially parathyroidectomy), joint lavage, and thyroxine replacement. Pseudogout is the most common cause of acute monoarthritis in the elderly. The knee is involved in more than half the episodes, but intense involvement

of the first metatarsophalangeal joint *(pseudopodagra)* is well recognized.

CHRONIC PYROPHOSPHATE ARTHROPATHY Chronic pyrophosphate arthropathy has a female predominance, affecting two to three times as many women as men, with a peak age of onset from 65 to 75 years. The knees are most commonly affected, followed by wrists, shoulders, elbows, and hips. In the hand, the second and third metacarpophalangeal joints are predilected. Features of this inflammatory arthritis include early-morning stiffness and multiple joint involvement. Functional impairment may be severe enough to suggest an elderly onset of rheumatoid arthritis; however, the lack of tenosynovitis, extraarticular features, and bony erosions help distinguish this group. Affected joints show certain features of osteoarthritis: bony swelling, crepitation, and limitation of movement; but the marked inflammatory features and history of acute attacks distinguish this disorder from osteoarthritis. The natural history of chronic pyrophosphate arthropathy is poorly documented, but most patients with small- and medium-sized joint involvement have a benign course.

ANALYSIS OF SYNOVIAL FLUID   Mean synovial fluid leukocyte counts in CPPD deposition disease are 20,000 cells per cubic millimeter, with overwhelming predominance of neutrophils. Gram stain and culture of joint fluid are essential to exclude infection. Blood-stained fluid is common, and other causes of hemarthrosis must be considered, including trauma, clotting disorders, and subchondral fractures.

ASSOCIATIONS WITH METABOLIC DISEASE Numerous metabolic associations with CPPD have been described. Many reflect the chance concurrences of age- related disorders, such as diabetes, uremia, Paget disease, and hypothyroidism. Strong associations have been found for hyperparathyroidism, hemochromatosis, hypophosphatasia, hypomagnesemia, and Wilson disease.

MANAGEMENT   The aims of treatment for pseudogout and chronic pyrophosphate arthropathy are to reduce symptoms, identify and treat associated illnesses, and maintain mobility. Joint aspiration alone may greatly relieve symptoms. NSAIDs reduce pain and inflammation but should be used judiciously in the elderly with known age-related reductions in hepatic and renal function. For involvement of single joints, with infection excluded, intra-articular steroids may preclude the necessity for systemic therapy. Oral colchicine is as efficacious for pseudogout as for gout. For polyarticular attacks unresponsive to these measures alone, systemic oral corticosteroids may be considered, although their efficacy is anecdotal. Treatment of metabolic disease associated with CPPD does not alter the arthropathy. Weight reduction, walking aids, education in joint usage, and improvement in muscle strength reduce mechanical stress and optimize patient mobility. Progressively disabling arthropathy, especially in weight- bearing joints, may require replacement of the joint.

Fibromyalgia

Fibromyalgia describes a chronic condition of unknown etiology characterized by widespread pain and tender points in the soft tissues. Associated complaints include sleep disruption and swelling of soft tissues that is not apparent on physical examination. Fibromyalgia predominantly affects women in the reproductive years, although its prevalence is difficult to ascertain, since the nature of the disorder is still uncertain. The previous term, *fibrositis,* has been abandoned because no evidence of inflammation has been found. The diagnosis is based solely upon clinical criteria as established by the American College of Rheumatology in 1990 (Table 15.4). The diagnostic workup should include tests to rule out more serious disorders. Screening tests include blood chemistries, a complete blood count, and an ESR. With clinical suspicion, ANA, RF, creatinine kinase, Lyme serology, or thyroid

Table 15.4   The American College of Rheumatology 1990 Criteria for the Classification of Fibromyalgia[a]

1. History of widespread pain

   Definition. Pain is considered widespread when all of the following are present: pain in the left side of the body, pain in the right side of the body, pain above the waist, and pain below the waist. In addition, axial skeletal pain (cervical spine or anterior chest or thoracic spine or low back) must be present. In this definition, shoulder and buttock pain is considered as pain for each involved side. "Low back" pain is considered lower segment pain.

2. Pain in 11 of 18 tender point sites on digital palpation.

   Definition. Pain, on digital palpation, must be present in at least 11 of the following 18 tender point sites:

   Occiput: Bilateral, at the suboccipital muscle insertions

   Low cervical: Bilateral, at the anterior aspects of the intertransverse spaces at C5-C7

   Trapezius: Bilateral, at the midpoint of the upper border

   Supraspinatus: Bilateral, at origins, above the scapular spine near the medial border

   Second rib: Bilateral, at the second costochondral junctions, just lateral to the junctions on upper surfaces

   Lateral epicondyle: Bilateral, 2 cm distal to the epicondyles

   Gluteal: Bilateral, in upper outer quadrants of buttocks in anterior fold of muscle

   Greater trochanter: Bilateral, posterior to the trochanteric prominence

   Knee: Bilateral, at the medial fat pad proximal to the joint line.

Digital palpation should be performed with an approximate force of 4 kg. For a tender point to be considered "positive," the subject must state that the palpation was painful. "Tender" is not to be considered "painful."

---

[a] For classification purposes, patients are said to have fibromyalgia if both criteria are satisfied. Widespread pain must have been present for at least 3 months. The presence of a second clinical disorder does not exclude the diagnosis of fibromyalgia.

SOURCE: Wolfe F, Smythe HA, Yunus MB, et al: The American College of Rheumatology 1990 criteria for the classification of fibromyalgia: Report of the Multicenter Criteria Committee. *Arthritis Rheum* 33:160–172, 1990. With permission.

function testing is indicated. Radiography of symptomatic areas or electrodiagnostic testing to evaluate paresthesias may be indicated.

Treatment of fibromyalgia includes education of patients on the chronic nature of the disorder and the lack of tissue damage. Beneficial therapy includes tricyclic antidepressants to restore restful sleep, but the lowest effective dose should be employed to avoid daytime somnolence and anticholinergic effects. In addition, NSAIDs are sometimes helpful despite the lack of inflammation. Aerobic exercise is also of benefit, although many patients are seriously deconditioned and must start at a low level. Judicious injection of tender points, biofeedback, massage, ultrasound therapy, and acupuncture may provide symptomatic relief. There is no role for narcotic analgesics.

SUGGESTED READINGS

CORMAN LC, BELL CL, EDWARDS NL, HARMON CE (EDS): *Rheumatology for the House Officer.* Baltimore, Williams & Wilkins, 1990.

KELLEY WN, HARRIS ED, RUDDY S, SLEDGE CB (EDS): *Textbook of Rheumatology,* 5th ed. Philadelphia, Saunders, 1996.

KLIPPEL JH, DIEPPE PA (EDS): *Rheumatology.* St Louis, Mosby, 1994.

McCARTY DJ, KOOPMAN WJ (EDS): *Arthritis and Allied Conditions: A Textbook of Rheumatology,* 13th ed. Philadelphia, Lea & Febiger, 1996.

SCHUMACHER HR JR, KLIPPEL JH, KOOPMAN WJ (EDS): *Primer on the Rheumatic Diseases,* 10th ed. Atlanta, Arthritis Foundation, 1993.

Chapter 16

Metabolic and Endocrinologic Disorders

Patrick P. Lin and Frank C. Wilson

GENERAL ASPECTS OF BONE METABOLISM

GENERAL ASPECTS OF BONE METABOLISM

The two most important functions of bone are structural support and maintenance of the metabolic balance of critical minerals, including calcium and phosphate. Occasionally, these two functions are incompatible. To preserve metabolic homeostasis, the structural integrity of bones may have to be compromised; conversely, diseases of bone may lead to metabolic derangements.

In spite of recent advances, there is still much to be learned about bone metabolism. While it is rare now to see a patient with rickets or a brown tumor, the most common metabolic bone disease, osteoporosis, is still a therapeutic mystery. New findings are challenging old notions; the actions of hormones are more complex than once thought; and the effects of growth factors and cytokines on bone have just begun to be elucidated. This chapter provides an overview of this evolving and expanding area of orthopaedics.

Ions

Calcium

Calcium is necessary for the function of many organs, including the heart, brain, and muscles. Normal total serum concentrations range from 8.5 to 10.7 mg/dL and vary with serum protein levels. Approximately 40 percent of calcium is bound to protein, principally albumin; 10 percent is complexed to small anions; and 50 percent is ionized. The ionized calcium concentration is the critical physiologic value and must be maintained within a narrow margin.

A steep calcium concentration gradient exists across cell membranes. Whereas the extra-cellular concentration of ionized calcium is $\sim 10^{-3}\ M$, the intracellular concentration is a thousandfold less, or $\sim 10^{-6}\ M$. High intracellular levels of calcium are toxic, and cells rapidly sequester excess calcium in organelles, such as mitochondria, or pump it out of the cell. This calcium gradient is important to cell functions. Fluxes of calcium are essential for propagating electrical impulses in nerves and muscles. In addition, transient fluxes of calcium across the cytoplasmic membrane signal numerous cell processes.

The skeleton is the major reservoir of calcium. The average adult possesses 1000 g of calcium, of which 99 percent is in bones. Calcium homeostasis reflects an interplay between the skeleton and the organs that absorb and excrete calcium, namely the intestines and kidney. A normal young adult is in neutral calcium balance, with no net daily gain or loss of calcium (Fig. 16.1). Approximately 500 to 1000 mg is ingested each day, of which 250 to 500 mg is absorbed in the duodenum and upper small intestine. Free phosphate ions probably have minimal effects on calcium absorption, but organic phosphates, such as phytates in bran, may form insoluble salts with calcium and impede its absorption.

Calcium is lost in sweat, feces, and urine. Fecal excretion is a combination of unabsorbed dietary calcium, which is highly variable, and secreted calcium, which is relatively constant (~ 100 mg/day). Renal excretion, like intestinal absorption, varies with metabolic needs. In the kidney, most of the filtered calcium is reabsorbed in the proximal tubule and thick ascending loop of Henle (Fig. 16.2). The fine control of reabsorption occurs in the distal convoluted tubule, under the influence of parathyroid hormone. Hypercalcemia, hypermagnesemia, and metabolic acidosis increase cal-

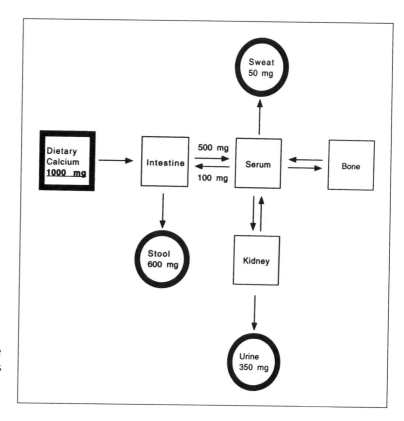

Figure 16.1 Calcium homeostasis. In a normal young adult, there is no net daily gain or loss. Approximately half of the ingested calcium is absorbed. Excess calcium is lost through the kidneys. The numeric figures are estimates and vary with dietary intake and metabolic needs.

cium excretion. Hyperphosphatemia and $1,25(OH)_2$ vitamin D_3 increase phosphate excretion. Loop diuretics, such as furosemide, diminish calcium reabsorption, whereas thiazides enhance it. The kidney cannot conserve all of the calcium, and obligatory losses vary from 20 to 200 mg/day. In states of hypercalcemia, the kidneys can excrete 800 mg/day or more by reducing reabsorption. No active secretion of calcium occurs.

It is not known how the ionized calcium concentration of serum is kept within tight limits. Although the kidney may play a role, it cannot be the sole regulator, since patients with renal failure are able to maintain stable calcium concentrations even during dialysis.

Bone is also involved in the minute-to-minute regulation of calcium levels. The surface area of bone canaliculi affords a large reservoir of easily mobilized calcium ions ideally suited to stabilize fluctuations in calcium concentrations, although their precise role in doing so remains a matter of speculation.

Another enigma of calcium metabolism is *mineralization.* Serum is a metastable solution, since calcium and phosphate are in relatively high concentrations. Without organic stabilizers in the serum, calcium phosphate would precipitate spontaneously. At the osteoid mineralization front, calcium and phosphate undergo transformation to the solid phase in a controlled manner, forming hydroxyapatite crys-

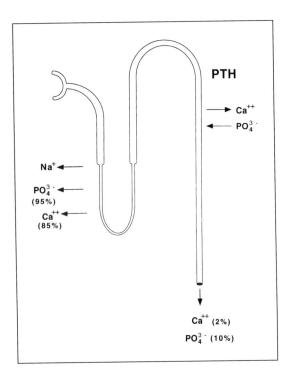

Figure 16.2   Renal reabsorption of calcium and phosphate. Most calcium and phosphate reabsorption occurs in the proximal portion of the nephron, including the thick ascending loop of Henle, and follows sodium reabsorption.

tals. The mechanism by which phase transformation occurs is incompletely understood, but it apparently relies on organic nucleation agents, which provide the seeds for crystal growth. The process of mineralization can be impaired if the *ion product* (calcium × phosphate concentration) is below 30 mg^2/dL^2, while metastatic calcification can occur in soft tissues if it exceeds 75 mg^2/dL^2.

Abnormalities of serum calcium concentration lead to a myriad of clinical findings. *Hypercalcemia* is characterized by headache, inability to concentrate, lethargy, weakness, and

hyporeflexia. Renal manifestations include polyuria, polydipsia, inability to concentrate urine, dehydration, nephrolithiasis, and nephrocalcinosis. Gastrointestinal effects are nausea, vomiting, constipation, pancreatitis, and peptic ulcers. Cardiovascular consequences include hypertension, bradycardia, and first-degree atrioventricular block.

The clinical manifestations of *hypocalcemia* are increased neuromuscular irritability, paresthesias, tetany, seizures, laryngospasm and bronchospasm. Positive *Chvostek* (twitching of facial muscles with light percussion of the facial nerve at its egress from the parotid gland) and *Trousseau* (sustained contraction of the forearm muscles with inflation of a blood pressure cuff) (Fig. 16.3) signs further support the diagnosis of hypocalcemia.

Phosphate

Phosphorus is ubiquitous in the body, occurring as phosphate esters, phospholipids, and nucleic acids. Eighty-five percent of the body's phosphorus is stored in the skeleton; 15 percent is in the soft tissues. Serum phosphate levels range from 2.5 to 4.5 mg/dL. The concentration is not regulated as tightly as calcium and may vary as much as 50 percent in one day. Phosphate is present in many foods, including dairy products and meats. The average daily diet includes about 800 to 1500 mg of phosphate, of which two-thirds is absorbed by the intestines. Vitamin D stimulates intestinal absorption of phosphate. The kidney is the principal regulator of phosphate concentration and has limited intrinsic ability to adjust phosphate levels. In addition, parathyroid hormone provides hormonal control of phosphate excretion by inhibiting reabsorption, which occurs primarily in the proximal tubule.

Acute hyperphosphatemia may induce hy-

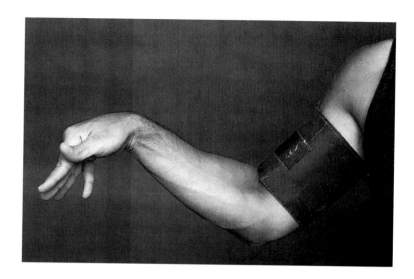

Figure 16.3 Trousseau
sign of hypocalcemia.

pocalcemia by forming insoluble complexes
with calcium. Tetany and neuromuscular irritability are the result of secondary hypocalcemia. In *chronic hyperphosphatemia,* patients
develop secondary hyperparathyroidism. Soft
tissue calcification may ensue if both phosphate and calcium levels become elevated. *Hypophosphatemia* is common in hospitalized
patients, although mild involvement is usually
asymptomatic. In severe cases, patients may
develop red cell and platelet dysfunction, neurologic symptoms, rhabdomyolysis, metabolic
acidosis, cardiomyopathy, and impaired renal
function.

Other Ions

Bone is a storehouse for the important cation
magnesium. Approximately two-thirds of the
25 g of magnesium in the body is in bone,
complexed to the surface of hydroxyapatite
crystals. Bone crystals contain many other
ions, including sodium, potassium, carbonate,
citrate and fluoride. The structural function of
these ions in bone is unclear; moreover, the

role of bone in the metabolism of these ions is
not well established. Nevertheless, metabolic
bone disease can have an impact on physiologic processes that depend upon these ions.

Hormones

Parathyroid Hormone

Parathyroid hormone (PTH) is a small protein
secreted by the parathyroid glands. Both high
serum calcium concentrations and high vitamin D levels inhibit the secretion of PTH,
whereas low concentrations of calcium stimulate its secretion. Parathyroid hormone increases the concentration of serum calcium by
increasing reabsorption from kidneys, mobi-
lizing calcium from bones, and activating vitamin D, which stimulates intestinal absorption of calcium.

In the kidney, PTH causes the distal tubule
to increase calcium absorption and phosphate
excretion. It also stimulates renal conversion
of 25(OH) vitamin D to the more potent form
$1,25(OH)_2$ vitamin D. The action of PTH de-

pends in part on the production of cyclic AMP in the distal tubule; in fact, measurement of urinary cyclic AMP levels provides an indirect assessment of the effect of PTH on the kidney.

The primary effect of PTH on bone is to increase resorption and release of calcium. Cortical bone seems to be affected to a greater degree than trabecular bone. Surprisingly, there are no receptors for PTH on mature osteoclasts, and the mechanism for osteoclastic activation is uncertain. Some believe that osteoclastic precursors are directly stimulated by the hormone, while others believe that PTH affects osteoblasts, which in turn activate osteoclasts. Parathyroid hormone receptors are present on osteoblasts, and PTH does stimulate osteoblastic activity and proliferation. Alkaline phosphatase levels rise in response to PTH, reflecting the increase in osteoblastic activity. Parathyroid hormone thus stimulates not only bone resorption but also bone formation. The net effect is an increase in the rate of bone turnover. A normal, basal level of PTH is vital to skeletal growth, and children with hypoparathyroidism exhibit disturbances of growth.

Vitamin D

"Vitamin" D is a misnomer, since the molecule is a steroid hormone and not a vitamin. The substance is produced endogenously by the skin after exposure to ultraviolet light, and there is no strict dietary requirement. The chief action of the molecule is to increase calcium and phosphate levels by stimulating intestinal absorption of these ions.

Many forms of vitamin D circulate in blood. Ultraviolet light activates 7-dehydrocholesterol to previtamin D_3, which isomerizes to vitamin D_3 (cholecalciferol). In the blood, it becomes active first by hydroxylation at the 25(OH) position in the liver, then at the 1(OH) position in the kidney (Fig. 16.4). The most active and biologically significant molecule is 1,25(OH)$_2$ vitamin D_3 (1,25-dihydroxyvitamin D_3 or calcitriol). The designations D_1, D_2, and D_3 refer to chemically related molecules with similar properties. Vitamin D_2 (calciferol) is the active ingredient in fortified milk and commercial vitamin preparations, but is not found naturally in humans. Vitamin D_1 was historically described first, but later found to be a mixture of compounds.

Vitamin D exerts self-regulatory behavior. It inhibits secretion of PTH, which reduces production of the potent 1,25-dihydroxyl form of vitamin D. In the kidney, vitamin D causes

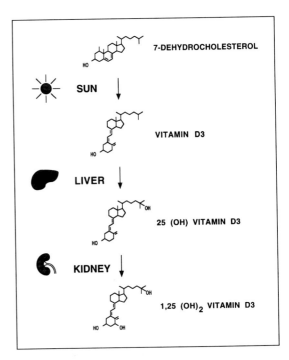

Figure 16.4 Endogenous production of vitamin D.

hydroxylation at the 24(OH) position instead of the 1(OH) position, resulting in the much less active molecule 24,25(OH)$_2$ vitamin D.

Like other steroid hormones, vitamin D regulates genetic expression via its DNA-binding receptor, which is present in nearly all tissues; thus, the actions of vitamin D are widespread. One unexpected finding is that vitamin D stimulates formation of multinucleated cells with bone-resorbing potential. The significance of this action is uncertain.

Calcitonin

Calcitonin is a 32–amino acid peptide secreted by the C cells of the thyroid gland in response to a high calcium level. The hormone directly inhibits osteoclastic bone resorption and causes osteoclasts to shrink. It may also stimulate osteoblasts. The biological requirement for calcitonin in humans is unclear, since thyroidectomy does not cause ostensible dysfunction of calcium metabolism. Levels are lower in females and in the aged.

Other Hormones and Influences

Bone is responsive to many influences, the best-studied of which are hormonal. Many of these hormones, like vitamin D, are steroid hormones, including estrogen, testosterone, and cortisol. Other hormones, like PTH, are proteins, including growth hormone and thyroid hormone. Deficiency or excess of these hormones may lead to disorders such as osteopenia, extraskeletal calcification, and stunting of growth in children. Other biological molecules that affect bone formation and resorption are growth factors, such as *bone morphogenetic protein, transforming growth factor β,* and *insulinlike growth factor,* which promote bone formation. In contrast, biological agents such as *interleukin-1, tumor necrosis factor,* and *prostaglandin E* increase resorption. The role of these *cytokines* in mineral metabolism is uncertain. It has been proposed that growth factors influence cellular events locally. For example, when resorption of bone is initiated, bone morphogenetic protein may be released, attracting osteoblasts and stimulating them to form osteoid in the areas excavated by osteoclasts.

Another important influence on bone, apart from hormones and growth factors, is mechanical stress. Weight bearing and physical activity are necessary to maintain the mineral content in bone (Fig. 16.5). The manner in which mechanical stress is detected by cells in bone is poorly understood but may involve electrical properties of bone.

Diagnostic Tests

Serum and Urinary Tests

Relevant serum tests for patients with suspected metabolic bone disease include calcium, phosphate, albumin, BUN, and creatinine levels. The total calcium level is affected by the albumin concentration; hence the ionized calcium level is more meaningful. BUN and creatinine screen for renal disorders. More specialized tests, which may be indicated in selected patients, include 25(OH) vitamin D and 1,25(OH)$_2$ vitamin D levels. Parathyroid hormone can be assayed indirectly by measuring immunoreactive peptides from the cleavage of the native molecule, which has a short half-life in serum.

Alkaline phosphatase is a nonspecific marker for osteoblastic activity. Its level in serum is elevated by increased bone formation.

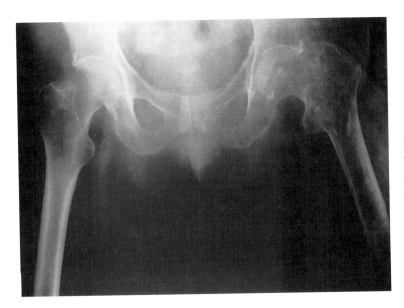

Figure 16.5 The effect of weightbearing and mechanical stress on bone density. This patient has had a left above-knee amputation; he does not use a prosthesis and bears weight only on the right leg. Note the relative osteopenia in the left femur.

Three genes for alkaline phosphatases have been identified: intestinal, placental, and tissue nonspecific, the latter of which is expressed in bone, liver, kidney, and other organs. Both normal (e.g., pregnancy) and pathologic conditions (e.g., bone or liver disease) may increase serum alkaline phosphatase levels.

Osteocalcin (bone Gla protein), a specific marker for osteoblastic activity, is produced solely by osteoblasts. Serum osteocalcin levels reflect new protein synthesis by osteoblasts rather than matrix breakdown. Osteocalcin makes up 10 to 20 percent of the noncollagenous proteins in bone. Its structure is unique in having three carboxylated glutamic acid residues that bind calcium. The function of osteocalcin is unknown, but it may be important in mineralization.

Urinary tests for many ions and metabolites are available, including calcium, phosphate, and magnesium. The indications for these tests are limited to certain situations. For example,

urinary calcium and oxalate levels may be checked in patients with nephrolithiasis and states of high calcium excretion; or urinary cyclic AMP may be measured to assess the responsiveness to PTH. Urinary *hydroxyproline* and *glycosylated hydroxylysine* reflect bone turnover. These molecules are amino acids unique to collagen and are released when collagen is degraded; however, urinary levels reflect total collagen breakdown and are not specific for bone. Furthermore, only 5 to 10 percent is excreted by the kidney; the rest is reused by the body.

Noninvasive Measures of Bone Density

Plain radiographs are highly insensitive for the measurement of bone loss, since there must be a 30 to 40 percent decrease in bone mineral to be appreciated. *Single-photon absorptiometry* was the first method developed to measure bone density (grams of mineral per unit area or volume) accurately. This technique is limited to certain areas, such as the distal radius, where soft tissue artifacts are minimal. A radioactive source delivers a beam of photons through the bone, and a detector measures the amount of energy absorbed. *Dual-photon absorptiometry* introduced dual-energy photon beams to cancel soft tissue artifacts, thus broadening the applicability of photon absorptiometry to all areas of the body, including the axial skeleton. The main disadvantage was the need for a radioactive source. *Quantitative digital radiography,* also known as *dual-energy x-ray absorptiometry,* utilizes two x-ray beams rather than photon beams and is the preferred method for measuring bone density. Radiation exposure is less than that with a routine chest radiograph. *Quantitative computed tomography* affords spatial resolution of cortical and cancellous bone. It is most useful in the lumbar spine, although scans can be made of the appendicular skeleton as well. Its main disadvantage is delivery of a higher dose of radiation.

Biopsy

Bone biopsy and histomorphometry are indicated in equivocal cases of metabolic bone disease, especially if osteomalacia is suspected. The technique usually involves double tetracycline labeling 10 to 20 days apart, which marks the mineralization front and allows the rate of mineralization to be measured. Many other parameters can also be monitored, including total trabecular volume, thickness of osteoid seams, and the number of active osteoblasts and osteoclasts. The biopsy specimen is usually obtained from the iliac crest. The main disadvantages of the procedure are its invasiveness and the possibility of sampling errors.

CLINICAL DISORDERS

Disorders of Parathyroid Hormone and Related Conditions

Hyperparathyroidism

Primary hyperparathyroidism is characterized by excessive, inappropriate secretion of PTH, whereas *secondary hyperparathyroidism* is a fitting response to a low serum calcium level. The prevalence of primary hyperparathyroidism is approximately 1 in 1000. Occurring most frequently in elderly women, it is the most common cause of hypercalcemia and, together with the hypercalcemia of malignancy, accounts for over 90 percent of cases of hypercalcemia. The full-blown skeletal manifestations of hyperparathyroidism *(osteitis fibrosa cystica)* consist of bone pain, pathologic fractures, deformities, and *brown tumors.* These nonneoplastic, lytic masses erode both cancellous and cortical bone. Today, few patients develop full-blown osteitis fibrosa cystica because of earlier recognition of hyperparathyroidism.

A solitary adenoma is responsible for 80 percent of cases of primary hyperparathyroidism. Hyperplasia of all four parathyroid glands accounts for 15 to 20 percent of cases and may be associated with multiple endocrine neoplasias. Adenocarcinoma of the parathyroid gland causes fewer than 1 percent of cases.

Findings in patients with symptomatic hypercalcemia include weakness, polyuria, and polydipsia. Nephrolithiasis and nephrocalcinosis occur in 5 to 20 percent of patients and can lead to renal embarassment. Hypercalcemia favors the deposition of calcium pyrophosphate dihydrate (CPPD) crystals in artic-

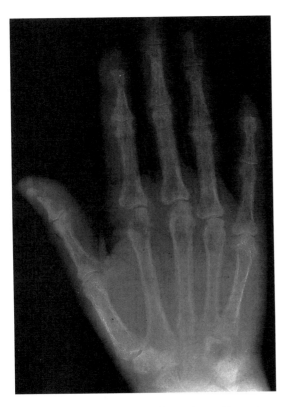

Figure 16.6 Hyperparathyroidism. Note the widespread subperiosteal erosions in the phalanges.

ular cartilage and menisci, sometimes resulting in pseudogout and acute arthritic attacks (see Chap. 15). Hyperparathyroidism has traditionally been associated with peptic ulcer disease, pancreatitis, and hypertension, but the relationship may be coincidental.

In most cases, osteopenia is the only radiographic finding. High-quality images of the hands often demonstrate subperiosteal resorption in the phalanges, especially along the radial aspect of the index and middle fingers, but endosteal, subchondral, and subligamentous

bone resorption may also be observed (Fig. 16.6). Brown tumors appear as larger, more focal lytic areas that can be confused with neoplastic or infectious processes (Fig. 16.7).

Increased serum levels of both parathyroid hormone and calcium are almost diagnostic of primary hyperparathyroidism. Phosphate levels are low to normal. Alkaline phosphate is high, reflecting increased turnover of bone. Urinary cyclic adenosine monophosphate (cAMP), calcium, and hydroxyproline are elevated. Radioimmunoassay for PTH helps dis-

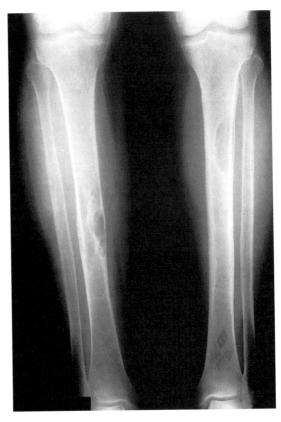

Figure 16.7 Hyperparathyroidism. Note the multiple brown tumors in the tibias.

tinguish primary hyperparathyroidism from the hypercalcemia of malignancy.

Biopsied bone shows fewer trabeculae, more osteoclasts, and replacement of the marrow by highly vascularized fibrous tissue, which constitute the classic triad of osteitis fibrosa cystica. Brown tumors, when examined histologically, are composed of giant osteoclasts and fibrous tissue; they may undergo necrosis and liquefaction, producing cysts.

Treatment of primary hyperparathyroidism usually entails surgical removal of the adenoma. The treatment of asymptomatic patients with hypercalcemia is controversial. If the serum calcium is more than 1 mg/dL above normal limits or if systemic manifestations such as nephrolithiasis are present, surgery is probably indicated. The *"hungry bone syndrome"* can occur after excision of the adenoma, with rapid deposition of calcium into bone. If patients cannot be treated surgically, they should not be placed on calcium-restricted diets, since this treatment exacerbates the hyperparathyroidism. No medical treatment has proven effective.

Hypercalcemia of Malignancy

The second most common type of hypercalcemia is that caused by malignancy. Two mechanisms may be responsible: direct osteolysis, as in breast cancer, or secretion of a protein, with PTH-like effects on bone. This molecule has been isolated and is homologous to the first 13 amino acids of PTH, which is the active portion of the hormone. Hypercalcemia of malignancy differs from primary hyperparathyroidism by having markedly elevated renal excretion of calcium, depressed urinary cAMP levels, depressed 1,25-dihydroxyvitamin D levels, and, most impor-

tant, diminished PTH levels by radioimmunoassay.

Hypoparathyroidism

Hypoparathyroidism is an uncommon disorder that results from diminished PTH secretion. Primary hypoparathyroidism stems from insufficient parathyroid function (usually after thyroidectomy or parathyroidectomy), whereas secondary hypoparathyroidism occurs in response to a high serum calcium level. Occasionally, hypoparathyroidism arises after irradiation of the neck. Only in rare cases does the disease arise from idiopathic causes, such as hypoplastic or absent glands.

The symptoms of hypoparathyroidism are those of hypocalcemia; they include irritability of the neuromuscular system, seizures, laryngospasm, and tetany. Patients with primary idiopathic hypoparathyroidism often have a constellation of findings: dental abnormalities (delayed eruption, pitting, and caries); moniliasis, caused by a defect in the immune system; endocrine disorders, such as adrenal insufficiency; and cutaneous manifestations, including alopecia, coarse hair, dry skin, and cataracts.

Radiographic findings are rarely helpful; however, laboratory tests are useful: immunoreactive PTH peptides are low or undetectable, serum calcium is lowered, phosphate is moderately elevated, and 1,25-dihydroxyvitamin D levels are low. Alkaline phosphatase is normal, but other parameters of bone resorption and turnover, such as urinary hydroxyproline levels, are low. The *Ellsworth-Howard test* is positive, with a marked increase in urinary cAMP and phosphate excretion after administration of parathyroid hormone.

Treatment is aimed at restoring serum calcium levels while avoiding hypercalciuria. Calcium and vitamin D supplements are given to maintain serum calcium in the low-normal range. Sometimes phosphate-binding antacids are needed to diminish the phosphate level, and thiazides may be used to reduce urinary calcium excretion.

Pseudohypoparathyroidism

Pseudohypoparathyroidism is clinically similar to hypoparathyroidism but is caused by resistance to PTH. These patients also have hypocalcemia and hyperphosphatemia, but the distinguishing feature is a high PTH level. The Ellsworth-Howard test fails to show an increase in urinary cAMP and phosphate excretion following a PTH challenge. Patients with pseudohypoparathyroidism have a constellation of musculoskeletal abnormalities known as *Albright's hereditary osteodystrophy,* which includes subcutaneous ossification, calcification of the basal ganglia, metacarpal and metatarsal shortening, premature physeal closure, exostoses, obesity, short stature, and round facies. Treatment is similar to that for primary hypoparathyroidism, with calcium and vitamin D supplements.

Pseudopseudohypoparathyroidism may represent a milder form of pseudohypoparathyroidism. Patients demonstrate characteristic findings of Albright hereditary osteodystrophy but are more responsive to PTH. Normocalcemia is the rule, often with normal PTH levels as well.

Disorders of Mineralization

Osteomalacia and Rickets

Osteomalacia is a disease of impaired bone mineralization. In childhood the disorder affects physeal growth and is called *rickets.* At the end of the nineteenth century, rickets became widespread because of the lack of exposure to sunlight that accompanied industrialization and urbanization. Cod liver oil was known at that time to prevent and sometimes reverse the stigmata of rickets. As a result, many early investigators favored the theory that rickets resulted from a dietary vitamin deficiency, failing to understand that vitamin D is a steroid hormone produced endogenously in response to sunlight.

Nutritional rickets is usually caused by a lack of *both* sunlight and vitamin D. Natural sources of vitamin D are few, the best being certain fish oils, but nutritional rickets is rare today because of routine fortification of milk with vitamin D. It occasionally occurs in breast-fed infants, since maternal milk is not fortified. In one U.S. study, there were fewer than 0.4 cases per 100,000 pediatric admissions; however, nutritional rickets remains a problem in the third world.

A low serum level of vitamin D results in poor intestinal absorption of calcium. Mineralization of osteoid is impaired, but the reason is unclear. The serum calcium concentration and the calcium-phosphate ion product often remain normal. It is possible that vitamin D affects mineralization directly; however, intravenous calcium alone can reverse the abnormalities of vitamin D deficiency. By some undetermined mechanism, the body is able to sense the diminished intake of calcium and slow the deposition of calcium into bones. It should be stressed that mineralization is not the result of osteoblastic activity. Osteoblasts continue to make osteoid more rapidly than normal, since bone resorption and turnover increase to sustain the serum calcium level. The histologic hallmarks of osteomalacia are widened, unmineralized osteoid seams (Fig. 16.8).

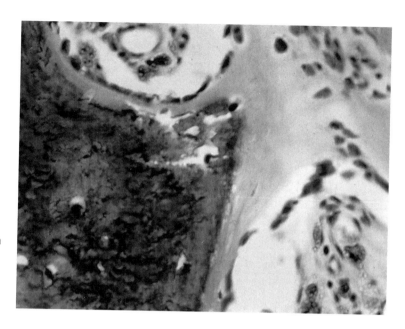

Figure 16.8
Osteomalacia. This uncalcified histologic section shows wide osteoid seams lined by plump osteoblasts. The calcium appears as black spots.

Poor dietary intake of calcium rarely causes osteomalacia and rickets. The body has a remarkable capacity to increase the efficiency of calcium absorption from the intestines and kidney, provided of course that vitamin D levels are normal. One important group of patients at risk for pure calcium deficiency are premature infants. Mineralization of the skeleton occurs at a very rapid pace during the third trimester. Premature infants have a higher daily calcium requirement than infants born at term, and the amount of calcium in regular formula may not suffice. Inattention to calcium intake, whether by oral feeding or parenteral nutrition, can lead to rickets.

Excluding renal osteodystrophy, over 75 percent of cases of osteomalacia are caused by gastrointestinal disorders, including malabsorption syndromes, hepatobiliary diseases, and pancreatic insufficiency. Partial or total gastrectomy is responsible for half of the cases. In a sense, patients have nutritional osteomalacia, since the absorption of calcium or vitamin D is impaired. The causes of calcium and vitamin D malabsorption include poor dietary intake, avoidance of dairy products, diarrhea, dumping syndrome, and anatomic changes in the gastrointestinal tract. The loss of biliary acids and steatorrhea reduce the absorption of fat-soluble vitamins, including vitamin D; moreover, excess fatty acids in the intestinal lumen bind calcium and impede its absorption.

The symptoms of osteomalacia and rickets include bone pain, weakness, and difficulty walking. Bone pain is usually dull and aching. Sometimes the pain is localized to a stress fracture. Weakness results from a myopathy of uncertain origin, possibly neurogenic, since biopsies have not shown primary disease of muscle. The gait is waddling and broadly based, with a short stride and wide trunk oscillation, which result from a combination of weakness, pain, and skeletal deformities.

The clinical picture is age-related. Rickets is typified by genu varum or bowlegs (Fig. 16.9). Other long bones may also be bowed. The *saber shin* results from the strong pull of the calf muscles. Eruption of teeth is delayed, and problems with dentition are common. The skull may exhibit *craniotabes,* which consists of frontal bossing, parietal flattening, and softening. Scoliosis occurs frequently. The term *rachitic rosary* refers to prominent costochondral junctions over the chest and upper abdomen, which arise from widened growth plates

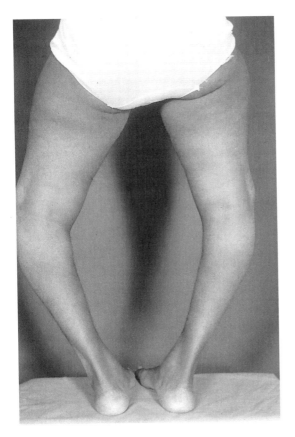

Figure 16.9   Rickets. Genu varum is pronounced in untreated rickets.

of ribs. *Harrison's groove* is an indentation of the lower ribs at the attachment of the diaphragm.

Radiographs in children characteristically show enlarged physes and widened metaphyses. The bone at the metaphyseal end appears osteopenic, frayed, and irregular. As the physes enlarge, the metaphyseal end becomes cupped, with a thin rim of bone extending around the epiphysis (Fig. 16.10).

The clinical findings of osteomalacia differ from those in rickets. Skeletal deformities are uncommon. Bowing of long bones does not occur, although patients may develop kyphosis of the thoracic spine and pectus carinatum. Radiographs most commonly show nonspecific osteopenia. The softened vertebrae often have a biconcave appearance from compression by the disks. Occasionally, *protrusio acetabuli* creates a *triradiate pelvis,* which imparts a trefoil shape to the pelvic inlet. Natural childbirth may be hazardous or impossible with such a pelvis. *Looser zones* or *pseudofractures* appear as radiolucent lines (osteoid seams) at right angles to the cortex (Fig. 16.11). Although suggestive of stress fractures, Looser zones behave differently and tend to be bilateral, symmetrical, and constant over long periods of time. They often involve bones that do not bear weight: ribs, pubic rami, scapulae, and the proximal ulna. Looser zones are not pathognomonic for osteomalacia, since they occasionally occur in other diseases, such as osteoporosis, fibrous dysplasia, and Paget disease.

Biochemical indices often aid diagnosis, but test results depend to a certain extent on underlying pathology. Calcium and phosphate levels are low to normal, but the alkaline phosphatase is characteristically high, reflecting greater bone turnover. Parathyroid hormone levels may be elevated as a result of hypocalcemia. In equivocal cases, bone biopsy with

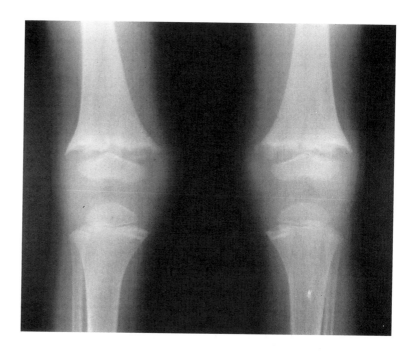

Figure 16.10   Rickets. Note the osteopenia, widened physes, and flared, irregular metaphyses of the distal femur.

tetracycline labeling is the best means of establishing a diagnosis.

Treatment depends in large measure on underlying disorders. Patients with malabsorption of fat, for example, usually require parenteral vitamin D or ultraviolet light therapy to raise levels of vitamin D. In general, patients should receive supplements of both calcium and vitamin D. For patients with normal intestinal absorption, vitamin D_2 (calciferol) usually suffices. For patients who need more potent preparations, calcifediol (as 25-hydroxyvitamin D_3) is safer than the more potent calcitriol [$1,25(OH)_2$ vitamin D], which is occasionally associated with serious side effects, including renal toxicity, hypercalcemia, nephrolithiasis, and increased bone resorption.

Vitamin D–Dependent Rickets

Vitamin D–dependent rickets is caused by an inborn error of metabolism. Children with this rare disorder develop rickets despite normal

vitamin D intake and exposure to sunlight. In type I disease, the renal 1-hydroxylase enzyme is deficient, leading to diminished levels of 1,25-dihydroxyvitamin D. In type II disease, there is a defect in the receptor for vitamin D, resulting in markedly elevated levels of 1,25-dihydroxyvitamin D. Treatment of type I disease is accomplished with physiologic doses of 1,25-dihydroxyvitamin D. Type II disease, more difficult to treat, may entail empiric trials of vitamin D analogues and high doses of calcium (1 to 3 g/day). In refractory cases, patients may benefit from intravenous calcium therapy.

Hypophosphatemic (vitamin D–Resistant) Rickets

Hypophosphatemic (vitamin D–resistant) rickets is an X-linked dominant disease that reduces renal tubular reabsorption of phosphate. Following the decline of nutritional rickets, hypophosphatemic rickets is now a

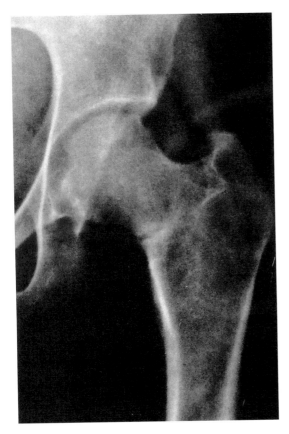

Figure 16.11 Osteomalacia. Note the Looser zone, or pseudofracture, at the base of the femoral neck.

and widening of the physis (Fig. 16.12). The disease is treated in childhood with aggressive phosphate replacement, 1 to 3 g/day. The risk of secondary hypocalcemia and secondary hyperparathyroidism is lessened by the addition of 1,25-dihydroxyvitamin D, which is more effective in this disorder than other forms of vitamin D. It is not known whether therapy should be continued in the adult.

Fanconi Syndrome

Fanconi syndrome embraces a diverse group of disorders that have in common a defect in proximal tubular transport in the kidneys. Os-

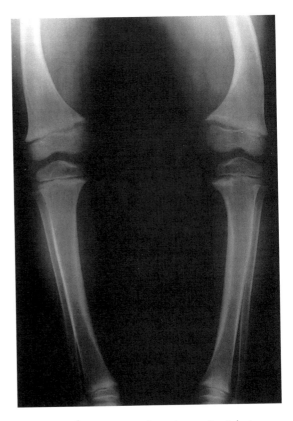

Figure 16.12 Hypophosphatemic rickets. Note the mild bowing and physeal irregularity.

more common cause of rickets in the United States. The reduction in phosphate level has a direct, adverse effect on bone mineralization. In addition, patients also have an abnormality of vitamin D metabolism. The classic triad of hypophosphatemia, lower limb deformities, and short stature most often affects males. Heterozygous females have impaired phosphate reabsorption, usually with minimal clinical sequelae. The severity of the disorder varies; many patients have subtle findings, and some exhibit genu valgum rather than genu varum. Radiographs often show only mild irregularity

teomalacia results primarily from impaired phosphate resorption but may also arise from defective vitamin D metabolism. Many molecules besides phosphate are excreted in excess, including calcium, glucose, bicarbonate, and amino acids. The syndrome may be inherited or, more commonly, caused by damage to the proximal tubule. Some patients fare better with phosphate replacement; others require vitamin D supplementation.

Renal Tubular Acidosis

In *renal tubular acidosis* (RTA), which is frequently caused by Fanconi syndrome, a defect in bicarbonate reabsorption leads to metabolic acidosis. Osteomalacia is not common but can result from metabolic acidosis, which impedes mineralization and promotes bone erosion. Other conditions that cause metabolic acidosis, such as ureteral diversion, can manifest a similiar picture. Administration of alkali usually leads to resolution of osteomalacia in these patients.

Hypophosphatasia

The term *hypophosphatasia* refers to a rare group of disorders that bear a certain resemblance to rickets but stem from a defect in alkaline phosphatase rather than a derangement of calcium, phosphate, or vitamin D metabolism. The prevalence of the disease is 1 in 100,000. The disorders have a wide range of expression, from a lethal, infantile form to a mild, adult form. Adults commonly develop stress fractures (especially of the metatarsals), chondrocalcinosis, and pseudofractures. Fractures are often slow to heal. Calcium, vitamin D, and PTH levels are normal. The alkaline phosphatase level is low and the phosphate level high. The pyridoxal 5'-phosphate level, a specific test for this disorder, is elevated. No effective treatment is available. Vitamin D and

mineral supplements may precipitate hypercalcemia and hypercalciuria.

Anticonvulsant Therapy

Anticonvulsant therapy produces a radiographic picture suggesting mild rickets in some 8 percent of epileptic children, but the bone disease is not well understood. Possibly, anticonvulsants stimulate hepatic enzymes, which increase catabolism of vitamin D. However, while phenobarbital is the most potent inducer of hepatic microsomal enzymes, phenytoin is the drug most commonly associated with bone disease. It is possible that the drugs have specific direct effects on the absorption of calcium and the mineralization of osteoid.

Disorders of Vitamin D and Calcium Excess

Milk-Alkali Syndrome

The mirror image of osteomalacia is a condition resulting from excessive intake of calcium and vitamin D, which can also lead to serious metabolic derangements. The milk-alkali syndrome arose from a diet introduced by Sippy in 1915 for peptic ulcers that involved ingestion of large amounts of milk with alkaline salts of calcium. Many patients developed toxic hypercalcemia and metabolic alkalosis as a result of the diet.

Sarcoidosis (Boeck Sarcoid)

Excessive vitamin D intake is occasionally iatrogenic, but certain diseases can cause inappropriate, extrarenal production of 1,25-dihydroxyvitamin D, including sarcoidosis, granulomatous diseases, and lymphomas. Patients show the usual manifestations of hypercalcemia. Approximately 10 percent of patients have bone pain, especially in the hands

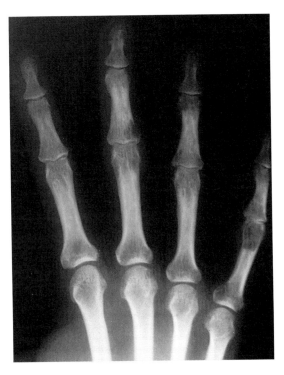

Figure 16.13 Sarcoidosis. Note the multiple lytic lesions and coarse trabeculae.

(Fig. 16.13). Macrophages in granulomas have been found to be responsible for the 1-hydroxylation of 25-hydroxyvitamin D outside the kidney. Gamma interferon, not PTH, stimulates macrophages to produce the hydroxylase. The macrophages are exquisitely sensitive to and inhibited by corticosteroids.

Renal Osteodystrophy

The term *renal osteodystrophy* refers to the derangements of bone and mineral metabolism that accompany chronic renal failure. The processes primarily responsible for this syndrome are osteomalacia and secondary hyperparathyroidism. Clinical manifestations are variable

and depend upon whether osteomalacia or hyperparathyroidism predominates.

Osteomalacia may result from impaired renal hydroxylation of vitamin D. The kidneys are progressively less able to convert 25(OH) vitamin D to 1,25(OH)₂ vitamin D. Another important cause of osteomalacia is aluminum toxicity, which impairs mineralization of osteoid. In the past, patients accumulated aluminum from impurities in dialysis solutions, but recognition of this problem has led to better water purification. Aluminum toxicity is now more likely to occur from ingestion of large amounts of antacids and phosphate-binding gels.

Secondary hyperparathyroidism is related to hyperphosphatemia, but its pathogenesis is obscure. One theory is that hyperphosphatemia inhibits renal production of 1,25(OH)₂ vitamin D, which normally suppresses secretion of parathyroid hormone.

Clinical findings in renal osteodystrophy include bone pain, skeletal deformities, growth retardation, dental abnormalities, fractures, and myopathy. In patients with severe hyperphosphatemia, soft tissue calcification can lead to numerous debilitating symptoms. Metastatic calcification becomes likely when the calcium-phosphate ion product exceeds 75. Calcific deposits in joints and tendon sheaths evoke an inflammatory response similar to that in pseudogout. In blood vessels, calcifications may lead to obstruction, vascular compromise, and even gangrene. Rarely, when calcifications reach massive proportions, *tumoral calcification* occurs (Fig. 16.14).

The most common radiographic finding in renal osteodystrophy is osteopenia, but lesions of both rickets/osteomalacia and hyperparathyroidism may coexist. Looser zones are typical of osteomalacia, and bowing of long bones

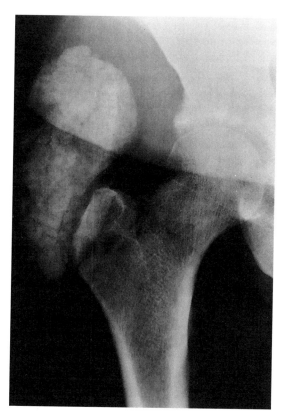

Figure 16.14 Tumoral calcinosis. The massive precipitate of calcium salts is caused by metabolic derangement rather than neoplastic growth.

malities. Calcium levels may be low, normal, or even high. Hyperphosphatemia worsens as the glomerular filtration rate diminishes. Hypermagnesemia can develop, especially with ingestion of magnesium-containing antacids, and alkaline phosphatase is usually elevated. Osteocalcin, a marker of osteoblastic activity, increases in secondary hyperparathyroidism but is a reliable test only in patients undergoing dialysis. Parathyroid hormone levels are elevated, and an inverse relationship exists between PTH levels and the glomerular filtration rate; however, PTH levels do not closely correlate with bone pathology or the severity of secondary hyperparathyroidism.

Bone biopsy is useful to assess pathologic processes in bone and to distinguish "low-turnover bone disease," generally attributed to osteomalacia, from "high-turnover bone disease," which is more characteristic of hyperparathyroidism. Osteomalacia exhibits increased osteoid thickness and a decreased rate of mineralization, while secondary hyperparathyroidism is associated with increased numbers of osteoclasts, Howship's lacunae, and fibrosis of the marrow. Bone biopsy is preferred for the diagnosis of aluminum toxicity, since serum levels of aluminum do not reflect total body stores.

Treatment of renal osteodystrophy is complex. The phosphate level must be controlled to remove the impetus for secondary hyperparathyroidism. Dietary restriction is difficult, since phosphate is widespread in foods and is abundant in meat and dairy products, and many find a low-phosphate diet unpalatable. Furthermore, patients on continuous ambulatory peritoneal dialysis need a relatively high protein intake to offset peritoneal losses of protein. Many patients take phosphate-binding gels to reduce secondary hyperparathyroidism.

and physeal widening suggest rickets. Subperiosteal erosions and large lytic areas follow hyperparathyroidism. A characteristic but enigmatic lesion of renal osteodystrophy is *osteosclerosis,* which usually involves the ribs, pelvis, or spine. Vertebrae may exhibit a *"rugger jersey"* appearance, with bands of sclerosis across the end plates. Another curious radiographic finding is *periosteal neostosis,* in which new periosteal bone formation occurs, favoring the femur and metatarsals.

Biochemical tests show a variety of abnor-

Aluminum hydroxide is commonly prescribed, but it is unclear how much can be given safely without causing aluminum-induced osteomalacia. The alternative is calcium carbonate or calcium acetate, but a large dose must be administered, typically 2 to 15 g/day, which is dangerous if the phosphate level is markedly elevated, since simultaneous hypercalcemia and hyperphosphatemia will precipitate extraskeletal calcification. Patients with persistent hypercalcemia and secondary hyperparathyroidism may benefit from partial parathyroidectomy or treatment with 1,25-dihydroxyvitamin D, which exerts an inhibitory effect on the parathyroid glands.

If phosphate levels can be controlled, calcium supplements (1 to 2 g/day) are added to ensure adequate intake. Hypocalcemia in the presence of normal phosphate levels suggests the need for vitamin D treatment, especially if PTH levels are elevated and secondary hyperparathyroidism is present. Biopsy-documented osteomalacia is another indication for vitamin D therapy, but osteomalacia caused by aluminum toxicity will not respond to vitamin D. If aluminum toxicity is present, calcium carbonate must be substituted for aluminum-based phosphate binders, and the concentration of aluminum in the water for dialysis must be kept under 10 μg/L. In severe cases, deferoxamine may be necessary for chelation of aluminum.

Endocrinologic Disorders

Cushing Syndrome

An important cause of osteopenia is excessive endogenous secretion of cortisol, which occurs in Cushing syndrome. More commonly, however, glucocorticoid excess is a result of long-term steroid therapy. Corticosteroids have multiple deleterious effects on mineral metabolism, including suppression of osteoblasts, stimulation of renal calcium excretion, and impairment of intestinal absorption of calcium. Parathyroid hormone levels increase to sustain serum calcium levels, leading to osteoclastic resorption of bone. The degree of bone loss is not strictly related to the steroid dose.

Clinical manifestations of bone disease may be few; in fact, a fracture following minor trauma is often the first indication of bone pathology. Radiographs usually demonstrate nonspecific osteopenia and trabecular bone loss. Serum calcium, phosphate, and vitamin D levels are normal. Alkaline phosphatase and osteocalcin usually decline, since less bone is formed.

As there is no effective way to increase osteoblastic activity, therapy must emphasize increased calcium intake, which causes PTH levels to decrease and the rate of bone resorption to diminish. To avoid nephrocalcinosis and nephrolithiasis, caution must be exercised in administering calcium and vitamin D. Patients with hypercalciuria may benefit from thiazide therapy prior to calcium supplementation.

Thyroid Disorders

Thyroid hormone is essential for skeletal growth and development. In children with *hypothyroidism,* the lack of thyroid hormone leads to *cretinism,* which is characterized by growth retardation, delayed maturation, and dental anomalies. Epiphyseal fragmentation and irregularities are common radiographic findings. In adults, bone changes are minimal, although bone density may increase as a result of decreased turnover.

Hyperthyroidism increases bone turnover and causes mild hypercalcemia, hyperphosphatemia, elevated alkaline phosphatase, and hypercalciuria. Thyroid hormone has a direct effect on bone metabolism independent of parathyroid hormone. While osteopenia, bone pain, and fractures occur in some patients, bone disease is usually not prominent.

Disorders of Growth Hormone

Growth hormone is essential for skeletal growth and has multiple effects on protein, carbohydrate, and mineral metabolism. Intestinal calcium absorption, bone formation, and excretion of urinary calcium increase in response to growth hormone. Patients are in positive calcium and phosphate balance, with more mineral absorbed than lost daily.

In children, a deficiency of growth hormone results in short stature, whereas an excess produces *gigantism.* In adults, overproduction of growth hormone stimulates periosteal bone formation and results in *acromegaly,* which is characterized by mandibular enlargement ("lantern jaw"), prominence of the forehead, coarsening of facial features, dental malocclusion, and enlargement of the skeleton. Arthritis is common because growth hormone promotes the synthesis of a friable cartilage matrix, which is prone to early degeneration.

Osteoporosis

Primary osteoporosis is a disease of generalized diminished bone mass unrelated to other diseases. Loss of mineral content weakens bones, and the incidence of fractures rises exponentially as bone density declines (Fig. 16.15). *Osteopenia* is a more general term referring to decreased bone density, but this con-dition may occur locally and be reversible, as in cast immobilization. While osteoporosis may occur in the young, the overwhelming majority of patients are elderly. Since bone mass decreases in all people after the third or fourth decade, osteoporosis entails *excessive* bone loss; however, there is no firm agreement on the distinction between normal and abnormal bone loss, which is sometimes made on the basis of fractures following minimal trauma.

In western societies, osteoporosis is the most common and the most costly metabolic bone disease. In the United States, approximately 1.5 million fractures are attributed to osteoporosis each year. The lifetime risk of a fracture of the hip is 15 percent for women and 5 percent for men. The costs for acute care of hip fractures exceed $7 billion annually, and the total cost is much higher, since many patients require extended nursing care.

Sex and race are important risk factors. Females are affected at an earlier age and to a greater degree than men. Vertebral fractures favor women by a 10 : 1 margin, while hip fractures predilect women by a 3 : 1 ratio. Blacks have greater bone mass than whites, who have more bone mass than Orientals.

Estrogen deficiency has clearly been linked to osteoporosis. The lack of sex steroids, either estrogen or testosterone, has an adverse effect on osteoblasts. Osteoporosis has thus been divided into two broad categories, postmenopausal (type I) and senile (type II). Women with postmenopausal osteoporosis exhibit a rapid loss of calcium in the years immediately following menopause. Women who undergo oophorectomy or become amenorrheic (as from excessive exercise or anorexia nervosa) develop essentially the same type of osteoporo-

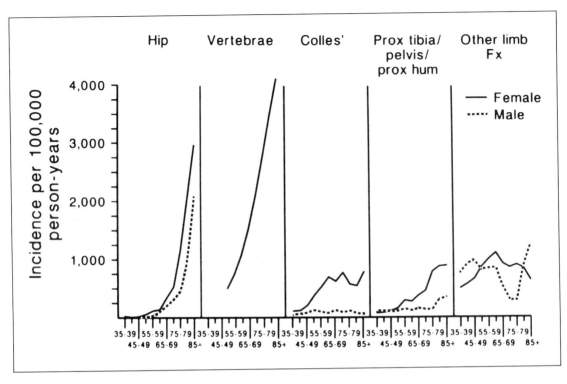

Figure 16.15 Osteoporosis. Relationship between the incidence of
fractures, age, and anatomic location. (Reprinted with permission from
Melton LJ and Cummings SR: Heterogeneity of age-related fractures:
implications for epidemiology. *Bone Miner* 2:321–331, 1987

sis. In contrast, senile osteoporosis is a slow,
age-related phenomenon that becomes symptomatic much later than postmenopausal osteoporosis and affects men as well as women.

The development of senile osteoporosis is
related to multiple factors. The efficiency of
intestinal absorption of calcium decreases with
age. Since most patients have normal vitamin
D levels, the decrease in absorption is probably
caused by an intrinsic intestinal problem. Dysfunction may be present in the kidneys as well;
despite the reduction in intestinal calcium absorption, the kidneys fail to decrease the rate

of calcium excretion. As a result, there is a net
negative calcium balance, with slightly more
calcium lost each day than is absorbed. Osteoblastic function appears to be compromised
in the elderly. The number of osteoblasts falls,
the ratio of osteoblasts to osteoclasts declines,
and osteoblasts are active for shorter periods
of time. Decreased physical activity may further contribute to bone loss, as do other conditions that reduce mechanical stress, such as
bed rest, weightlessness, and immobilization.

The early stages of osteoporosis are usually
asymptomatic; however, with rapid postmen-

opausal bone loss, multiple vertebral compression fractures cause back pain and progressive deformity. Collapse of the vertebral column leads to diminished height, abdominal protrusion, and apposition of the costal margin to the pelvic brim, which can be painful. Increased thoracic kyphosis gives rise to the *dowager's hump.*

Most cases of osteoporosis come to attention following an acute fracture. Not all bones are equally affected (Fig. 16.15). Osteoporosis has a distinct predilection for the distal radius, proximal femur, and thoracolumbar spine. Fractures of the distal radius occur at an earlier age than fractures of the hip or spine because loss of trabecular bone is more pronounced in the distal radius. As the disease involves cortical bone to greater degrees, fractures of the hip become more likely. Although such a fracture is usually a dramatic event, some individuals ambulate with stress fractures of the hip or nondisplaced fractures for weeks before seeking medical attention.

Radiographic findings in osteoporosis are often only those of bone loss. The spine may show *codfish vertebrae,* with concavities of the end plates (Fig. 16.16). In long-standing cases, anterior vertebral collapse leads to increased thoracic kyphosis, and occasionally flattening of entire vertebrae occurs. Both types of vertebral failure result from stress fractures.

Laboratory tests, such as serum calcium, phosphate, and alkaline phosphatase, while usually within normal limits, are useful to exclude other causes of osteopenia. Patients with equivocal serum and urine tests may benefit from a bone biopsy after tetracycline labeling to exclude osteomalacia. Patients with rapidly worsening osteoporosis and multiple vertebral fractures are also candidates for biopsy. The most characteristic microscopic finding is a de-

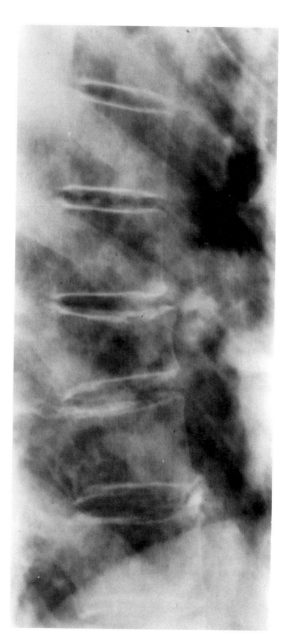

Figure 16.16   Osteoporosis of the thoracic spine. Note the anterior collapse of a vertebra, collapse of end plates (codfish vertebra), and osteopenia.

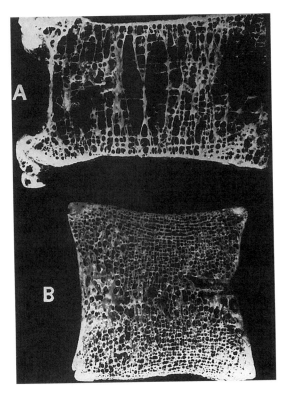

Figure 16.17   Osteoporosis. Macroscopic section of a vertebral body from a patient with osteoporosis shows *(A)* loss of trabeculae and gross flattening of the bone compared to *(B)* a normal young adult. (Reprinted with permission from Barzel US (ed): *Osteoporosis.* Orlando, FL, Grune & Stratton, 1970.)

therefore been placed upon prevention. One strategy is to maximize peak bone mass. If more bone mineral were accrued during childhood, more calcium would have to be lost before bones became significantly weakened, which might delay or avert osteoporosis. Several studies have suggested that increased dietary intake of calcium during childhood and adolescent years increases peak bone mass, while calcium supplementation maintains peak bone mass from early to middle adulthood. The current recommendation for calcium intake in adults is 1000 to 1500 mg/day (Table 16.1). Most people do not ingest this much calcium and need supplements. Calcium carbonate is absorbed better in an acid environment and should be taken with food. Calcium citrate is more readily absorbed but more expensive than calcium carbonate.

Although adequate dietary calcium intake is important, it is ineffective in preventing and treating postmenopausal osteoporosis. Estrogen replacement therapy is superior to oral calcium alone and is most effective when started at the time of menopause. Estrogen does not reverse bone loss and is therefore less effective when begun long after menopause. Progestins are usually added to avoid endometrial hyperplasia. The advantages of estrogen replacement include a protective effect against ischemic heart disease and relief of menopausal symptoms. Disadvantages include recurrent menses and a possible increase in blood pressure. The effect on the risk of breast cancer is uncertain, but no clear relationship has yet been demonstrated. Compliance is a problem for many women, since therapy must be lifelong. Discontinuation results in rapid loss of bone mass.

Alternatives to estrogen therapy are cur-

crease in trabecular bone volume (Fig. 16.17). Cortical bone does not show increased porosity but is thinner, owing to endosteal bone erosion. Other histomorphometric parameters are normal.

Most treatments for osteoporosis stabilize bone mass but do not achieve significant increases in bone mineral content. Emphasis has

Table 16.1   Recommended Daily
Calcium Intake

Pediatric patients	Calcium Intake, mg/day
0–6 months	400
6–12 months	600
1–5 years	800
6–10 years	800–1200
11–24 years	1200–1500
Males	
25–65 years	1000
>65 years	1500
Females	
Lactating or pregnant	1200–1500
25–50 years	1000
50–65 years, on estrogen	1000
50–65 years, not on estrogen	1500
>65 years	1500

rently under investigation. *Fluoride* has a well-known but poorly understood ability to increase bone mass. It has not yet been proven to prevent fractures. The therapeutic window for fluoride is narrow. A low dose results in an unpredictable increase in bone mass, whereas a high dose may cause *fluorosis,* a painful disease characterized by osteosclerosis, osteoarthritis, exostoses, and neurologic complications.

Calcitonin inhibits osteoclasts and stabi-

lizes bone mass but has not yet been shown to decrease the risk of fractures. *Biphosphonates* also stabilize bone mass by inhibiting resorption. Older medications, such as sodium etidronate, inhibited mineralization significantly and had to be given on a cyclical basis. Newer medications, such as alendronate, have much less effect on mineralization and do not need to be given cyclically. Alendronate has been approved by the FDA for use in osteoporosis. Various preparations of *vitamin D* have been used in clinical trials. Calcitriol, or 1,25-dihydroxyvitamin D, is the most potent form, but its efficacy in osteoporosis is uncertain. Patients should be monitored for hypercalcemia and hypercalciuria. *Anabolic steroids* are synthetic derivatives of the androgen testosterone. These compounds increase bone mass significantly, but they are associated with liver dysfunction, elevation of low-density lipoproteins, hirsutism, acne, and hoarseness.

The most serious complication of osteoporosis is death following a fracture. The risk of death in patients who sustain a fracture of the hip is 15 to 20 percent above age-matched controls during the first year after fracture. In the absence of major medical illnesses, surgery is relatively safe and avoids the complications of fluid stasis attendant upon prolonged bed rest.

Sclerosing Dysplasias of Bone

Numerous metabolic bone diseases result in excessive bone formation, but they are rarer than disorders that cause osteopenia, and they are not usually associated with significant disturbances of calcium and phosphate metabolism. *Myositis ossificans progressiva* (also known as *fibrodysplasia ossificans progressiva*) is an inherited disorder that produces

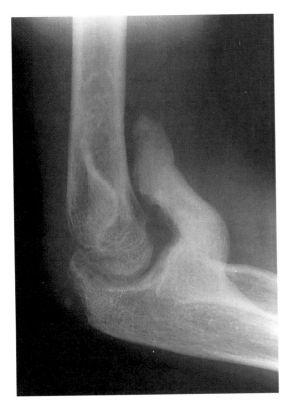

Figure 16.18 Heterotopic ossification in the brachialis muscle following a dislocation of the elbow.

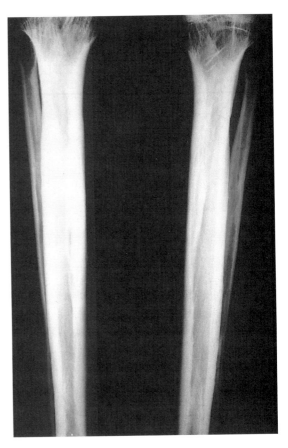

Figure 16.19 Engelmann disease. Note the cortical thickening in both tibias.

widespread ectopic ossification and ankylosis of joints. Excision is followed promptly by massive recurrence. The disease is distinct from *heterotopic ossification,* which is a common, localized sequela of trauma and surgery (Fig. 16.18). *Progressive diaphyseal dysplasia (Engelmann disease)* is an autosomal dominant disease characterized by symmetrical, fusiform swelling of the shafts of long bones (Fig. 16.19). Both osteoblastic and osteoclastic activities are increased. Abundant disorganized bone replaces lamellar bone and obliterates the medullary cavity, causing secondary anemia. In addition to Engelmann disease, many other curious disorders are characterized by increased bone formation in various patterns (see Chap. 17).

Osteopetrosis

Osteopetrosis, also known as *marble bone disease* or *Albers-Schönberg disease,* results from a failure of osteoclasts to resorb bone. Although bones appear more dense, they are structurally brittle and weak because of a defect in the remodeling of immature, woven

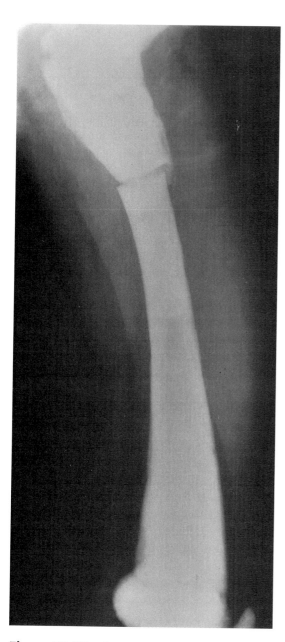

Figure 16.20 Osteopetrosis. Note the radiodense bone lacking a medullary canal. Despite the solid appearance, the bone is quite brittle, and a transverse fracture has occurred.

bone to mature, lamellar bone. Obliteration of the medullary canal confers a striking radiographic appearance (Fig. 16.20).

At least five different types of the disease have been described. The two major types include an autosomal dominant "benign" form and an autosomal recessive "malignant" form. The benign form is often asymptomatic, whereas the malignant form is fatal in childhood if untreated. Early manifestations of the malignant variety include nasal stuffiness, cranial nerve palsies, delayed eruption of teeth, fractures, genu valgum, and failure to thrive. Bone marrow failure causes bleeding, anemia, and recurrent infections. Treatment entails bone marrow transplantation, which is not uniformly successful, perhaps reflecting the heterogeneity of the disorder.

SUGGESTED READINGS

AVIOLI LV, KRANE SM (EDS): *Metabolic Bone Disease and Clinically Related Disorders.* Philadelphia, Saunders, 1990.

BROADUS AE, MANGIN M, IKEDA K, ET AL: Humoral hypercalcemia of malignancy: Identification of a novel parathyroid hormone–like peptide. *N Engl J Med* 319:556–563, 1988.

COCCIA PF, KRIVIT W, CERVENKA J, ET AL: Successful bone-marrow transplantation for infantile malignant osteopetrosis. *N Engl J Med* 302: 701–708, 1980.

COE FL, FAVUS MJ (EDS): *Disorders of Bone and Mineral Metabolism.* New York, Raven Press, 1992.

CUMMINGS SR, KELSEY JL, NEVITT MC, O'DOWD KJ: Epidemiology of osteoporosis and osteoporotic fractures. *Epidemiol Rev* 7:178–208, 1985.

FAVUS MJ (ED): *Primer on the Metabolic Bone Diseases and Disorders of Mineral Metabolism*, 2d ed. New York, Raven Press, 1993.

KOOH SW, FRASER D, REILLY BJ, ET AL: Rickets due to calcium deficiency. *N Engl J Med* 297: 1264, 1977.

RIGGS BL, MELTON LJ III (EDS): *Osteoporosis: Etiology, Diagnosis, and Management.* New York, Raven Press, 1988.

NIH CONSENSUS DEVELOPMENT PANEL ON OPTIMAL CALCIUM INTAKE: OPTIMAL CALCIUM INTAKE. *JAMA* 272:2942–2950, 1994.

Chapter *17*

Developmental Disorders

Edmund R. Campion and Frank C. Wilson

GENERALIZED DISORDERS

Paget Disease (Osteitis Deformans)

Osteosclerosing Disorders
   Caffey Disease (Infantile Cortical Hyperostosis); Melorheostosis; Osteopoikilosis; Osteopathia Striata

REGIONAL DISORDERS

Disorders of Alignment in the Lower Limbs
   Physiologic Genu Varum; Physiologic Genu Valgum; Femoral Torsion; Tibial Torsion

Flat-Foot Deformities
   Flexible Flat Foot (Pes Planovalgus); Tarsal Coalition

Metatarsalgia

Hallux Valgus

Mallet Toe, Hammer Toe, and Claw Toe

Palmar Fibromatosis (Dupuytren Disease)

Plantar Fibromatosis (Lederhosen Disease)

The musculoskeletal system requires an exquisitely orchestrated balance of internal and external influences for normal growth and development. Disorders of structure and alignment result from internal perturbations of the normal developmental process or from external forces acting over time. Bowed legs (genu varum) and knock-knees (genu valgum) are examples of the former and are caused by derangements of growth; hallux valgus, which reflects the influence of footwear, typifies the latter.

GENERALIZED DISORDERS

Paget Disease

Paget disease *(osteitis deformans)* is an idiopathic, nonneoplastic condition characterized by disordered modeling of bone, with an increase in both resorption and formation. The condition was first described by Sir James Paget in 1877 and can be localized to one bone

(monostotic) or widely disseminated. Favored sites of involvement are the skull, spine, pelvis, femur, and tibia. The disease tends to affect the elderly, and its prevalence rises with age. In the United States, 3 to 4 percent of the population over 45 years of age have the disease, while 8 percent of people over 80 are affected. Men are affected more often than women, and people of Anglo-Saxon or European descent are especially at risk. The disease is rare in Africa and Asia, but African-Americans are affected to a significant degree.

Paget disease develops through three phases. In the initial osteolytic phase, osteoclasts resorb bone in an aggressive, haphazard manner. In the active or osteoblastic phase, osteoblasts rapidly form osteoid to fill the newly excavated sites, while osteoclastic activity continues. Abundant woven bone is produced in a disorganized mosaic pattern (Fig. 17.1). With time, the bone becomes thickened, deformed, hypervascular, and prone to pathologic fractures. In the final inactive or "burned out" phase, bone turnover diminishes and the

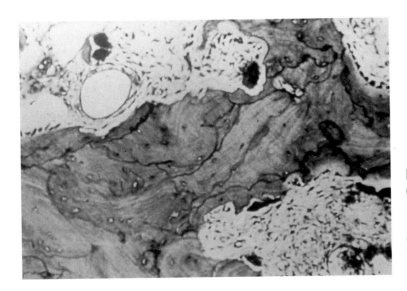

Figure 17.1   Paget disease (active phase). Note *(upper right)* the osteoclasts resorbing bone and osteoblasts forming bone. The mosaic pattern is characteristic of the disorder.

bone becomes sclerotic. Since pagetoid bone does not remodel to form normal lamellar bone, it remains very dense, hard, and brittle.

Nuclear and cytoplasmic inclusions that resemble the nuclear capsids of the respiratory syncytial and measles viruses have been demonstrated within the osteoclasts of pagetoid bone. These observations point toward an infectious cause, but, despite these tantalizing findings, no clear etiologic agent for the disease has been confirmed.

Many patients are asymptomatic and do not seek medical attention. Others have specific symptoms referable to an affected bone. Local warmth results from hypervascularity. Involvement of the femur or tibia results in progressive enlargement, bowing, and an abnormal gait (Fig. 17.2). Secondary degenerative changes often occur in joints, limiting movement and provoking pain. Disease of the spine can cause impingement upon nerve roots, spinal stenosis, and kyphosis. Enlargement of the skull induces frontal bossing and may cause irritation of cranial nerves, especially the acoustic nerve. Rarely, basilar skull invagination and brainstem compression occur.

Laboratory tests reflect increased bone turnover. The alkaline phosphatase level is a sensitive indicator of disease activity and may be elevated to 10 times normal. Urinary hydroxyproline and osteocalcin are also increased as a result of osteoclastic and osteoblastic activity respectively. Calcium levels are usually normal.

Radiographs show distinctive changes in each of the three phases. In the osteolytic phase, radiolucencies can be appreciated in affected bones. *Osteoporosis circumscripta* refers to a well-demarcated area of osteopenia in the cranial vault. Long bones often demonstrate a "blade of grass" or advancing "flame" of osteolysis extending from the epiphysis. In

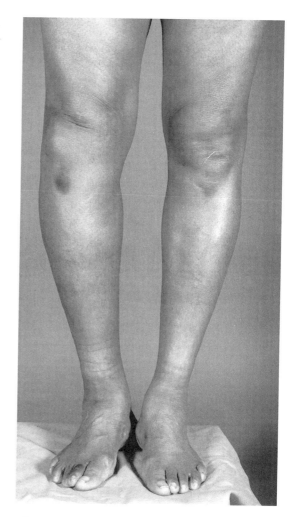

Figure 17.2 Paget disease of the right tibia. Note the bowing and enlargement of the leg.

the active phase, focal or patchy radiodensities become apparent, trabeculae coarsen and thicken, and deformities occur (Fig. 17.3). In the inactive phase, bones become osteosclerotic. The cranium often has a "cotton wool" appearance (Fig. 17.4), while vertebral bodies may resemble solid ivory or a picture frame.

The treatment of Paget disease varies with

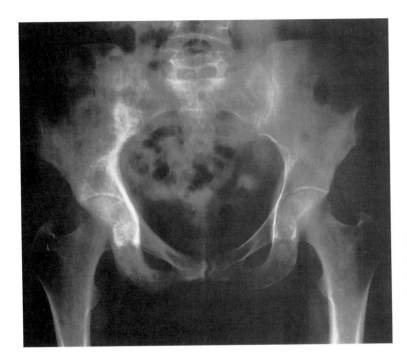

Figure 17.3   Paget disease of the right pelvis. Note thickening of the pubic ramus and ilium. The bony trabeculae are coarser and more radiodense than the uninvolved left pelvis.

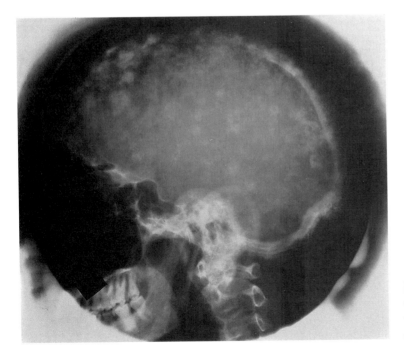

Figure 17.4   Paget disease of the skull. Note the "cotton wool" appearance of the outer table.

its severity. Most patients have mild symptoms and may be successfully managed with analgesics and observation. Treatment of severe cases involves prolonged therapy, which often produces prominent side effects. Although biochemical indices can be improved in two-thirds of patients by treatment, it is unknown whether fractures and other complications can be averted.

For patients with bone pain, biphosphates are tolerated better than other drugs. These medications are pyrophosphate analogues that inhibit bone resorption. Diarrhea, a common side effect with some of the older medications, is managed by withholding the drug for a few days.

Calcitonin directly targets disordered osteoclastic activity. By decreasing bone resorption through inhibition of osteoclastic activity, calcitonin can produce symptomatic relief in less than 2 weeks. Salmon calcitonin is given by subcutaneous injection, starting with 100 units per day, but after a few months, the dose may be reduced to 50 units every other day. Decreased urinary hydroxyproline excretion and serum alkaline phosphate levels parallel the clinical response. Common side effects include flushing and nausea, which are disconcerting but do not necessitate cessation of therapy. After several months, salmon calcitonin may lose its effectiveness, possibly because of downregulation of receptors or an immune response. Human calcitonin is available but is less potent than the salmon preparation.

Plicamycin (mithracin) is a toxic but potent drug that rapidly reduces biochemical indices of bone turnover. Plicamycin is reserved for severe cases, such as those with acute spinal stenosis or brainstem compression, which may mandate emergent surgical decompression. Other indications for surgery include fractures

or arthritis. Joint replacement has been effective in relieving symptoms of degenerative joint disease.

In fewer than 1 percent of patients, the pagetoid lesion undergoes sarcomatous change, usually to osteogenic sarcoma but occasionally to fibrosarcoma or chondrosarcoma. Another uncommon complication is high-output heart failure, stemming from arteriovenous fistulas that occur in pagetoid bone.

Osteosclerosing Disorders

There are a number of rare but interesting skeletal disorders characterized by different patterns of increased bone density. Since these conditions are often asymptomatic, they are usually discovered as unexpected findings on radiographic examinations. These conditions are sometimes hereditary or familial, but no specific causative factors have been identified.

Caffey Disease (Infantile Cortical Hyperostosis)

Caffey disease is a rare and highly unusual hyperostotic lesion seen in children under 5 months of age. This entity was first described by Caffey and Silverman in 1945 and has since been noted in all ethnic groups, without gender preference. The hallmarks of the disorder are periostotic new bone formation and adjacent soft tissue swelling (Fig. 17.5). Caffey disease usually begins with the abrupt onset of fever, soft tissue swelling, and irritability. Any bone can be involved as an isolated finding or as one of multiple foci. The most common sites are the mandible, clavicles, and ribs; the phalanges, tarsal and carpal bones, and vertebrae are the least common. The clinical and radiographic changes subside over a period of months to a few years in most patients, but

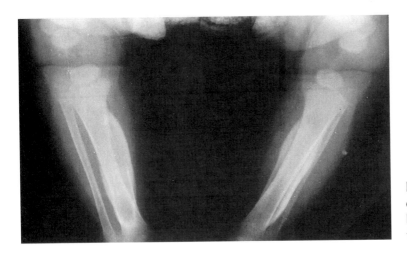

Figure 17.5 Caffey disease. Note the impressive bilateral periosteal bone formation in the tibia.

active disease can persist into later life, with resultant developmental delay and deformity. Fever, elevation of the erythrocyte sedimentation rate, and acute inflammatory changes seen in the periosteum hint at infectious etiology, but no viral or bacterial agents have been identified. Given the usual complete resolution of this disorder, its main importance lies in differentiating it from other entities with which it may be confused. Scurvy may resemble Caffey disease clinically and radiographically, but the onset is later in life. Osteomyelitis and leukemia are distinguished by their distinctive laboratory findings.

Melorheostosis

Melorheostosis is a rare bone disorder distinguished by its unique radiographic appearance (Fig. 17.6). Hyperostoses develop in the long bones as wavy, sclerotic densities that have the appearance of wax flowing down the side of a candle. In flat bones, the hyperostotic lesions are manifest as rounded, sclerotic patches. A second distinctive feature of melorheostosis is its predilection toward involvement of a single limb, in which one or more bones may be affected. No causative factor for melorheostosis has been described. Clinical manifestations are usually minimal and consist of pain, swelling of joints, and limitation of motion, all of which are more common in adults than in children. Deformity and disability occasionally result from limb-length inequality, angulation, and joint contracture.

Osteopoikilosis

In osteopoikilosis, or *spotted bones,* small areas of condensation give the affected bones a speckled radiographic appearance (Fig. 17.7). Involving primarily the metaphyseal and epiphyseal regions of the bone, lesions are composed simply of thickened trabeculae in the spongiosa. Symptoms are infrequent, and no treatment is known or necessary.

Osteopathia Striata

The osteosclerosis seen in osteopathia striata takes the form of longitudinal striations or

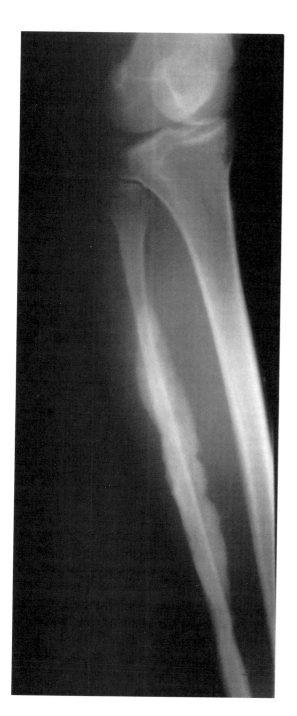

streaks that eventually extend the entire length of the bone (Fig. 17.8). Other than hereditary and familial occurrence, the cause is unknown. The absence of clinical manifestations makes treatment unnecessary.

REGIONAL DISORDERS

Disorders of Alignment in the Lower Limbs

The alignment of mature lower limbs evolves through a process that begins in utero and is finalized by late adolescence. It involves sequential changes in both rotation and angulation of the limbs, many of which, while normal, are also common causes of parental concern.

Bowing of the lower limbs, involving both the tibia and femur, is normal in the early months of life (Fig. 17.9). The varus positioning in utero gradually "corrects" sometime between the 16th and 24th month, when neutral alignment is achieved. This normal developmental swing into more valgus continues until about 4 years of age, when valgus may reach 15°. From then until completion of growth, there is a progressive decrease in physiologic valgus until normal adult alignment of 7 to 8° valgus is reached. Slightly more genu valgum is normal for mature women, which is related to the greater width of the female pelvis.

Figure 17.6   Melorheostosis. Note the hyperostotic lesions of the fibula, resembling wax flowing down the side of a candle.

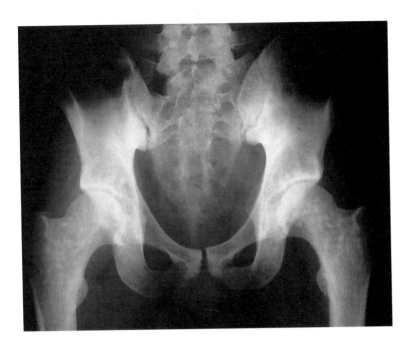

Figure 17.7
Osteopoikilosis. Note the punctate radiodensities in both proximal femurs.

Physiologic Genu Varum

Pathologic varus alignment of the knee is discussed in detail in Chap. 9. In reassuring families that the bowing of early childhood is normal, it is important to differentiate between physiologic or developmental varus and pathologic varus, which is likely to persist or progress. The metaphyseal-diaphyseal angle of Drennan is helpful in this regard (Fig. 9.9). Patients with a Drennan angle of less than 11° are unlikely to develop the changes associated with Blount disease. Other pathologic causes of tibia vara, including rickets, infection, trauma, and bone dysplasias, must also be excluded.

Reassurance, primarily parental, is the only treatment needed for physiologically bowed legs. Radiographs are unnecessary other than in cases of extreme malalignment, and there is no evidence that bracing enhances or hastens correction; but bowed legs can be very disturbing to parents and understanding their concern is an important part of caring for the child.

Physiologic Genu Valgum

Valgus alignment of the knee is a normal finding after 2 years of age (Fig. 17.10). The valgus reaches its peak around 4 years of age and approaches its mature position by age 8. Persistent valgus, especially when combined with obesity, can lead to slowing of lateral growth in the femoral and tibial physes, with progression of deformity beyond the physiologic range. The progression of deformity is best documented by assessing the *intermalleolar distance,* which is the distance between the medial malleoli when the child is standing with knees touching. The likelihood of progression is extremely low unless the intermal-

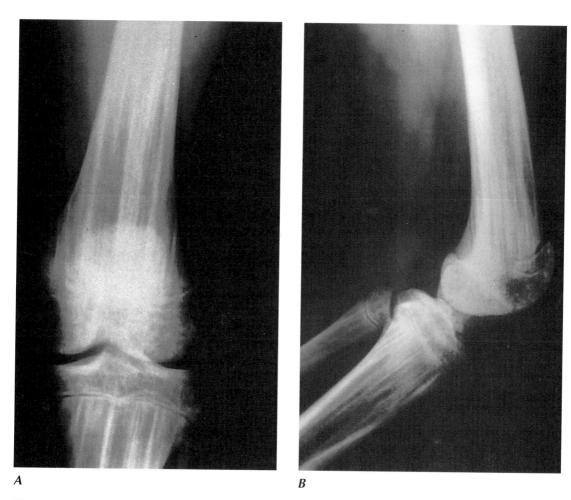

A   *B*

Figure 17.8   Osteopathia striata about the knee. Note the linear radiodensities that typify this entity.

leolar distance is greater than 7.5 cm at age 11 to 12 years.

Persistent genu valgum can lead to an awkward gait with pronated feet, contraction of the iliotibial band, and a propensity to lateral subluxation of the patella. Tibiofemoral and patellofemoral degenerative changes are potential long term sequelae.

The management of most patients with genu valgum is observation. Bracing has never been shown to be efficacious. Should the intermalleolar distance remain greater than 7.5 to 10 cm in adolescence, a medial tibial and/or femoral hemiepiphysiodesis should be considered if adequate growth remains. If not, a varus-producing osteotomy affords an alternative

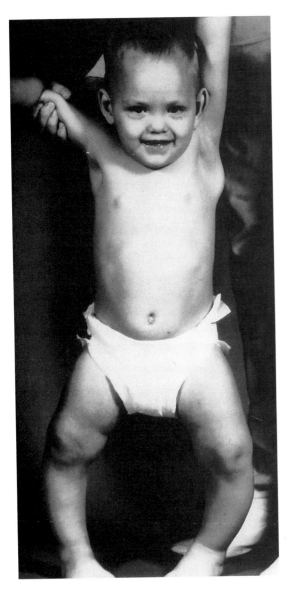

Figure 17.9 Physiologic genu varum. Despite the degree of bowing, there was complete resolution with growth.

means of correction. Since the femur is usually more profoundly involved than the tibia, it is the usual site of operative intervention (Fig. 17.11).

Femoral Torsion

Rotational alignment of the lower limbs evolves throughout childhood in concert with angular development. The commonly encountered complaints of in- toeing and out-toeing are the result of contributions from the foot, tibia, and femur. The combination of these influences is reflected in the *foot-progression angle*, which is defined as the difference between the long axis of the foot and the line of progression during gait (Fig. 17.12). From the onset of walking until maturity, the mean value of this angle is slightly external; however, the range of two standard deviations from the mean (from a slightly in-toeing posture to external rotation of 15°) is within normal limits. In the assessment of an abnormal foot-progression angle, it is important to determine the alignment of the foot as well as that of the tibia and femur.

As illustrated in Chap. 5, femoral torsion is the angular difference between the transcervical and transcondylar axes. In the neonate, the femoral shaft is usually internally rotated approximately 40° with respect to the neck. This degree of *femoral anteversion* decreases gradually to 10 to 15° of anteversion at maturity. While there are roentgenographic techniques for precise measurement of femoral version, it can be estimated with reasonable accuracy by rotation of the hips. With the child prone and the knees flexed to a right angle, the legs are allowed to fall into maximum internal and external rotation. As a rule of thumb, internal rotation should be in the 40 to 50° range and external rotation 40 to 60° throughout child-

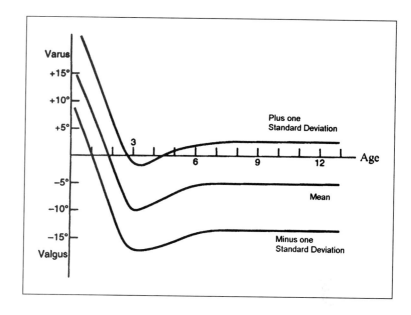

Figure 17.10 The evolution of normal limb alignment. Note the initial bowing, maximum valgus alignment near 4 years of age, and final alignment after age 8.

hood. When excessive femoral anteversion is present, internal rotation of the hips exceeds external rotation. When external rotation is increased and internal rotation decreased, *femoral retroversion* exists.

Management of abnormal femoral version by control of the sleeping, sitting, or walking activities of children is ineffective and frustrating; nor are braces or splints effective. Persistent femoral anteversion is often familial and less likely to correct spontaneously during growth than rotational deformities of the tibia. If, after 8 years of age, internal rotation of the hip is more than 85° and lateral rotation less than 10°, femoral anteversion should be measured by biplane radiography or computed tomography. When it exceeds 50°, rotational osteotomy of the femur should be considered if the clinical indications—such as awkwardness of gait, frequent tripping, and esthetics—are also present. There is no evidence to suggest that abnormal femoral ver-

sion leads to degenerative changes in the hip or knee.

Tibial Torsion

Tibial torsion refers to the contribution of the tibia and fibula to the rotational profile of the leg and is reflected by the angle between the long axis of the foot and the long axis of the thigh. With the knee flexed to 90°, a line is drawn between the midpoints of the tibial and fibular malleoli. The angular deviation between a right angle to that line and the long axis of the thigh is the *transmalleolar axis* (Fig. 17.13). At maturity, normal alignment is near 20° external (lateral) torsion, a gradual progression from the normal 5° of lateral torsion during the first year of life. Isolated internal or medial tibial torsion is uncommon and usually occurs in combination with metatarsus adductus and/or genu varum. Each of these factors contributes to the in-toeing that brings parents to a physician after the

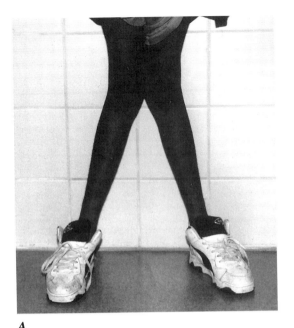

A

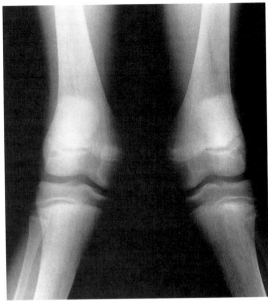

B

C

Figure 17.11   Genu valgum. *A.* With knees touching, the intermalleolar distance is 30 cm. *B.* Underlying renal disease has caused marked deformity in the distal femurs. *C.* Correction was obtained through varus-producing distal femoral osteotomies.

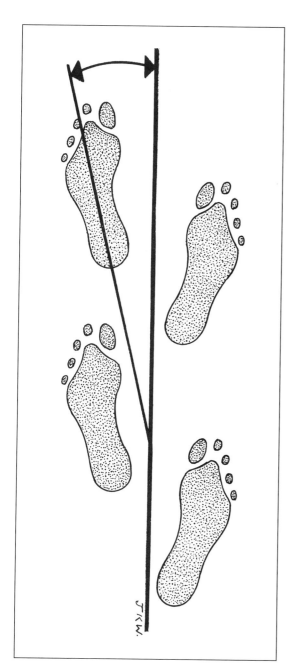

Figure 17.12   Foot-progression angle. The angle formed by the long axis of the foot and the line of progression during gait.

child begins weight-bearing. Casting, splints, braces, and "special shoes" have never been shown to affect tibial rotation, but each of these treatment modalities can *cause* secondary changes, such as flatfoot or genu valgum. In the rare instance of excessive medial tibial torsion persisting at maturity, a derotational osteotomy may be considered.

Flat-Foot Deformities

Flexible Flat Foot (Pes Planovalgus)

The developmental flatfoot is one of the most common and overtreated entities in medicine. Decreased height of the medial longitudinal arch is present in approximately 15 percent of normal adults. Although there is an increased prevalence among patients with diffuse ligamentous laxity and connective tissue disorders (e.g., Ehlers-Danlos syndrome), it is well to remember the prevalence of this condition in the normal population.

The terminology used to describe flat feet reflects the confusion surrounding this subject. The primary deformity includes valgus alignment of the heel and abduction of the forefoot (Fig. 17.14). This alignment gives the appearance of a pronation deformity; in actuality the forefoot is supinated relative to the hindfoot. Correction of the hindfoot deformity makes the supination of the forefoot apparent. For centuries, a relative weakness of the tibialis posterior was posited as the etiology of idiopathic flat feet, and strengthening of this muscle (along with the intrinsic toe musculature) was prescribed as a remedy. Although the tibialis posterior *is* elongated in individuals with pronounced flat feet, there is no evidence that muscle strengthening diminishes or reverses the deformity. It is true, however, that laceration or rupture of the tibialis posterior tendon is the most common cause of an acute acquired flat foot.

Idiopathic tightness of the heel cords is usually associated with flat feet. It is unclear whether this contracture is primary, causing the heel to evert, or secondary to a preexistent valgus alignment of the hindfoot. Idiopathic flat feet that are painful are more commonly associated with pronounced tightness of the heel cords.

The medial longitudinal arch is barely detectable in most newborns, largely due to the fat pad in the midfoot. Over the first 6 years of life, the arch develops a configuration approximating adult alignment. Elegant studies have shown that although bracing can hold the foot in a corrected position, bracing and orthotics have *no* impact on the development of the arch. Customized shoes, orthotics, and bracing do not affect development of the feet but may be effective symptomatic treatment for painful, profoundly malaligned feet.

The customary reasons for treating flat feet are pain or excessive shoe wear. In either instance, a combination of heel-cord stretching, strengthening of secondarily weak inverters, and orthotics will usually suffice. Surgery is rarely indicated for idiopathic flat feet.

Radiographs are almost never necessary in patients with flat feet unless there is pain or marked restriction of motion. If obtained, standing anteroposterior radiographs show an increase in the talocalcaneal angle; but, in contrast to such pathologic causes of flat feet as tarsal coalition and congenital vertical talus,

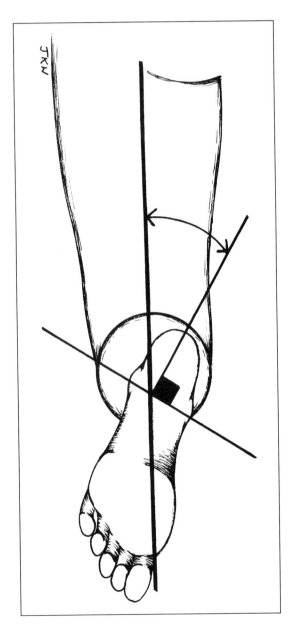

Figure 17.13 Transmalleolar axis. The angle is defined by the long axis of the thigh and a line drawn at 90° to the line connecting the midpoints of the tibial and fibular malleoli. (Redrawn with permission from Staheli LT: The lower limb, in Morrissy RT (ed): *Lovell and Winter's Pediatric Orthopaedics,* 3d ed. Philadelphia, Lippincott, Chap. 20, "The Lower Limb," p 744.)

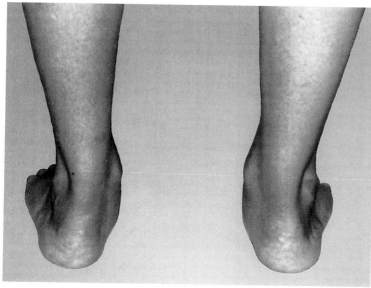

A

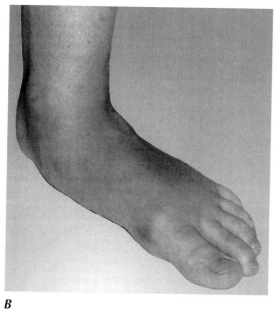

B

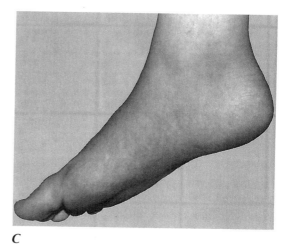

C

Figure 17.14   Flexible flatfoot. Note *(A)* the valgus alignment of the heel
with weight-bearing; *(B)* loss of the medial longitudinal arch. When the
foot is unloaded *(C)*, the arch is reconstituted

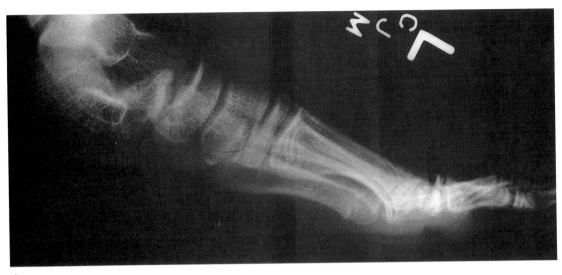

A

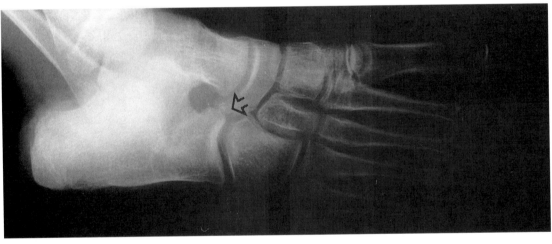

B

Figure 17.15   Tarsal coalition. *A*. The lateral radiograph does not clearly
show the coalition, but the oblique radiograph *(B)* demonstrates a
calcaneonavicular bar *(arrow)*. *C*. CT reveals the bony and fibrous nature
of the coalition *(arrows)*.

these radiographic abnormalities can be corrected by passive positioning of the foot. Another hallmark of a flexible flat foot is the normal appearance of the medial longitudinal arch
when it is not bearing weight.

Other potential causes of flat feet must be
ruled out. Neuromuscular diseases, such as
spina bifida and cerebral palsy, are usually apparent by history and physical examination.
Congenital vertical talus is detectable by the

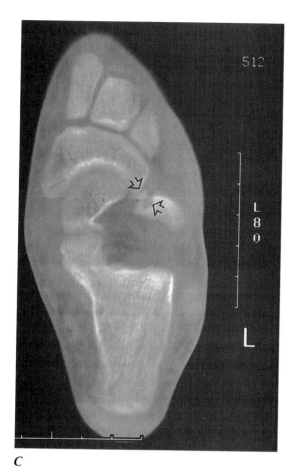

C

Figure 17.15   Continued

pronounced rigidity of the deformity and distinctive radiographic changes (see Chap. 8). When hindfoot mobility is markedly restricted, particularly if accompanied by pain, a congenital tarsal coalition must be considered.

Tarsal Coalition

The most common cause of a rigid flat foot is fusion of the tarsal bones, which probably dates from fetal life. The intertarsal connection is usually cartilaginous in the young child,

thereby allowing slight motion. As the child approaches adolescence, the cartilage begins to ossify, creating increased stiffness, a tendency to ankle sprains, and pain. The typical presentation is that of an adolescent with a stiff flat foot, pain, and a history of recurrent ankle sprains. Sometimes the classic *peroneal spastic flat foot* will be seen, in which spasm in the peroneal tendons contributes to limitation of motion and pain.

Tarsal coalitions are present in nearly 6 percent of the population, with the most common locations between the calcaneus and the navicula and the talus and the calcaneus. Tarsal coalition can usually be diagnosed by examination and plain radiographs. Oblique radiographs are particularly helpful for the recognition of calcaneonavicular bars, but computed tomography is the most helpful modality for mapping the deformity (Fig. 17.15).

About half of the calcaneonavicular bars and 20 percent of talocalcaneal bars are asymptomatic well into adulthood, in which case no treatment is indicated. Cast immobilization may benefit the acutely symptomatic foot, but persistent or recurrent pain suggests the need for surgical intervention. Excellent results can be expected from excision of a calcaneonavicular bar and interposition of muscle or fat if the resection is sufficiently extensive. Excision of a talocalcaneal bar is less likely to be successful if more than 50 percent of the subtalar joint is involved. If resection is unsuccessful and a painful, malformed foot persists, triple arthrodesis may be necessary.

Metatarsalgia

Metatarsalgia refers to pain in the region of the metatarsophalangeal (MTP) joints, but the term has no specific diagnostic implications, since numerous conditions can cause the disorder. Painful callosities are associated with plantar prominence of the metatarsal heads. Although pain and callus formation are most often located beneath the second metatarsal head, this picture usually occurs as a consequence of a problem elsewhere in the foot. Metatarsal fractures can lead to prominence of a metatarsal head because of either increased plantar or dorsal angulation of the broken metatarsal. In the former event, findings are localized beneath the head of the fractured bone, whereas in the latter, they occur beneath adjacent metatarsals *(transfer metatarsalgia)*. Claw toes and hallux valgus, which are discussed below, can also cause plantar prominence of the metatarsal heads and secondary metatarsalgia. Any condition that causes unloading of one region of the foot can result in increased weight-bearing in another area, with resultant metatarsalgia.

If there is underlying deformity, its correction is integral to treatment of the metatarsalgia. When pain is caused by inappropriate footwear or repetitive trauma, as in long-distance runners, attempts are made to relieve the pressure under the involved region by distributing weight-bearing over the rest of the foot, which can be accomplished by metatarsal pads (placed proximal to rather than directly under the metatarsal head) and/or other orthotics. Paring of the callosities accelerates symptomatic relief.

Hallux Valgus

Hallux valgus, in its most simplistic description, consists of lateral deviation (valgus) of the great toe (hallux). In reality, the deformity is much more complex and includes an abduction contracture of the MTP joint, medial prominence of the distal metatarsal *(bunion),*

and attenuation of the medial capsule. There is a familial predisposition to hallux valgus, but no clear genetic link has been delineated. The valgus deflection of the hallux caused by shoes with pointed toes is compounded by the addition of high heels, which suggests an explanation for the more frequent occurrence of hallux valgus in females. Other etiologic factors are pronation of the foot and increased medial angulation of the first metatarsal, although whether the latter is cause or effect has been debated. Certainly, as the great toe drifts laterally, the head of the first metatarsal is forced into a more divergent (varus) alignment relative to the second metatarsal. When this intermetatarsal angle exceeds 10°, *metatarsus primus varus* exists, which, if progressive, is paralleled by an increase in the valgus deformity of the hallux (Fig. 17.16).

Progression of the valgus deformity forces the sesamoids laterally from beneath the first metatarsal head; as a result of this displacement, the sesamoid tendons, which are attached to the proximal phalanx, cause medial rotation, or pronation of the great toe. Once lateral soft tissue contracture and bony rotation have occurred, the altered biomechanics of the first MTP joint precludes normal weight-bearing along that ray, with subsequent transfer of weight to the lateral metatarsal heads, producing transfer metatarsalgia.

Nonoperative measures constitute the first line of treatment for hallux valgus. Since inappropriate footwear is a primary causative factor, changing to a shoe with a wider toe box and a lower heel may ameliorate symptoms and, if done early enough, may halt progression of the deformity. Strapping, taping, and orthotics may also benefit a patient who is not a surgical candidate.

If sufficient pain and deformity are present,

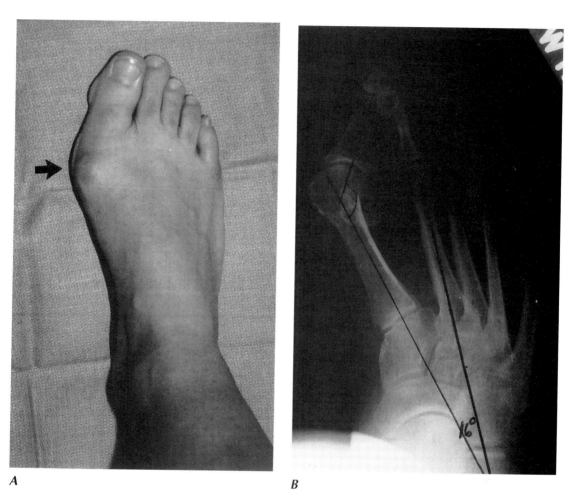

A   *B*

Figure 17.16   Hallux valgus. *A.* Bunion *(arrow). B.* Metatarsus primus varus
   with hallux valgus. The (increased) angle between the first and second
   metatarsals measures 16°.

operative realignment of the first ray may be
undertaken. Numerous procedures have been
described, which have in common the goals of
removing the medial eminence (bunion), rea-
ligning the hallux, and decreasing abnormal
splay between the first and second metatarsals.
The factors that predispose to recurrence are
inadequate bony correction of the intermeta-

tarsal angle or inattention to the details of soft
tissue reconstruction about the first MTP joint.

Mallet Toe, Hammer Toe, and Claw Toe

The causes of deformities of the lesser toes are
usually neurologic or traumatic. If the claw toe

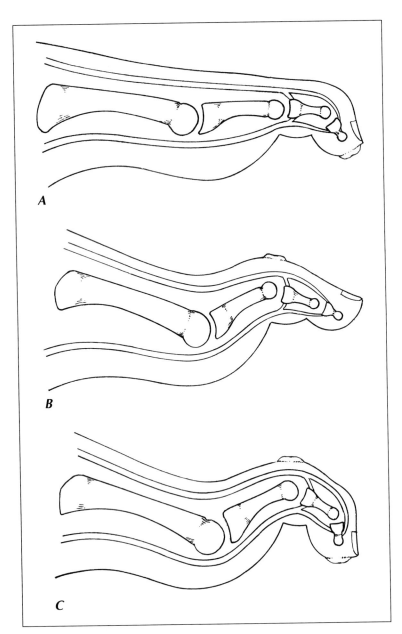

Figure 17.17 *A.* Mallet toe; note the flexion of the DIP joint. *B.* Hammertoe; note the flexion deformity of the PIP joint and mild hyperextension of the MTP joint. *C.* Claw toe; note the flexion deformities of both IP joints and hyperextension deformity of the MTP joint.

deformity is generalized, the possibility of a systemic neurologic disorder, such as Freidreich ataxia or Charcot-Marie-Tooth disease, should be investigated.

The terminology for deformities of the lateral toes is confusing. A mallet toe, which most commonly involves the second toe, consists of a fixed flexion deformity of the distal interphalangeal (IP) (Fig. 17.17*A*) joint. It is, however, a painful callus on the tip of the toe, rather than the deformity, that usually causes the patient to seek consultation. Small adhesive "donut" pads can be obtained that may provide adequate symptomatic relief. If not, release of the flexor digitorum longus tendon, with or without arthrodesis of the distal IP joint, is curative.

A hammer toe consists of a flexion deformity, fixed or flexible, of the proximal IP joint and a mild, flexible hyperextension deformity of the MTP joint (Fig. 17.17*B*). Painful calluses on the tip of the toe or over the dorsum of the proximal interphalangeal joint are the major complaints, although pain beneath the metatarsal heads may also be present. Nonoperative treatment includes metatarsal pads or bars and trimming and padding of tender calluses. Shoes in which the height of the toe box is increased are also beneficial. If these measures do not provide symptomatic relief, arthrodesis of the proximal interphalangeal (PIP) joint is a simple and effective procedure. If the extension deformity of the MTP joint is fixed, PIP arthrodesis is accompanied by dorsal release of the MTP joint.

A claw toe deformity includes the elements of both mallet toe and hammer toe deformities: MTP extension with flexion of both IP joints (Fig. 17.17*C*). Claw-toe deformities are more likely to be severe and fixed than hammer toe

deformities. The chief complaint is usually pain related to shoe pressure on a tender callus over the PIP joint, although pain beneath prominent metatarsal heads may result in tender calluses in this region as well. Nonoperative management includes a shoe with an adequate toe box and a metatarsal bar, which usually suffice for less severe and nonfixed deformities. The need for surgical treatment is suggested by failure of nonoperative measures. The same procedure is carried out as that used for mallet toe deformities, although dorsal capsular release of the MTP joint is always necessary.

Palmar Fibromatosis (Dupuytren Disease)

Dupuytren disease is a nodular contracture of the palmar and digital fascia that predilects men over the age of 50 (Fig. 17.18). Among northern Europeans, there is a strong familial predisposition with a dominant mode of inheritance. In addition to genetic factors, conditions such as alcoholic cirrhosis, seizure disorders, and repetitive (particularly vibrational) trauma, contribute to the development of the disease.

The pathologic changes consist of nodular fibroblastic proliferation of the fascia of the hand. The early or proliferative stage of Dupuytren disease is marked by the development of highly cellular and vascular nodules; it precedes joint contracture. The second stage of the disease, the involutional or active stage, is characterized by fascial contracture and palpable nodules in the hand. The tissue at this stage contains numerous myofibroblasts, which are laden with contractile elements that appear to be important in the de-

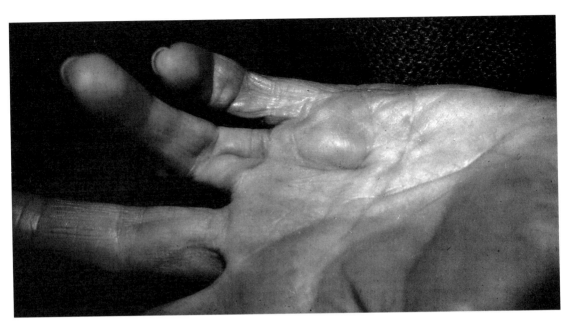

Figure 17.18   Dupuytren disease. Involvement of the palmar and digital fascia of the small and ring fingers has produced nodules, cords, and contractures. The photograph was taken with attempted finger extension, demonstrating the restriction of movement.

velopment of deformity. Marked contractures and prominent palmar cords are present in the residual or advanced stage of the disease. During this stage the involved tissue is relatively acellular.

There is no effective nonsurgical treatment for Dupuytren disease. Physical therapy, massage, vitamin E, ointments, and steroid injections may appear beneficial early but have not been shown to alter the course of the disease. Surgical intervention is recommended when contracture of the interphalangeal joints occurs or when skin care becomes problematic. Recurrent deformity and extension of the disease are common after simple release, so more ex-

tensive procedures involving excision of palmar fascia and skin are usually necessary. Even with these measures, deformity may recur.

Plantar Fibromatosis (Lederhosen Disease)

Nodular fasciitis of the plantar fascia is less common than that of its palmar counterpart. It is histologically identical to Dupuytren disease, with the same clinical stages, but resultant deformities of the toes or foot and involvement of surrounding structures are much less marked, which creates less need for operative intervention.

SUGGESTED READINGS

GREEN DP (ED): *Operative Hand Surgery,* 3d ed. New York, Churchill Livingstone, 1993.

MORRISSY RT (ED): *Lovell and Winter's Pediatric Orthopaedics,* 3d ed. Philadelphia, Lippincott, 1990.

TACHDJIAN MO: *Pediatric Orthopedics,* 2d ed. Philadelphia, Saunders, 1990.

WENGER DR, RANG M: *The Art and Practice of Children's Orthopaedics.* New York, Raven Press, 1993.

WILSON FC (ED): *The Musculoskeletal System: Basic Processes and Disorders,* 2d ed. Philadelphia, Lippincott, 1985.

Chapter **18**

Orthopaedic Terminology

Frank C. Wilson

Abduction: movement of a body part away from the midline.

Adduction: movement of a body part toward the midline. (For lateral movements of the hand and foot, the reference midlines are the middle finger and the middle toe, respectively.)

Ankylosis: stiffness of a joint caused by bridging bone, cartilage, or connective tissue.

Antalgic: literally, "against pain." Applied commonly to gait disorders, the term refers to a short stance phase occasioned by the pain of weight-bearing.

Anteversion: term applied to a bone, usually the femur, to reflect (abnormal) internal torsion in that bone.

Arthrodesis: operative fusion of a joint.

Arthroplasty: operative procedure to mobilize a joint.

Calcaneus: dorsiflexed position of the ankle.

Cavus: excessive height of the longitudinal arch of the foot.

Comminuted: fracture in which more than two bone fragments are present.

Compound: old term for a fracture that extends through the skin (see *Open*, below).

Contraction: reversible shortening of a muscle during the performance of work (physiologic).

Contracture: fixed shortening of a muscle that results from scarring of its fibrous elements (pathologic).

Coxa: hip.

Dislocation: complete separation of a joint, i.e., no contact between the articular surfaces.

Equinus: plantarflexed position of the ankle.

Genu: knee.

Greenstick: an "incomplete" fracture occurring in children in which only the cortex subject to tension forces is seen to be broken. Often occurs in combination with a torus fracture (see below).

Hallux: great toe.

Impacted: fracture deformity in which one fragment is driven into the other, conferring a degree of stability.

Kyphosis: posterior curvature of the spine.

Lordosis: anterior curvature of the spine.

Malunion: bone healing with deformity.

Nonunion: failure of fractured or osteotomized bone ends to unite.

Open: Preferred term for a fracture that extends through the skin (see *Compound*, above).

Osteotomy: operative division of a bone.

Pes: foot.

Planus: flattening of the longitudinal arch of the foot.

Pronation: rotational movement of the forearm that results in the palmar surface of the hand being turned downward.

Recurvatum: extension of the knee beyond 0°.

Retroversion: a term applied to a bone, usually the femur or humerus, to reflect (abnormal) external torsion in that bone.

Segmental: term referring to two or more fractures involving the entire width of a bone, which produces three or more full-thickness "segments" of the bone.

Spondylolisthesis: slippage, usually forward, of a vertebra upon a subjacent vertebra.

Spondylolysis: uni- or bilateral defect in the pars interarticularis; if bilateral, spondylolisthesis may occur.

Spondylosis: degenerative disease of the spinal articulations.

Sprain: incomplete tear of a ligament.

Strain: incomplete tear of a muscle.

Stress fracture: a fracture, usually undisplaced, that results from repetitive rather than single trauma.

Subluxation: partial displacement of a joint in which the joint surfaces, while displaced, retain partial contact.

Supination: rotational movement of the forearm that results in the palmar surface of the hand being turned upward.

Tenodesis: fixation of the proximal end of a tendon to bone, which converts the tendon to a ligament.

Tenotomy: operative division of a tendon.

Torus: an "incomplete" fracture occurring in children in which the concave cortex, subject to compression forces, buckles. Often seen in combination with a greenstick fracture (see above).

Valgus: abnormal angulation of a limb in which the distal part is directed away from the midline.

Varus: abnormal angulation of a limb in which the distal part is directed toward the midline.

Index

*Page numbers followed by an 'f' or a 't' refer to figures or tables, respectively.